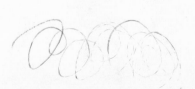

66

Printed in United States of America
Press of the Wolfer Printing Co., Inc.
416 Wall Street, Los Angeles, California 90013

The
ART and SCIENCE
of
BARBERING

66

Printed in United States of America
Press of the Wolfer Printing Co., Inc.
416 Wall Street, Los Angeles, California 90013

Contents

Alphabetically Listed

If

'If you think you are beaten, you are;
   If you think you dare not, you don't;
If you think you'd like to win, but you can't.
   It's almost a "cinch" you won't;
If you think you'll lose, you've lost,
   For out in the world you'll find
Success begins with a fellow's will—
   It's all in the state of mind.

"Full many a race is lost
   E'er even a race is run.
And many a coward fails
   E'er even his work's begun
Think big, and your deeds will grow,
   Think small and you fall behind,
Think that you can, and you will;
   It's all in the state of mind.

"If you think you are outclassed, you are;
   You've got to think high to rise;
You've got to be sure of yourself before
   You can ever win a prize.
Life's battle doesn't always go
   To the stronger or faster man;
But sooner or later, the man who wins
   Is the fellow who thinks he can."

Edgar A. Guest

Foreword

The aim of this book is to set forth a graphic, comprehensive study of barbering. An endeavor has been made to deduce from a huge mass of facts and details a practical, concrete, and simplified approach to the subject. There is need for a book that comes directly to the point, a book that explains and clearly illustrates the material to be learned. Emphasis has been placed on readability. The manner in which the book is written makes the points of importance readily observable. The salient points are PEDESTALIZED.

This book contains more than 700 pictures, illustrating styles, techniques, and other phases of barbering.

Art and science are interrelated in modern barbering. One supplements the other. Graceful ways of working and pleasing, complimentary results comprise the art; and the proven methods of working and the knowledge of the hair and skin comprise the science. The most successful barber is both scientific and artistic.

Most of the chapters on the related sciences, such as nerves, muscles and circulation, are in two parts. Part I deals with the aspects of such subjects closely related to barbering and Part II with other aspects. Part I should be sufficient, but Part II is included for those states and countries that still require the other aspect. **The current trend is away from so many details of the related sciences and places more emphasis on the fundamentals. The author hopes that state boards will discontinue examination questions on the subject of bones and on so much of the either irrelevent or remotely related material in Part II of the related sciences in this book. Too much time is being spent teaching students such material.**

Students should not be expected to learn the exact step-by-step procedure of every shampoo, every scalp treatment and every facial. They, however, should know the high points of the procedure of many such services, even if it is in their own words.

The Author

Sanitation

The importance of sanitation in barbering cannot be over-emphasized. Barber shop services bring the barber in direct contact with the skin of his clientele. The practice of sanitation insures the prevention of the spread of contagious diseases from one person to another. The barber, therefore, should know the best methods of practicing sanitation, and he should practice sanitary procedures rigorously.

Sanitation defined: Sanitation is complete cleanliness. The word "sanitation" comes from the Latin word **sanitas,** which connotes health and translated, means the science of maintaining healthful conditions.

Main purpose of sanitation: To prevent the spread of disease. Disease can be spread (1) from the customer to the barber, (2) from the barber to the customer, and (3) from customer to customer.

Four basic steps of sanitation:

1. Wash your hands with soap and water just before serving a patron.
2. Place a towel or neck-strip between the haircloth and neck.
3. Immerse in a disinfectant solution the implements or parts thereof to be used that contact the patron, **immediately before using them.**
4. Use only clean linen or paper towels on each patron.

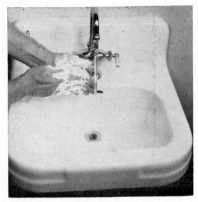

Fig. 1
Washing Hands

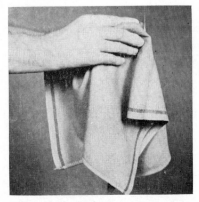

Fig. 2
Dry Hands Thoroughly

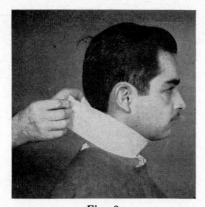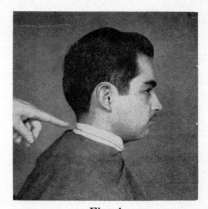

Fig. 3   Fig. 4
Protect Skin of Neck With Either Neck-Strip or Towel

Additional steps of sanitation:

1. Keep clean towels in a closed compartment.
2. Discard used towels immediately after serving patron.
3. Deposit used towels in a container after serving patron.
4. Do not use the same towel on the next patron until laundered.
5. Use clean towel or paper on head-rest for each patron.
6. Wear a clean smock or apron while serving patrons.
7. Keep finger nails short and clean.
8. Refrain from putting your fingers into your nose or pockets or on your face.
9. Sanitize clipper blades regularly.
10. Refrain from putting any implement into your pocket.
11. Clean any implement or part thereof before disinfecting it (Such agents as alcohol, kerosene or soap and water may be used.)
12. Change disinfectant solution daily or whenever needed.
13. Keep tools in a closed compartment or in an approved solution when not in use. Usually, permitted exceptions are strops, electric clippers, and shaving mugs and lather brushes. When certain tools are kept in a solution, only the parts that make contact with patrons are immersed, such as the blades of razors and clippers.
14. Remove creams from jars with a spatula, end of comb or razor blade.
15. Recover cream jars immediately after each use.
16. Use styptic or alum in powder or liquid forms to stop bleeding from minor cuts.
17. Keep implements and equipment clean. Pass a used towel over your work-stand and bowl several times daily and dust off chair after each patron.

18. Keep adequate disinfecting solution in the container to cover implements or parts thereof being disinfected.

19. Wash your hands before and after going to the toilet.

20. Do not permit the haircloth or shampoo cape to come in contact with the skin of the patron's neck.

Responsibility for sanitation at chair and in shop:

1. Each barber is responsible for sanitation at his chair.

2. The manager must provide the necessities for shop sanitation.

Disinfectant Chemicals: There are many already prepared chemical disinfectants on the market. Boards of Health and Barber Examiners publish lists of acceptable disinfectants. Your barber supply dealer will be glad to tell you about them. Use the ones recommended by the barber board or the board of health or an equivalent accepted by these boards. Some of the chemicals used are:

The following is a list of some disinfectants on the market. For convenience, they are classified into three groups. Manufacturers of these products provide instructions for their use and testing materials.

Group No. 1:

Ster-i-chlor	Chlor-o-zol
Chlorazene	Bacilli Killi

Solutions made from Group No. 1 are tested by a white starched potassium iodide paper. If of proper strength, the paper will turn purple or dark blue.

Group No 2:

Herpicide Sterilizing Tabs	Micro-Merc
Merax	Ra-Caps

Red litmus paper is used to test the solutions made from Group No. 2. Solutions of proper strength will turn the paper blue.

Group No. 3:

Amicide	Barbicide
Herpicide Disinfectant Tabs	

Solutions made from Group No. 3 can be tested by Marshall Test Paper-A or Hymine Testabs. If of proper strength, the paper will turn green.

Group No. 4:

Danco Germicidal Oil
Phenosterazine "Clipper Dip"

Solutions made from Group No. 4 are used for sterilizing clipper blades. Testing materials may be obtained from manufacturers of these products.

Testing disinfectants: The testing of disinfectants differs according to a particular disinfectant. There are many disinfectants on the market, and each manufacturer gives instruction on testing his product. A **chlorine solution** can be tested by a white paper strip that is a **starched potassium iodide paper**. The proper strength solution should turn the paper purple or blue.

Requirements of a good disinfectant: While it is true that **bacteria can be destroyed by chemicals, strong acids, and alkalies,** and by both dry and wet heat, it does not necessarily follow that all of these and all kinds of chemicals are practical or desirable. For examples, the expense, inconvenience of preparing, and unpleasant odors rule out phenol, L.C. com-

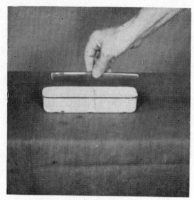

Fig. 5
Immersing Comb

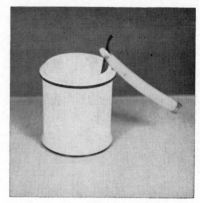

Fig. 6
Immersing Razor

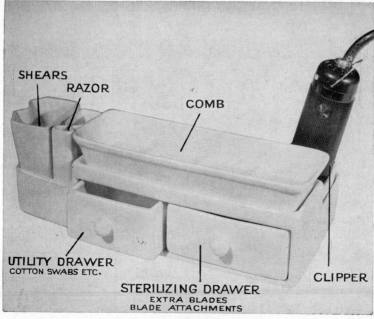

Fig. 7
Ultra Wet Sterilizer

pound, and formaldehyde in a barber shop. Likeswise, moist heat (boiling water) and dry heat (burning in an oven) are not practical. A good disinfectant should be:

1. Quick acting.
2. Non-corrosive.
3. Odorless or almost so.

4. Convenient to prepare.
5. Economical.
6. Non-harmful to skin.

Skin antiseptics: There are innumerable face antiseptic lotions on the market. Here is a list of four.

1. Witch Hazel
2. Bay Rum

3. Boric Acid Solution
4. Lilac Vegetal

Implements difficult to sterilize: Brushes of all kinds are difficult to sterilize, especially the hair brush. Neck dusters are in this category. It is scarcely possible to go beyond antisepticizing these items by washing them with soap and water. Substitutes have been invented for dusters and electric latherizers for shaving brushes.

Sanitation terms used interchangeably: While technically there is a difference between disinfection and sterilization, quite commonly the terms are used interchangeably, and so are **disinfect** and **sterilize**. "Sterilize" is more widely used. Sterilization is the widely accepted term for all processes of destroying germs. In the popular sense in which it is used, sterilization is a matter of degrees; its shades of meaning range from mild antiseptics to potent solutions deadly to all bacteria. Sterilize may be used as a synonym for sanitize, clean, disinfect, and even antisepticize. One hears: "He sterilizes his implements faithfully." Likewise **disinfectant, bacteriacide, parasiticide,** and **germicide** to mean the same thing.

Antiseptic, disinfectant, and sterilization defined:

1. An antiseptic is an agent that **retards** disease germs.
2. A disinfectant is an agent that **kills** disease germs.
3. Sterilization **destroys all germs,** infectious and otherwise.

A longer definition is: Sterilization is the process that makes an object germ-free by destroying all microorganisms, infectious or otherwise.

Some other sanitation terms:

1. Sterile—a condition free from disease germs.
2. Sterilize—to make sterile.
3. Germicide—an agent that kills disease germs.
4. Deodorant—an agent that destroys odors.
5. Spatula—a cream spoon to remove cream from jars.
6. Asepsis—a condition free from disease germs.
7. Sepsis—a poisonous condition where disease germs are active.

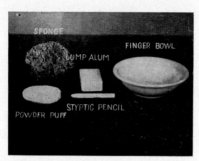

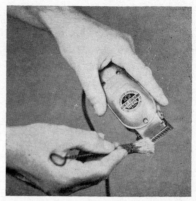

Fig. 8
Five Items Not to Use

Fig. 9
Brushing-Off Clipper Blades

Five items NOT to use in shop: In former days there were five items which seemed indispensible to the practice of barbering. These were the sponge, lump alum, styptic pencil, powder puff, and the finger bowl. The use of these items has been discontinued for sanitary reasons—each is a carrier of germs that spread disease and all but the finger bowl cannot be satisfactorily sterilized. The sponge was used to wash the face and neck and to remove lather; lump alum was used to give the finger tips a non-skid ability to stretch the skin; the styptic pencil was used to stop bleeding from nicks; the powder puff was used to powder the face; and the finger bowl was used to hold water for the second time over. These items have either been replaced by sanitary items or have been found unnecessary. The sponge has been replaced by clean towels; the lump alum is made unnecessary by shaving "clean" as you go, leaving no traces of lather to prevent holding the skin firmly; instead of a styptic pencil, liquid or powdered alum or styptic powder is used; the towel is manipulated to take place of the powder puff; and the finger bowl has been replaced by a water bottle or a water faucet near the chair (Fig. 8).

Three categories of sanitation: (1) Antiseptics, (2) disinfectants, and (3) sterilization.

Methods of sterilization: There are five methods of sterilization. Vapors and Rays are listed with reservation, since they mainly keep already sterilized implements sterile. These methods are:

1. **Immersion in chemicals.** This is the **most practical** and commonly used method in barber shops. A list of usable chemicals are given in this chapter, but there are numerous prepared chemicals on the market for barber shop use.

2. **Moist heat.** This method involves boiling or steaming under pressure. Boiling in water for 20 minutes is an effective method, but, like steaming, it is not practical for barber shop use.

3. **Dry heat.** An example is baking in an oven; it is not applicable for barber shop use.

4. **Vapors.** One formula is a tablespoonful of borax to a like amount of formaldehyde. Saturate a blotter with such a solution or put it in a small tray and place it in the bottom of an air-tight cabinet. The vapors only keep sterilized tools sterile.

5. **Rays.** Ultra-violet ray lamps are built into cabinets. Such lamps only keep sterilized tools sterile; they do not effectively sterilize.

The fact remains that some state boards approve such lamps as meeting the sterilization requirements. The use of these lamps impresses customers.

General types of sterilizers:

1. Wet sterilizer. Examples: Boiling water and immersion in chemicals.
2. Dry sterilizer. Example: Vapors.

Personal cleanliness aspect of sanitation: This aspect applies to the hands, finger nails, teeth, breath, body, clothing, shoes, and face.

Implements in pocket: Never put implements into your pocket.

Routine upon completing a service: Immediately upon completing a service and discharging the customer, discard used towels, clean and return all implements used to their proper places. (Do not leave implements lying on the workstand between customers.)

Obsolete and Objectionable Disinfectant Chemicals: Alcohol is too expensive and the other chemicals here listed give off undesirable odor.

1. Phenol (Carbolic acid). 　　　3. Liquor Cresolis.
2. Formaldehyde. 　　　　　　　4. Alcohol.

Formulas for making disinfectants from these chemicals are:

1. For a 5% phenol solution, mix one part phenol with 19 parts water.
2. For a 25% formalin solution, mix 2 parts formalin with 5 parts water and one part glycerine. (The use of glycerine is to prevent corrosion.)
3. For a 4% liquid cresolis compound solution, mix one part compound to 24 parts of water.
4. For an alcoholic solution, use 70% alcohol.

How To Be A Successful Barber Student

Every student should resolve to be as successful as possible to avail himself of the maximum benefits of the course. While the school has a responsibility to the student, a great deal depends upon the student, such as his determination, cooperation, and effort. The following is a list of suggestions on how to be a success as a barber student. Some of these could be incorporated into school regulations, but the student who desires to be a success will follow them voluntarily and willingly.

1. Make a firm resolve to be a successful student.
2. Be willing to go more than fifty percent of the way to get along with people. Your success depends largely on your ability to get along with others. Do not say everything you think. Do not condemn a person even though he is wrong. Agreeableness is an important factor of success.
3. Be cheerful. It is a long accepted philosophy that "smile and the world smiles with you; frown and the world frowns at you."
4. Emphasize good personal appearance. The first thing customers notice about you is your appearance.
   (1) Wear immaculately clean clothes.
   (2) Wear only a freshly laundered uniform.
   (3) Wear suitable clothes.
   (4) Keep your shoes well shined.
   (5) Keep your finger nails short, well trimmed, and clean.
   (6) Shave daily and early in the day. Do not shave yourself during the first nor last half hour of your shift, when a substantial number of students are in class, nor during the lunch periods when of course a large percentage of students are at luncheon.
   (7) Have your hair cut every ten days at least.
   (8) Develop a good posture. Stand erect when greeting or thanking a customer.
   (9) Wear an easy cheerful countenance.
   (10) Wash your hands frequently.
5. Invite instructors to help you. Do not over-do this privilege.
6. Do not monopolize class by questions or comments.

7. Do not spread your grievances among other students. Discuss them only with the instructor or manager.

8. Cultivate the habit of socializing with customers.

9. Do not carry on a conversation with anyone else when you are serving a customer.

10. Learn how to modulate and regulate your voice. Speak clearly and cheerfully when greeting and thanking customers. At the chair cultivate a low voice for conversation with the patron.

11. Adopt the home study plan. Have a regular time and place to study your asignment. Good study habits are important.

12. Develop good work habits. The proper time and place to develop such habits are at the school. Give your last customer of the day the same courteous and complete service as any other customer. Do not try to pick the customers you prefer to service. For the utmost development learn to serve all kinds of customers.

13. Restrict your personal friends or relatives to momentary (60 seconds) visitation.

14. Guard against bad breath or body odor. Both of these are offensive to customers. Use mouth wash and deodorants to prevent these offenses.

15. Do not smoke while serving a customer.

16. Keep "breaks," rest and lunch periods within the stipulated time allowed. Such time out should be by permission only, unless specified on your schedule.

17. Be willing to serve any customer the instructor assigns.

18. Do not try to correct an instructor even though in your opinion he is doing something wrong.

19. Do not ask for or receive any service from another student during either the first or the last half hour of your shift, or during lunch periods, or on Saturdays. (The instructor may grant exceptions.)

20. Never leave the premises without permission and do not ask for such permission when several other students have a like permission. Be willing to wait upon request of the instructor.

21. Bear in mind that you will probably complete only one course of barbering, and so endeavor to get the most possible out of it.

22. Give an excuse for every absence or tardiness. If you cannot attend, notify the college.

23. Be punctual. Punctuality is the mark of nobility.

24. Reduce to a minimum personal telephone calls to the college. Make any such calls short, about one minute.

25. Be courteous at all times—to other students, to the public, and to the instructor.

26. Cooperate with the instructor. Be cognizant of the fact that he desires to give you the utmost in training. No instructor can be at his best unless the student cooperates. Do not argue with the instructor. Pay strict and undivided attention to his instruction. Do not expect your instructor to be perfect. The student who analyzes his own habits and actions with the intent to improve himself will have fewer reasons to criticize his instructor. He should concern himself more about how to be a good student than trying to find something wrong with his instructor. If you will treat the instructor the way you would like to be treated were you an instructor, you will be the one who benefits most.

27. **Do not loiter around in the school.** Stay at your assigned chair.

28. Do not brood over the possible fact that the owner or owners of the college are making money. They have to make money in order to keep the college open. Bear in mind that you have come to the college too learn to be a barber. Whether or not the college makes any profit on your enrollment should not enter your mind other than that you should do your part as a student to meet your obligations, so that the college can meet its own. Concentrate on your own problems—not those of someone else. Sleep over your "beef feeling" before mentioning it to the instructor or manager.

Your Career Is In Your Hands

The acts of barbering cannot be performed without the hands. They are indispensable. Just what kind of hands should a person have to be a barber? Usually a discussion of hands centers around their size and shape. Probably the size and shape do have a relation to certain kinds of vocations, but only remotely to barbering. The type of work the barber performs with his hands is not delicate; but the implements which he uses do perform delicate, precision work.

No hands are drawn in this chapter to show the most suitable type. The basis upon which to determine whether or not a person has the proper hands are as follows:

1. Each hand should have a thumb and preferably all the fingers. The little finger is the least important.
2. The hands should have dexterity.
3. There should be good mental direction behind the hands.
4. There should be determination behind the hands.
5. The hands should be soft and smooth.
6. The fingers should be flexible.
7. The fingers should have **eye-hand coordination.**

The hands can be made soft and smooth by soaking them in warm water, thoroughly cleaning them, and massaging them with a lanolin preparation. This should be continued as long as necessary, giving about a half hour for the whole process daily.

Flexibility can be developed by the acts of barbering, but finger exercises are recommended. Apply a tissue cream or any good lanolin preparation and massage them about fifteen minutes daily until the hands are soft and pliable.

1. Open and close the hands slowly, and then gradually increase the speed of opening and closing.
2. Close one finger at a time, then two fingers, then three and four. Close and open the thumb separately.
3. Communicate with the fingers. This means to develop **mind-hand coordination.**
    (1) Place the open right hand on a table or stand, direct various fingers to rise and return to original position.
    (2) Interlock the fingers of both hands, then open and close each finger separately, directing various fingers out of sequence.

Implements

Implements are the tools used to perform the acts of barbering, whereas equipment is the facilities of the shop, such as barber chairs, bowls, mirrors, latherizers, etc.

Use good quality tools. The student especially needs good tools while he is learning. Inferior tools, such as a razor that has a crumbly edge or shears that dull quickly discourage the beginner. It is said that a workman is known by his implements.

Important things to know about implements are:

1. How to sterilize.
2. Names.
3. Structural parts.
4. Types.
5. Sizes.
6. Care.
7. How to identify good tools.
8. Proper use.

This chapter deals with implements under most of the above categories. Their proper use will be explained in the phases of barbering in which they are mostly used. For example, the techniques of using the shears, combs, and clippers will be explained in the chapter on haircutting.

Classification of implements:

1. Cutting implements. These are shears, razors, and clippers. (Also known as "primary" implements, but improperly so.)
2. Accessory implements. Some of these are combs, strops, mugs, brushes, hones, vibrators and tweezers.

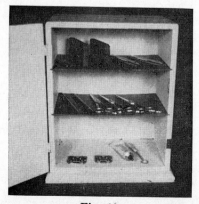

Fig. 10
Tool Layout in Cabinet

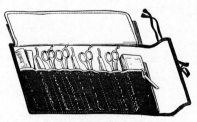

Fig. 11
Implement Kit

Layout of tools in cabinet: Tools should be arranged neatly and orderly and where they can be easily picked up. They may be separated and arranged according to their general use. On one shelf place the razors, hones, tweezers, and styptic powder; on another shelf place the plain shears, thinning shears, and combs. The extra clipper blades, oil, grease, clasp, and clipper brush may be placed with the shears, but preferably on a separate shelf or in a separate compartment.

Implement kit: This kit is designed to carry the more delicate and difficult implements to pack. It was formerly known as a "razor roll."

HAIRCUTTING SHEARS

Shears used in barbering are made especially for haircutting. They are manufactured in many countries, among which are the United States, England, Sweden, Japan, and Germany.

Types of haircutting shears: There are two general types of such shears.

1. French. (It has a finger brace.)
2. German. (It is without a finger brace.)

The French type is most commonly used. With such a brace, the shears can be held more securely and with minimum firmness.

Sizes of shears: Shears are made according to a definite size in length. The various sizes are indicated by inches, such as 6 inch, 6½ inch, 7 inch and 7½ inch. The size most widely used is the 7½ inch. The length from the blade to the finger brace determines the size.

Sizes of shanks: The shank is that part of the shears between the pivot and the finger grips. Shears come with short, medium, and long shanks. Barbers develop their own preferences for the various sizes of shanks, of blades, and of shears. Individual fancies account for some choices, but

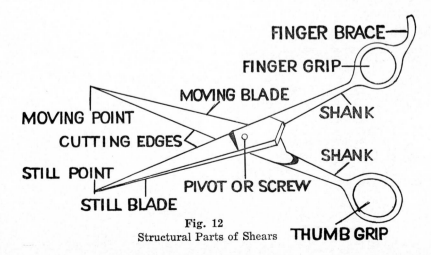

Fig. 12
Structural Parts of Shears

the size of the shank should be selected according to the size of the hand —long shanks for the large hand and short shanks for the small hand. For the barber with an average size hand, there is no size problem.

Types of grinds: The grind of shears is the kind of cutting edge. There are two kinds of grinds.

1. Plain grind. (This is a knife-like edge.)
2. Corrugated grind. (This is a furrowed or alternating ridge edge.)

The plain grind is most widely used. Such an edge may be fine, medium or coarse. The fine edge is called "razor edge." The preferred plain grind is medium.

Likewise, there are fine, medium, and coarse corrugated edges. Both blades may be corrugated, but a combination grind consists of one plain grind blade and one corrugated blade.

Temper of shears: The temper is the degree of hardness of the steel. Shears may be too soft or too hard. A medium temper is preferred. The temper of good manufacturers is usually correct.

Set of shears: The "set" is the tension of the blades and the way they are slanted. Without the right set, shears will not cut properly.

Structural parts of shears: In studying the structural parts of shears it will be noted that they have one movable and one still blade. The general theory is that only the movable blade moves and the still blade remains still. The shears should be used in this way to achieve maximum precision. It will also be observed that the modernly designed shears have a "cut away" shank which lessens the hazard of pinching the ear with the shanks. The names of the various parts of shears are given in the diagrammatical drawing (Fig. 12).

Use of rubber shear pads: Shear pads are made for both the finger and thumb grips. Unless one's finger and thumb are exceptionally small, such pads are not needed. The finger or thumb should never be tight in the grips since this would stiffen the hand and wrist and thereby lessen the flexibility necessary to facilitate proper manipulation of the shears. The thumb, for example, should not be fully inserted into the thumb grip.

THINNING SHEARS

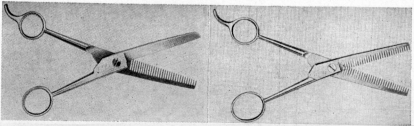

Fig. 13
One Notched Blade

Fig. 14
Two Notched Blades

Thinning shears are used primarily to reduce the thickness of hair. They may also be used for end-thinning, a method of tapering, but this is not recommended for general practice. The latter is recommended only when the hair presents a problem due to some irregularity. Thinning shears have most of the structural parts of plain shears. Either one or both of the cutting edges of the blades may be notched (serrated). The serrations on the cutting edge of the blade resemble the toothed edge of a saw. The number of these teeth varies widely in the various brands, running from 22 to 46. The more numerous the notched formations, the finer the hair can be thinned. The purposes of thinning shears are:

1. To thin hair.
2. To blend stubborn end-hair—terminal-blending.

COMBS

There are various types of combs, such as shingling combs, hairdressing combs, fine combs, coarse combs, pocket combs, and handle-combs.

Some types of combs:

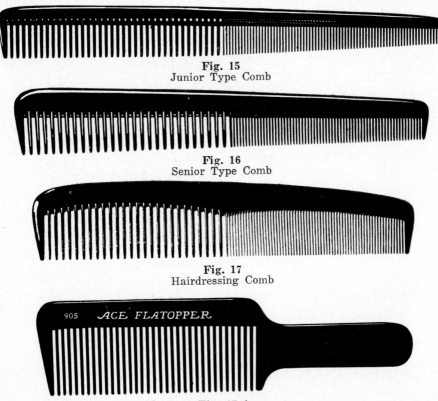

Fig. 15
Junior Type Comb

Fig. 16
Senior Type Comb

Fig. 17
Hairdressing Comb

Fig. 17-A
Flattopper Comb with Handle

Haircutting combs are used as a gauge as to how much hair to cut off, to put the hair into a cutting position, and to assist in checking evenness.

The design of the regular shingling combs may be classified as senior and junior. The senior design has slightly coarser and longer teeth than the junior design. The senior design is preferred for general shingling and cutting, and the junior design is preferred for the base of the arch and for cutting hair closer to the scalp. Hairdressing combs are sturdier and have longer teeth than regular shingling combs. They may be used for general combing, to hand the customer who desires to comb his own hair, and for scalp treatments.

Requirements of good comb:
1. The teeth of the comb should be shaped so that they feed into and through the hair. To do this, they must be smoothly tapered, neither too wide nor too close, and of the proper length.
2. The teeth should not be sharp, but tapered and round. Sharp teeth irritate the scalp.
3. The teeth should be flexible—capable of bending under strain without breaking.
4. The comb should be sturdy—capable of lasting a reasonable time.

Composition of combs: The best combs are made of hard rubber. Some are made from metal, bone, celluloid or plastic. Clean rubber combs in tepid, soapy water—hot water warps them.

Structural parts of comb:
1. The teeth. Except for specially designed combs, each comb has a combination fine and coarse tooth section.
2. The bar. The bar is the base of the comb apart from the teeth. Its function is to hold the hair picked up by the teeth of the comb.

CLIPPERS

A clipper is a haircutting implement with two blades. The top blade is known as the cutting blade, since it moves back and forth, and the lower blade is known as the still blade, since it does not move. The idea of using clippers to cut human hair originated from their use in cutting horse hair, in the latter part of the 19th Century.

General types of clippers: There are many makes of clippers, but they fall into two general types.
1. Hand clippers.
2. Electric clippers.

Designs of electric clippers: There are three designs of electric clippers; namely, (1) the non-adjustable, (2) the adjustable (with a lever to adjust the blades to various degrees of fineness or coarseness), and (3) the detachable blade design.

Types of electric clippers: There are two types.

1. Magnetic electric clippers.
2. Motor electric clippers.

The **magnetic type** is a compact vibrating mechanism whose principal part is a coil set according to a certain cycle, either 50 or 60 cycle.

The **motor type** is motor driven, and it will operate on either 50 or 60 cycles. The blades on this kind of clipper are usually detachable.

Sizes of blades: The sizes of blades are indicated by ciphers or numbers. Hand clipper blades usually range from 000 to #1, while electric clipper blades include such sizes as 0000, 000, 00, 0, 0A, 1, 2, and 3.

Cutting lengths of blades: Each size blade cuts a different length—size 0000 cuts the closest; #3, the coarsest. The cutting length of the 000 blade is estimated at 1/100th of an inch; #1 at 1/8th of an inch.

Why clipper blades pull hair: Dullness, dirtiness, need of oil, or need of adjustment can cause blades to pull hair. Blades may be cleaned by running them immersed in kerosene. Use clipper oil daily but sparingly. Two or three drops may suffice.

Blade attachments: There are several sizes of blade attachments, sometimes called slip-ons or comb attachments. These are attached to the blade so as to gauge the clipper blade and keep it the desired distance from the scalp. They are widely used for such special cuts as butches, crew cuts, and flat tops (Figs. 18-19).

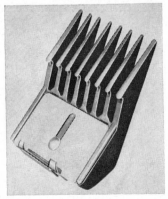

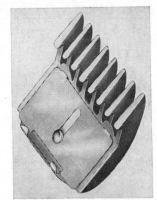

Fig. 18   Fig. 19

Blade Attachments

Pointers on use of hand clipper:

1. Place the index finger of the left hand on the set screw to steady it.
2. Make a full stroke with the movable handle.

3. Place the thumb along the still handle, and on the thumb rest.
4. Grasp the movable handle at about the first joints. The guide should be between the first and second fingers.
5. Move the clipper into the hair slowly.

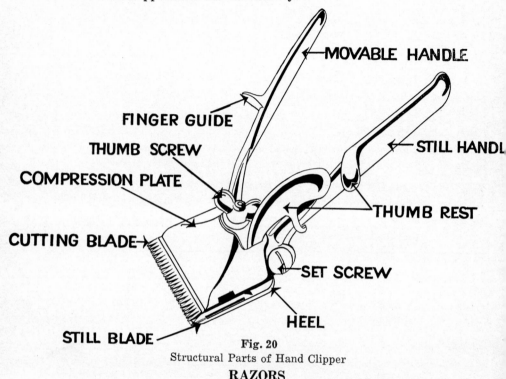

FINGER GUIDE
THUMB SCREW
COMPRESSION PLATE
CUTTING BLADE→
MOVABLE HANDLE
STILL HANDL
THUMB REST
SET SCREW
HEEL
STILL BLADE

Fig. 20
Structural Parts of Hand Clipper

RAZORS

The use of razors of some description dates back to the early days of Egypt and China. Early man used any hard, sharp material for shaving, such as bits of flint, shell fragments, and shark's teeth. The modern razor is considered the sharpest cutting instrument in the world.

The straight razor of early modern times was made of steel which had a wedge-shaped section, with straight sides tapering to a sharp edge. Early in the 19th century, the practice of hollowing out the sides of the blade by grinding was introduced to facilitate sharpening the blade and to improve the fineness of the cutting edge. The full hollow blade is thinner in the center than near the cutting edge. Hollow-grinding is performed by using grinding wheels of successively diminishing diameters. The processes of the production of the blade are: forging under the hammer, marking the name of maker, drilling the hole for the pin, then hardening and tempering of the blade. Finally, the blade is etched, fitted with handle, and whetted to a sharp edge. In this way the razor is made from many small pieces of steel welded together under terrific heat and pressure.

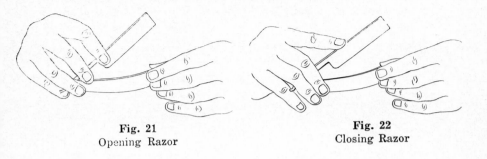

Fig. 21
Opening Razor

Fig. 22
Closing Razor

Structural parts of razor:

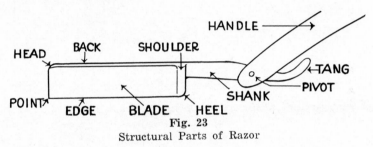

Fig. 23
Structural Parts of Razor

Seven points to know about razors:

These points are the (1) length, (2) width, (3) style, (4) grind (hollow ground or wedge), (5) balance, (6) finish, and (7) temper.

Straight razors: The discussion in this chapter will be confined to straight razors. This is the kind of razor that is used professionally by barbers to serve the public. It is not inconceivable, however, that its use will some day be supplemented by some other type or types of razor.

Grinds of razors: There are two general grinds of razors—**hollow** grind and **wedge.** The hollow grind is also known as concave. The concave costs more to produce and costs more on the market. Its flexibility and disposition to facilitate sharpening make it the more preferred type. Many barbers, however, still prefer wedges, although it is usually conceded that the hollow-ground is the most widely used. (Figs. 24 and 25, Page 20.)

Wedge razors have no concavity. Both sides of the blade form a sharp angle graduating to the edge. The concensus is that wedge razors are more difficult to sharpen, but they are capable of an excellent edge. Besides the full wedge type razor, there are the 1/4 wedge and 1/2 wedge.

Sizes of razor blades: Size refers mainly to the width of the blade. Sizes are indicated by fractions of an inch. Some of the specific sizes are 4/8, 9/16, 5/8, 6/8, and 7/8. Nine-sixteenths and five-eighths are the sizes most used. (Fig. 26, Page 21.)

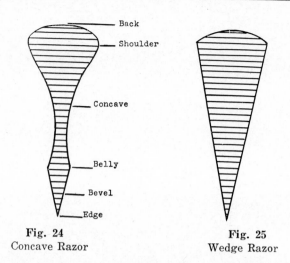

Fig. 24
Concave Razor

Fig. 25
Wedge Razor

Length of razor: Razors run fairly uniform in length. The standard length of a five-eighths hollow-grind razor is nine and one-half inches.

Styles of razors: The style of a razor refers to its shape and design. The pre-modern razor was designed very much like the modern razor except it had a round point. The modern razor has a straight back and edge parallel to each other, a round heel, a square point, a flat or slightly round handle. To prevent the square point from scratching the skin round it off slightly by drawing it over the side of a hone, the back leading.

Handles of razors: Most razor handles are made of hard rubber, but some are made of celluloid, bone, metal, or plastic. Transparent handles are made of plastic. Handles incorrectly installed or warped by such atmospheric factors as heat and dampness may cause the blade to strike against the handle and destroy its edge. Rubber handles may be adjusted by running hot water over them, or by gently tapping the pivot pin towards the shank on the side on which the blade touches the handle. Rest the pin on the square corner edge of a piece of iron. Use a small hammer to tap. The **tension** of handles is important. It should not be so tight that the handle is hard to move, nor so loose as to move of its own accord. The tension should be such that a little pressure is necessary to open or close the razor.

Balance, Finish, and Temper of razors:

1. **Balance.** The balance of a razor means that the weight of the handle is about the same as that of the blade.
2. **Finish.** The "finish" of the blade means its surface or polish. The polished steel finish is best, because it lasts longer and does not hide the quality of steel. This kind of finish is also known as **Crocus** or **Rouge** finish, since such a finish is achieved by this means. Nickel

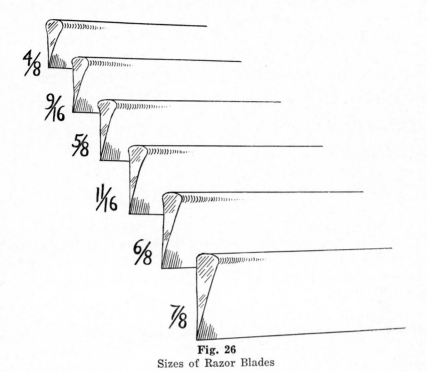

Fig. 26
Sizes of Razor Blades

or silverplated blades are often made of inferior steel. The cutting edge may be too soft to last or so hard it chips easily. The three kinds of finish are plain steel, polished steel, and metal plated (nickel or silver).

3. **Temper.** The temper of the blade means the degree of hardness of the steel. Proper temper is assured by reputable manufacturers. Temper is drawn by a process of heating and cooling. The temper of razors runs fairly uniform, but the temper of some razors are soft, medium, or hard. Medium and hard tempered blades are preferred since they hold their edge longer.

Regrinding razors: A razor can be reground. Regrinding is the process of grinding a razor down to a smaller size to make a new cutting edge. Razors can be successfully reground, but many times they are not up to par. Much depends on the grinder. Regrinding is occasioned by a razor being chipped beyond honing, or by the edge being worn out.

Razor's edge: The razor's edge, as studied under a microscope leads to much theorizing and controversy. True, its edge has been likened to the teeth of a saw, but only for the want of a better analogy. At best the comparison is a very broad one. Strictly speaking, the razor's edge does not have teeth like a saw. If the term "teeth" is used at all to describe the cutting edge, it should not be taken literally, for it is only an attempt to describe the elevated formations made by honing.

A sharp or freshly honed edge has temporary formations which resemble "hills and valleys." The "ups" and "downs" across the edge neither slant or point uniformly in any direction, nor are they even pointed.

It is reasonably accurate to say the razor's edge has teeth. When such formations are completely gone, the edge has lost its keenness and has become dull. These surface elevations are necessary to give the edge the proper cutting ability. New teeth are made by honing.

Razors are hot forged under drop hammers from high carbon steel. This steel is furnished by the mills in the form of bars and are then heated until they are red hot. When they have reached this stage the steel is then pounded under terrific pressure by the drop hammer in which the forging dies roughly shape out the razor blank. (After this process comes the tempering, grinding, and polishing.) This method applies to both hollow ground and wedge razors.

It is noteworthy that teeth set by a honing stroke in one particular direction are easily distorted and broken off by a honing stroke in the opposite direction. Uniformity in the angle of honing strokes is recommended to achieve a perfect cutting edge.

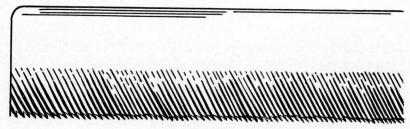

Fig. 27
Razor's Edge Under Magnification

HONES

A **hone** is a smoothly shaped, wearable solid with abrasive ability to cut steel. Hones are generally prepared in the form of flat slabs or small pencils or rods, but some are designed for a special implement. A razor hone is usually a rectangular block.

Purpose of hone: The purpose of any hone is to sharpen something. Some are used to sharpen scythes or mowing machines. The purpose of a razor hone is to sharpen razors.

Classification of hones: There are many kinds and makes of hones. They are classified according to their source, and there are two sources.

1. Manufactured. These are also known as **synthetic,** because they consist of more than one kind of substance. The swaty and carborundum hones are examples.

2. Natural. These are made from natural stones and examples of these are the Belgian and water hones.

Cutting ability of hones:

1. Water hones cut the slowest.
2. Carborundum hones cut the fastest.
3. All synthetic hones cut faster than natural hones because of their abrasiveness.
4. The cutting ability of hones can be increased by using water or lather on them.

Swaty hones: The swaty is a synthetic hone. Common on the market are swaty hones made in America or Austria. These hones have a medium fast sharpening ability, and they may be used either wet or dry. The new swaties are made by present day manufacturers and the old ones were made by an Austrian chemist. None of the old original swaty hones are on the market. The old swaty is different from the new swaty in that it is slightly harder, slower cutting, slightly thinner, has a lighter shade of brown, and it is about 1/64 of an inch shorter. If the finger nail is drawn across the surface of an old swaty, it will leave no mark. Whether the old swaty is superior to the new one is debatable, but some barbers will pay a fancy price for an old swaty.

Two-line and three-line swaty hones: These terms refer simply to the number of lines of words in the engraving. Some have two lines and some three. It is believed that the oldest old swaties were three-lined.

Where and by whom swaty was first made: The first swaty hones were made in Austria by an Austrian chemist. The story runs that he first made such hones to sharpen axes, and, finding the hones so successful, he conceived the idea of making them for sharpening razors. When he died the formula was not on record, so it is thought; but his son then made the hones, although he may have used a slightly different formula. Those made by the son are likely the two-line old swaties. The swaty is believed to be the **first manufactured hone.**

Carborundum hones: Carborundums are **synthetic** hones. They are manufactured in the United States. These composition hones contain carbon and silicon. Such hones may be used dry or wet. Carborundums are made in varying degrees of coarseness and are designated by such numbers as 79, 101, 102, 103, 118, 152, and 159. Number 118 is very popular.

Belgian hones: The Belgian hone is a **natural** hone. It is primarily a wet hone—use water, lather, or oil. It is slow-cutting but faster than the water hone. This hone is quarried from natural rock formed by alkali deposits in crevices deep in the earth. It is a two-toned natural stone with a yellowish top and a reddish slate base.

Water hones: The water hone is a **natural** hone and one of the oldest. It is usually imported from Germany. This accounts for the fact that it is sometimes called the German hone. This hone is a natural gray slate stone that has a very fine cutting surface. It cuts so slowly it is almost impossible to over-hone with it. An edge put on by a water hone will outlast an edge put on with any other hone. The water hone is a "wet" hone—use water or lather. It is the **slowest** cutting hone.

Cleaning hones: Hones may be cleaned with creamy lather and the palm of the hand. A pumice stone dampened with water may also be used. Keep your hone clean. New hones should be cleaned before using. After wet honing, always clean the hone to remove the fine particles of steel that adhere to it.

Combination hones: A combination hone consists of two kinds of hones, most often a carborundum and swaty.

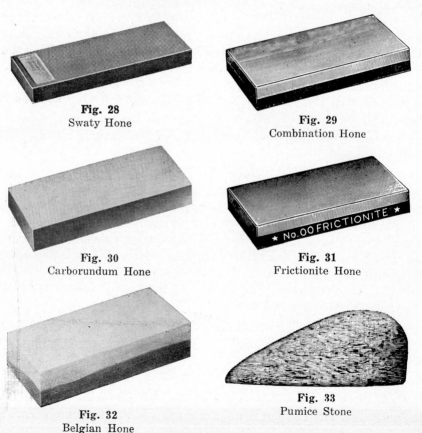

Fig. 28
Swaty Hone

Fig. 29
Combination Hone

Fig. 30
Carborundum Hone

Fig. 31
Frictionite Hone

Fig. 32
Belgian Hone

Fig. 33
Pumice Stone

STROPS

A razor strop is made of flexible durable material that is processed to a smooth surface. Its finish must be perfect to accommodate the delicate edge of a razor.

Noteworthy points about strops:

1. Purpose of stropping—to bring the razor to a smooth, whetted edge.
2. General classification of strops: (1) Leather and (2) Canvas.
3. A properly broken-in strop is preferred to a new one.
4. Animals that provide strop leather:

   (1) The pig.
   (2) The bear.
   (3) The cow.
   (4) The horse.
   (5) The seal.
   (6) Sheep.

5. Russian strops and Russian shells. Russian strops are made from cowhide. "Russian" as a term applied to strops refers to the system of tanning, which originated in Russia. The Russian **shell** is a leather strop that comes from the rumps of horses.
6. Composition of canvas strops: They are made of linen or silk. They vary in texture from fine to coarse.
7. Swivel: The hook or latch apparatus that fastens two strops together is called swivel.
8. Padding: A leather should not be used separately. Place another strop under it for padding.
9. Requirements of a good strop:

   (1) Very smooth, finished surface.
   (2) Proper thickness and uniform in thickness. Proper thickness runs from medium to very thick. Some barbers like thin strops, others like thick strops.
   (3) Medium texture—not too soft nor too hard. Barbers prefer a strop with a little "pull." A very soft leather has too much pull; a very hard one too little.
   (4) Capable of putting on a velvet-like edge.

10. The **swivel** is the metal attachment by which the strop is fastened to a stationary place for use, and by which the two strops are held together.
11. Breaking in a leather strop. There are several good ways to break in a leather strop. Some new strops need only to be cleaned with creamy lather and the palm of the hand. Others need to be treated by rubbing a dry pumice over them and then rubbing creamy lather in with a pumice. The finishing touch is to rub a smooth glass bottle over a strop to which has been applied fresh creamy lather. (Break in canvas by this latter method.)
12. **Care of strops:** Keep the strop clean. Rich creamy lather and the palm of the hand usually suffice.
13. A **combination strop** consists of a leather and canvas.

LATHER BRUSHES

A lather brush is used to make and spread lather for shaving. Although the lather brush is still widely used, it is gradually being replaced by other means of making lather and in some areas its use is prohibited by board rule or law. Other ways of making lather are (1) the electric latherizer, (2) shaving cream tubes, and (3) atomized latherizer.

Source of lather brush bristles: The bristles most commonly used come from boars. These bristles are largely imported from China, Korea, France, and Russia. Some come from the United States. The razor back hogs in some Southern states have bristles suitable for brushes. The choice bristles from boars are taken from underneath the chin and from the leg pits. Bristles are also made from badgers. The badger brush is very expensive.

Sizes of brushes: The size of brushes are indicated by numerals, such as 2, 3, 4, 5, and 6. Numbers 3 and 4 are used most.

Handles of brushes: Handles are made of celluloid, wood, and aluminum.

Breaking in a lather brush: Unless a lather brush is broken in correctly, it will swirl and throw lather. Soak the bristles of a new brush thoroughly with moist lather; then roll the bristles up in a wet face towel. Now, fold over the unused portion of the towel, and bind with a string or strong rubber band. Leave it thusly over night. Follow the same procedure for two or three nights. When properly broken in, the bristles will all slope in one direction (Figs. 34-35).

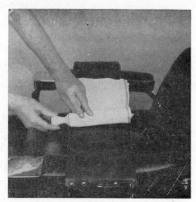

Fig. 34
Rolling up Lather Brush

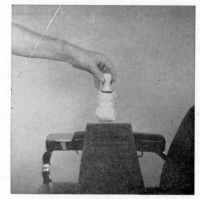

Fig. 35
Brush Correctly Bound

ELECTRIC LATHERIZERS

Electric latherizing machines are becoming increasingly popular. An electrically produced lather service appeals to the public psychologically. It signifies to the public an emphatic stress on sanitary standards. While there is nothing inherently unsanitary about the use of a lather brush, it does not provide the uniqueness of individualized sanitary measures. One important feature of a lather making machine is that its spout should

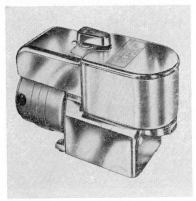

Fig. 36
Electric Latherizer

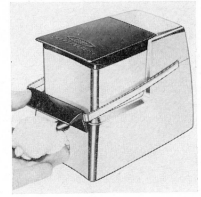

Fig. 37
Electric Latherizer

be scientifically designed so as to prevent any foreign matter from getting into the lather. Some merits advanced by the manufacturers of electric latherizers are as follows:

1. Greater uniformity in the consistency and temperature of lather.
2. The ever-readiness of lather saves time.
3. More economical—less soap and water.
4. Higher sanitary standard.
5. Added shop distinction in equipment.

DUSTERS

A duster is used to remove loose end-hairs occasioned by haircutting. On sanitary grounds, several substitutes have been devised, such as the use of the towel specially manipulated, individual paper hair removers, and electrical hair vacs. The evil of hair dusters has been exaggerated, since disease-producing germs would not choose to habitate in a duster as it is frequented with talcum powder and kept dry. However, these special devices have some merit and they are psychologically good.

A hair duster should be cleaned frequently by soaking in thick lather, and washing it out in luke-warm water. Roll about twenty bond paper around the duster, and use a rubber band or string to hold the paper in place. Allow it to dry naturally or dry it under an electric dryer.

Composition of hair dusters: Dusters are made largely from horsehair. While the hair comes mainly from the tails of horses, some come from their mane. Nylon dusters are also **made**.

Towel as duster: A duster is not indispensable. A small towel can be manipulated to dust off loose hairs. Fold the towel lengthwise, and then fold it again so as to bring the two ends together. Gather the towel into

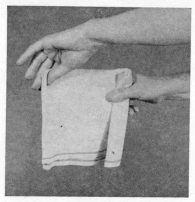

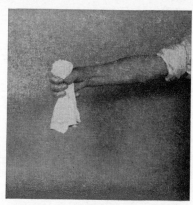

Fig. 38
Beginning

Fig. 39
Finish

Towel Used As Duster

the right hand completely. The feeding and holding should be between the third and fourth fingers. Having completed the gathering, sift powder on to the free ends and proceed in the same manner as with a duster (Figs. 38, 39).

ELECTRIC HAIR VACUUMS

Electric hair vacuums remove loose cut ends of hair. They may be used instead of dusters. The chief merit of such machines is increased sanitation. They have a good psychological appeal to the public. But clean and sanitized hair dusters are not transmitters of germs.

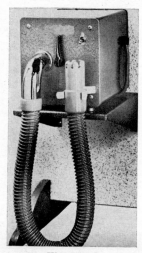

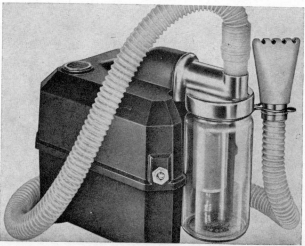

Fig. 39-A

Fig. 39-B

TWEEZER

Uses of the tweezer:

1. Pulling out ingrown hairs in the neck and face.
2. Removing blackheads.
3. Plucking stray eyebrow hairs.

Extracting ingrown hair with tweezer:

1. Set it astride the hair to be extracted.
2. Pull slowly to keep from breaking off the hair. Begin slowly to gain the proper tightness and then execute quickly to lessen or minimize the pain.
3. Hold skin tight at point of extraction.

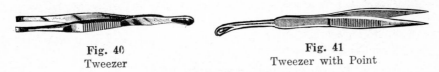

Fig. 40
Tweezer

Fig. 41
Tweezer with Point

VIBRATORS

Electric vibrators are used for massaging. There are several makes and designs on the market. Such machines enable the barber to massage and manipulate the tissues of the scalp, face, and neck without tiring the hands, and perhaps to do a better job. The use of vibrators also impresses the customer.

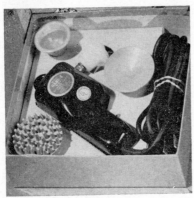

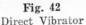

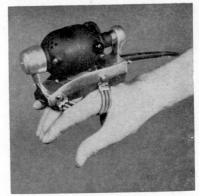

Fig. 42
Direct Vibrator

Fig. 43
Indirect Vibrator

Types of vibrators: There are two general of vibrators:

1. **Direct.** A vibrator of this type comes with a set of applicators. Their use brings them into direct contact with the skin.

2. **Indirect.** The indirect type is attached to the back of the hand and only the finger tips come in contact with the skin.

Many barbers prefer the indirect vibrator. They like the "finger" contact better than the "cup" contact. The fingers are more versatile than applicators and can massage small or large areas, and the fingers are easier to sanitize than rubber applicators. The indirect type is also known as "hand vibrator" and the direct as "cup vibrator."

LATHER MUGS

A lather mug is a specially designed receptacle in which to make lather. The bottom of the mug is usually made to accommodate a cake of soap. Lather mugs are made of glass, earthenware, plastic, or aluminum.

CARE OF IMPLEMENTS

The true artisan not only has a kit graced with the finest implements, he takes great pride in caring for them. He keeps them clean, ready for use, and protected against corrosion. The razor is the most tarnishable and it should be dried with a soft towel each time it is placed in the cabinet; the shears are the next most tarnishable.

When carrying tools, they should be very carefully packed. An implement kit is recommended for packing the shears, razors, combs, tweezers, clasp and hone. Razors may be packed in razor boxes and the blades of shears may be inserted in a shear sheath. Clippers are best packed in the clipper box. Place the guard over the blades and give extra protection by folding and tying heavy cardboard over the guard. Hones are very breakable. They are safest when wrapped generously with soft cloth, although they are fairly safe in hone boxes if lid is held on by a rubber band. Roll the strop with the usuable surface inside — do not roll tightly.

While tools should be cleaned whenever they need it throughout the day, they should have a general thorough cleaning regularly and systematically. Even though tools are thoroughly cleaned, they should be disinfected before using. All implements should be kept thoroughly clean, but emphasis should be placed on the ones that come in direct contact with the skin of the patron, such as the razor, shears, clipper, and comb.

Shears: Always lay down closed. Never use them to cut string, paper or cloth. Do not put oil in the pivot; if they squeak, run hot water over the pivot. Oil on the pivot would collect hair and bind the blades. Clean shears with a brush and a solution of soapy water, boric acid, or baking soda.

Combs: Combs may be cleaned as prescribed for shears. A stiff brush is best. Finish by running a strong stream of cold water over them.

Clippers: Brush the blades off before placing them in the cabinet, and before disinfecting them. There is a special clipper brush. The blades may be cleaned as prescribed for shears, although immersing them in a shallow jar or pan of kerosene while the clipper is running is recommended. Keep them immersed long enough to wash out the dirt and hair — a few seconds suffice. After cleaning the blades, be sure to oil them with a recognized clipper oil. Hang the clipper with the blades downward so that any excess oil will run to the teeth and not back into the clipper and on to the coil. Never put or hold the clipper under a water faucet. There is a danger of electric shock, and water will rust the blades. Do not hold the clipper when turning the water faucet on or off, or when the water is running. Occasionally clean the clipper as a whole. Although the clipper has a ring-hook by which it can be hung up, it is a much better system to lay it in a drawer of some kind, and thereby lessen the probability of missing the hood and dropping or knocking it down. The blades should be tilted downward. Be sure to keep a record of the serial number of the clipper.

Razors: Always lay the razor down closed. Never close it without first drying the blade. Clean around the pivot with a string. It is permissible to oil the pivot. The blade and handle may be cleaned with the same solutions suggested for cleaning shears, but use a soft cloth. A strong stream of hot water usually suffices. Do not attempt to remove stains of long standing. Do not use friction material to polish, such as steel wool. A shear grinder can professionally polish razor blades.

Hones: Never run hot water over a hone — it would crack. Wipe off the hone with the palm of the hand before each use. Clean it daily, using rich creamy lather and the palm of the hand.

Strops: Pass the palm of the hand over the strop before each use. Never clean a leather strop with water because water drys and hardens. Use thick lather and the palm of the hand. A canvas, however, may be cleaned with a soapy water solution. Strops should be kept thoroughly clean. They should have a general cleaning, including the swivel, once weekly. There are some good strop cleaning preparations that are purchaseable.

Mug and lather brush: Rinse off the mug before each use. Give both the mug and the handle of the lather brush a good cleaning daily.

Immediately after serving a customer, clean all implements used and return them to their proper places. (Do not leave implements on the work-stand between customers.)

Honing and Stropping

Honing and stropping are a knack as well as a science. There are therefore different theories about each of these processes. The beginner should be guided by the established techniques. The student should use a dummy razor to practice honing and stropping. He may use his good hone, but he should use either an old strop or a canvas.

HONING

Definition of honing: Honing is the process of sharpening a razor on a hone.

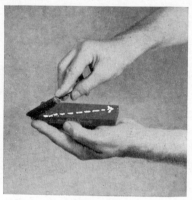

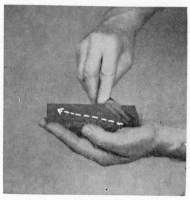

| Fig. 44 | Fig. 45 |
| Starting Position | Return Position |

Pointers on honing:

1. Draw the blade diagonally across the hone, from the heel to the point, and towards the cutting edge.
2. The honing strokes should be of equal length to assure regularity in the new teeth formation.
3. Keep the blade flat on the hone in all strokes.
4. Apply equal pressure in all strokes on each side of the razor.
5. Pressure on the hone should be from light to moderate.
6. The time required for sharpening depends upon the condition of the edge, the newness of the razor, the kind of hone, the rate and length of the strokes. The required number of strokes run from five to

ten unless it is a case of reconditioning the razor. A new razor requires fewer strokes than an old one. Discretion will have to be employed when using a fast or slow cutting hone. One will learn by a kind of "mysterious draw" when the razor is taking an edge; he will sense a suction effect. This effect acts as a signal to stop.

7. The strokes should be about three-fourths the length of the hone.

8 Begin the strokes at the farther end of the hone, making sure to have the heel on the hone.

9. Stop on each stroke with about one-half the blade left on the hone to allow for accurate turning of the razor in preparation for the next stroke. At the end of a stroke, turn the razor over and at the same time slide it up to a position which corresponds to the original starting position at the other end of the hone.

10. Turn the razor over at the end of each stroke with the fingers only, without moving the wrist. Using the fingers makes for quickness and gracefulness.

11. Special pointers on holding and turning the razor while honing:

   (1) Hold the razor firmly, but not tightly.

   (2) Set the handle almost in line with the blade.

   (3) For the take off, lay the razor flat near the end of the hone, place the ball of finger one on the shank just behind the shoulder, the ball of the thumb directly in front of the pivot, the ball of the second finger directly behind the pivot, and bend the other two fingers around the handle to hold it steady and to aid in turning.

   (4) Turn the razor at the end of the first stroke, simply roll the razor over to the right, keep the back in contact with the hone by use of all the fingers including the thumb. By turning the razor in this way, it will be discovered that the razor is rolling over in the fingers instead of the fingers rolling over it. In position for the next stroke, the first finger will over-lap the front of shank somewhat, the thumb will be almost at the back of the pivot, the first joint of the second finger will brace the front pivot section of the handle, and the other two fingers will have closed in just a little more.

   (5) On returning to the original end of the hone, if more honing is to be done, turn the razor back to the "take-off" position.

   (6) Always end the stroke at the same end of the hone that the first stroke began.

   (7) Strokes should never be too fast and jerky. Make them long, smooth, even, rhythmical, and graceful.

12. A razor should not be honed unless it is dull. A properly honed razor is good for several shaves. It should not be necessary to hone after each shave. The edge is preserved by the manner in which it is used.

13. The most common error in honing is to over-hone.

14. Removal of over-honed effects:
    (1) Hone with the back of the blade leading instead of the cutting edge. In other words, hone with a stropping stroke.
    (2) Pull the cutting edge over a bar of soap.
    (3) Drag the cutting edge over a very soft piece of pine wood.

15. Testing the edge of a freshly honed razor:
    A freshly honed razor is best tested by drawing it over a moistened thumb nail (Fig. 46). The real test however is in the actual shaving. One can develop the knack of knowing when the honed edge is right. He knows the disposition of his razor and knows about how many honing strokes to make. It is a misconception that the ability of a razor to split a single hair proves that it has a perfect cutting edge. Of course a dull razor will not split a hair, but a razor that has a rough, over-honed edge if manipulated correctly will split a hair, yet its edge would be too rough and wire-like for a smooth shave and it would produce a burning effect on the face. The hair-splitting ability of a razor indicates one or two conditions — one, that it has a rough, wire-like sharp edge, and the other is that it has a proper cutting edge.

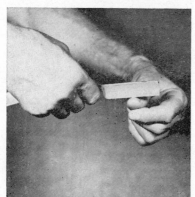

Fig. 46
Testing Off Hone

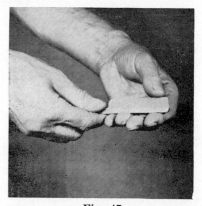

Fig. 47
Testing Off Strop

16. Sensations indicating condition of the razor's edge:
    (1) A slight dragging but somewhat smooth sensation indicates a keen, perfect edge. (Ready for stropping).
    (2) A very smooth sliding sensation indicates dullness and blunt-needs more honing).
    (3) A decided digging in, grating sensation indicates a rough, coarse over-honed edge.
    (4) An unevenness of sensation indicates faulty honing or a defect in the razor through dropping, over-use, etc.

(5) A harsh, biting sensation in one particular place indicates the presence of a nick or gap. (Needs more honing, perhaps a general honing).

17. Use lather or water on hone: The use of water or lather on a hone hastens sharpening. The use of lather is recommended to remove nicks or to recondition a very dull razor.

STROPPING

Definition of stropping: Stropping is the process of smoothing the edge of a razor on a strop. Stropping gives the razor a whetted edge.

Pointers on stropping razor:

1. When to strop a razor. The best answer is to strop it whenever it needs it. Theoretically, it is stropped (1) before the first stroke, (2) about half-way through a shave, (3) before shaving the second time over, and (4) before arching over the ears and shaving sides of neck.

2. The razor is stropped with the back of the blade leading. The direction of the blade in stropping is the opposite of that in honing.

3. The angle of the stroke is about the same as that for honing.

4. Make stropping strokes long, from six to ten inches.

5. Keep the razor entirely flat on the strop. It is advisable to lift up just a little at the shoulder of the razor so as to make doubly sure that the point comes in full contact with the strop. The general tendency is to ride the base line near the heel and thereby slight the point.

6. Pressure on the strop should be moderate, but more than on the hone. Too much pressure, especially if its a full hollow ground type of razor, bends the blade so that the point does not receive full benefit from the stropping.

7. Hold the strop rigid so that there is practically no give, to avoid cutting the strop and prevent too much pressure on the point.

8. Strop noiselessly. Do not pound the strop with the razor.

9. Never lift the razor off the strop during the process of stropping—contact is not broken.

10. Strop less after honing than at any other time, because the freshly honed edge is more sensitive and responds quickly to anything that comes into contact with it, and because the very edge is easily disturbed.

11. A freshly honed razor is stropped on a leather strop only. A canvas strop is too coarse for the razor in this sensitive condition.

12. After using the razor, strop on the canvas first if a canvas and leather combination strop is used.

13. The standard number of stropping strokes runs from ten to twenty.
14. Do not make the strokes too fast or too slowly. The tempo should be between these two extremes.
15. The strokes should be rythmical, long, angular, of little pressure and graceful.
16. Hot water on razor. It seems to add to the cutting ability of a razor to run hot water over the blade just before using it. It is a known fact that warm steel cuts more easily than cold steel, and then a cold razor is uncomfortable to the skin.

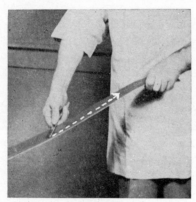
Fig. 48
Starting End

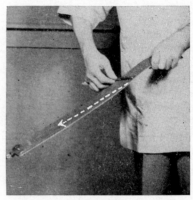
Fig. 49
Return End

Linen Uses In Common

There are some uses of linen that are employed in two or more services. Only such uses will be discussed and illustrated in this chapter. The uses that are particular to a given service are in connection with that service.

Spreading and folding haircloth:

1. Pick up folded haircloth by inserting the index finger of the left hand in the neck piece (Fig. 50).
2. With finger so inserted, lift the haircloth upward and shake it slightly so that it will unfold naturally (Fig. 51).

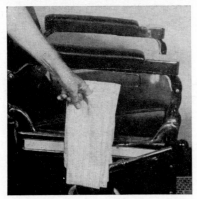

Fig. 50
Pick Up Haircloth

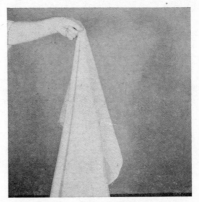

Fig. 51
Unfolding Haircloth

3. Hold the haircloth on each side of the neck piece, stand on he right side of the chair, and make a graceful wide swing so that the haircloth will fall gently upon the patron (Fig. 52).
4. The haircloth should not touch the skin of the patron's neck (Fig. 53).
5. Remove haircloth gracefully. Step to the right side of the patron, grasp with the left a gathered section of the haircloth on the left side about where it touches the patron's knees, and likewise with right hand. Lift upward and join with the respective sections near the top of the haircloth. Lift haircloth off patron (Figs. 54, 55).
6. After use, fold the haircloth neatly and replace it on the chair so that the neck piece shows. Fold the haircloth lengthwise, then midwise, and then fold it twice more (Figs. 56 to 59).

Small Towel (Also called face towel) :

1. To unfold a small towel, grasp any corner of it with the thumb and first finger of the left hand. The weight of the towel will cause it to unfold of its own accord (Figs. 60, 61).
2. Arranging face towel across front and sides of neck.

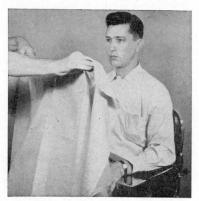

Fig. 52
Spreading Haircloth

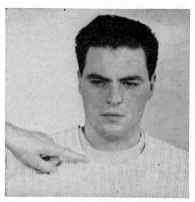

Fig. 53
Completed Spread

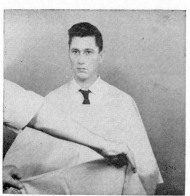

Fig. 54
Removing Haircloth
(First Step)

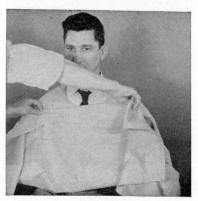

Fig. 55
Removing Haircloth
(Second Step)

(1) Unfold face towel and lay it diagonally across patron's chest.
(2) Tuck left corner section over and inside shirt collar, using a gentle sliding movement of the forefinger of the left hand to smooth it out.
(3) Cross lower right corner section of towel over to left side of neck and arrange same as on right side, but use **right forefinger** to smooth out.

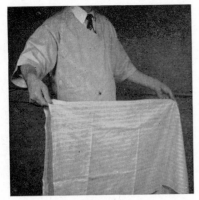

Fig. 56
Folding Step No. 1

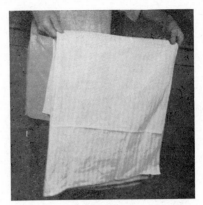

Fig. 57
Folding Step No. 2

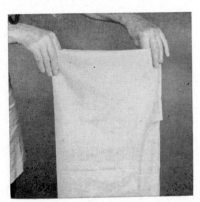

Fig. 58
Folding Step No. 3

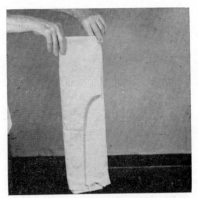

Fig. 59
Folding Final Step

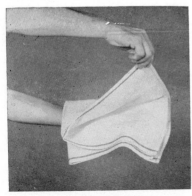

Fig. 60
Picking Up Face Towel

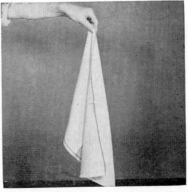

Fig. 61
Unfolding Face Towel

(4) Do not reach over patron's face while arranging this towel. Stand at same place, and at right side.

(5) With both hands smooth out portions of towel lying across patron's chest.

(6) Lower edge of towel should be straight across chest at right angle.

(7) A **double thickness** of the small towel may also be used. It is especially appropriate for a facial to give double protection to the customer's clothing. Simply make a small diagonal fold at each corner of the towel to be tucked over the collar, and proceed as just explained.

3. Blotting face with small towel. Fold the towel lengthwise once. This gives the correct padding for pressure in blotting. Lay the towel across the sides of the face and neck. Place the finger tips of each

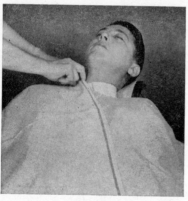
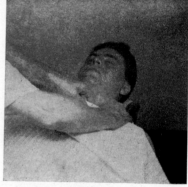

Fig. 62   Fig. 63

Making Linen Set-up for Shave or Facial

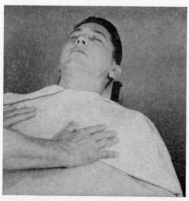
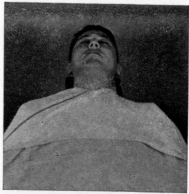

Fig. 64   Fig. 65
Smoothing Out Towel   Complete Set-up

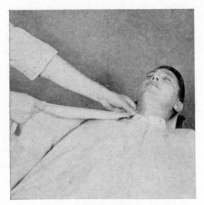

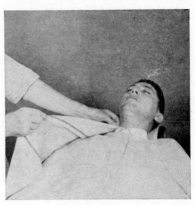

Fig. 66
A Single Thickness Set-up

Fig. 67
A Double Thickness Set-up

hand together at the chin and slide them firmly over the towel, spreading the fingers gradually. Proceed so as to cover the entire face and neck (except forehead). Then lift the towel to one side of the face and place it over the eyes and forehead. Apply pressure with the finger tips, gently over eyes and firmly over forehead (Figs. 68, 69).

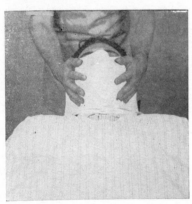

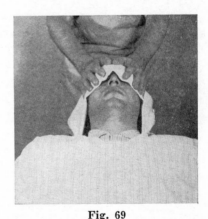

Fig. 68

Fig. 69

Blotting Face with Towel

4. Fanning face with small towel. Fold the towel lengthwise and make the back and forth motion with the right hand, while the left hand is held stationary (Figs. 70, 71).

5. Wiping face with small towel. The towel is first folded lengthwise. Grasp one end of the towel with the thumb and first finger of the left hand and at about four inches from the other end grasp it with the first two fingers of the right hand. Manipulate the hands so as to bring the towel diagonally across the palm of the right hand and

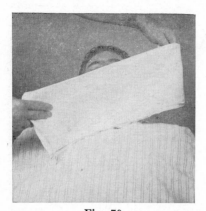

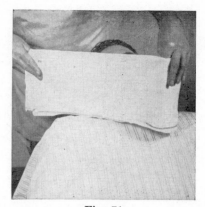

Fig. 70   Fig. 71

Fanning Face with Towel

around to the back of the right. Twist the loose end of the towel, bring it around the thumb and place it between the thumb and first finger of the right hand. Now tuck the overlapping portion of the towel between the second and third fingers. Completed, the result is a soft, neat pad for wiping the face. Make sure that the exact portion of the towel to be used to wipe the face is smooth. If powder is to be applied with the towel, re-wrap the towel after turning it around or over so as to assure a dry surface for the powder (Figs. 72-78).

Wrapping Face Towel Around Hand
Standard Method

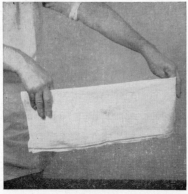

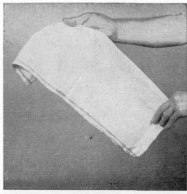

Fig. 72   Fig. 73

Wrapping, Step No. 1   Wrapping, Step No. 2

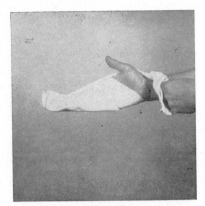

Fig. 74
Wrapping, Step No. 3

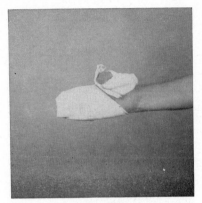

Fig. 75
Wrapping, Final Step

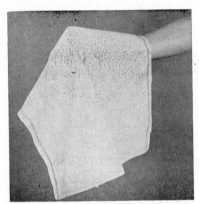

Fig. 76
Step No. 1

Vacuum Wrap

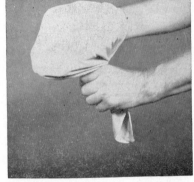
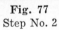

Fig. 77
Step No. 2

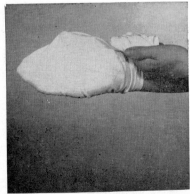

Fig. 78
Final Step (Vacuum)

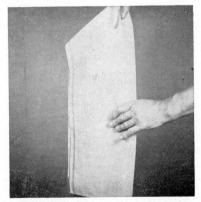

Fig. 79
Quick End Wrap, Step No. 1

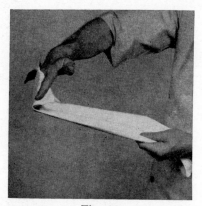

Fig. 80
Quick End Wrap, Step No. 2

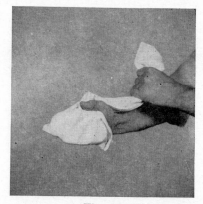

Fig. 81
Quick End Wrap, Final Step

Powdering face: There are two good ways to powder the face (Figs. 82, 83).

1. Sift powder onto the small towel after it has been wrapped around the hand in the same manner as for wiping the face.
2. Sift powder directly into the palm of the left hand and then distribute it over the finger tips of both hands.

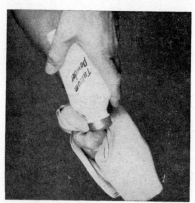

Fig. 82
Powdering with Towel

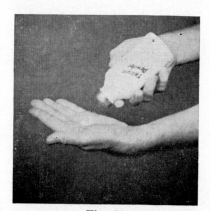

Fig. 83
Powdering with Hands

Steaming scalp with steam-towel: Carry a folded steamer in the left hand to a point just above the left ear. The closed edge of the towel should be down; this assures a straight and neat looking edge around the head. Grasp each end of the towel, unfold and wrap around the head so that the right end overlaps the left. While the left end is being held on the head it serves as a brace so that the left hand can tighten the steamer and complete a thoroughly tight wrapping (Figs. 84, 87).

Steaming Scalp

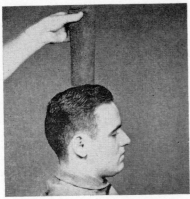

Fig. 84
Wrapping Steamer, Step No. 1

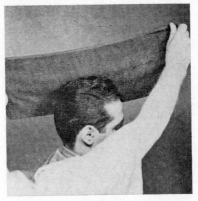

Fig. 85
Wrapping Steamer, Step No. 2

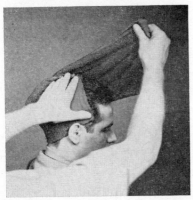

Fig. 86
Wrapping Steamer, Step No. 3

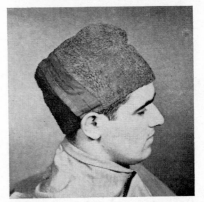

Fig. 87
Wrapping Steamer, Final Step

Preparing steam towel (Figs. 88 to 91).

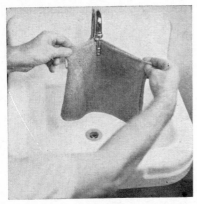

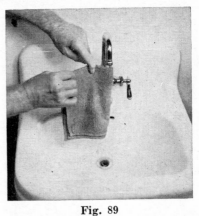

Fig. 88
Fig. 89
Wrapping Steamer Around Faucet

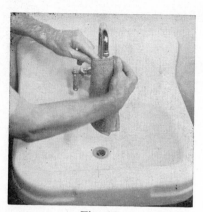

Fig. 90
Wrapping Steamer Around Faucet

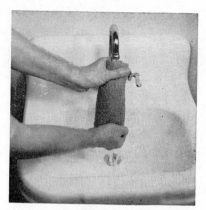

Fig. 91
Heating Steamer

1. Fold it lengthwise, and again lengthwise, bringing the ends together. At mid-point hook it on the faucet and manipulate it into a roll. Saturate it thoroughly with moderately hot water. While water is running through the towel, grasp the bottom of the rolled towel with the right hand and manipulate the towel up and down so as to facilitate water distribution.

2. Wring the towel out especially well.

Steaming the face "plain." Plain steaming is done with steam towels (Figs. 92-95).

1. The steam-towel should be carried folded in the left hand to the chin. Unfold it at the chin and allow it to fall gently and naturally over the face as the ends are brought to the forehead where the **right end is placed over the left.** The towel should be lax so that it will take the shape of the face. A tautly spread towel is ropey.

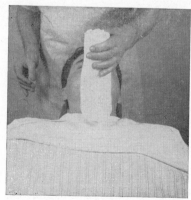

Fig. 92
Applying Steamer, Step No. 1

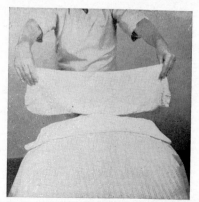

Fig. 93
Applying Steamer, Step No. 2

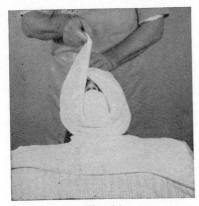

Fig. 94
Applying Steamer, Final Step

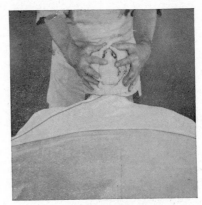

Fig. 95
Pressing Steamer

2. When the placement of the steamer on the face is complete, spread the fingers of both hands and place them over the towel, the thumbs resting over the eyes, the first two fingers over the mouth and on the chin, and the other two fingers along the sides of the neck Press down gently and firmly about three seconds. ow remove the hands from the towel. **Do not pat the towel** (Fig. 95). Now lift the hands from this position and place them over the forehead so as to press down gently over the eyes with the cushion tips of the first two fingers and at the same time press down firmly for about three seconds over the forehead with the portions of the hands that fall naturally upon it

Removing steamer from face: When a second steamer is to be applied immediately the earlier steamer may simply be lifted from the face.

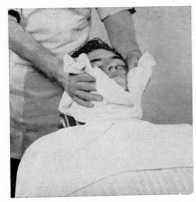

Fig. 96
Gathering Up Steamer

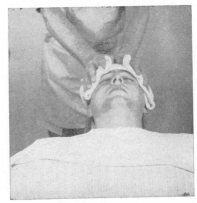

Fig. 97
Soothing Eyes—Forehead

1. When there is lather or excess cream to remove from the face, gather the steamer up into the hands as it is being removed so that it does not fall over the towel across the neck (Fig. 96).

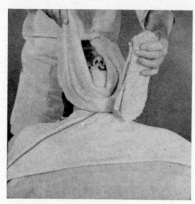

Fig. 98
Lifting First Steamer Off

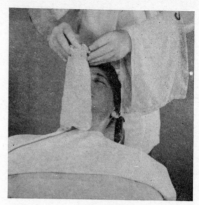

Fig. 99
Starting Second Application

Haircutting

Haircutting is both an art and science. The finished hair cut reveals the barber's mood as well as his artistic abilities. The true artist has a yen for accomplishment and he gets a thrill out of adding becomingness to someone else. The successful barber envisages such resultants every hour. A person's style of hair cut is definitely a part of his personality and so through this medium the barber has an opportunity to make an invaluable contribution.

Haircutting is an art in so far as it involves the principles just mentioned. The "eyeball perception" refers to the artistic phase of shaping and cutting hair. This is the phase on which two or more persons do not always entirely agree, but it is the phase all appreciate. The science of haircutting consists of the established techniques of performances, such as the scientific use of the comb, shears, and clippers. The mechanics, then, constitute the science of haircutting, whereas the adaptations, variations, designing, styling, and individual touches represent the art. The learning of the science is comparatively simple. The art is never completely accomplished. The artisan continues to grow, improve and progress. One does not have to be an artist to be a good hair cutter; but an outstanding hair cutter is artistic. The "knacks" of haircutting are the result of individual abilities, but the general scientific and artistic principles of haircutting are explainable, illustrative and learnable.

Definition of haircutting: Haircutting is the process of cutting and shaping hair according to a pattern. (It is not simply an act of cutting off hair. The cutting must result in an artistic creation. This process includes blending, tapering, shingling, designing, styling, and hair tailoring.)

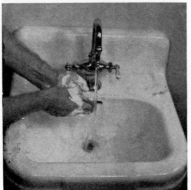

| Fig. 100 | Fig. 101 |

Washing and Drying Hands Just Before Serving Patron

Prerequisites of haircutting:

1. Knowing how to use the necessary implements. (Study the chapter on implements in conjunction with this chapter.)
2. Understanding the principles of haircutting.
3. Having mental images or pictures of the various styles.
4. Potential dexterity, patience, confidence, imagination, diligence, and determination.

Dressing patron for hair cut:

1. Spread haircloth gracefully. The haircloth should not touch the skin of the patron's neck or face (Figs. 102 to 103).
2. Ways of protecting skin of patron:
   (1) **Neck-strip set-up:** Carry a neck-strip in the left hand around the side of the neck to the front, and arrange it around the neck, over-lapping it in back. Arrange the U-shaped part of the

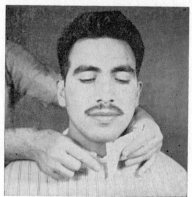

Fig. 102
Placing Neck-strip

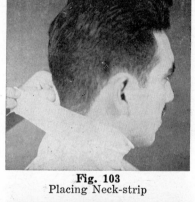

Fig. 103
Placing Neck-strip

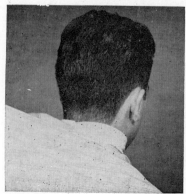

Fig. 104
Overlapping & Fastening
Haircloth

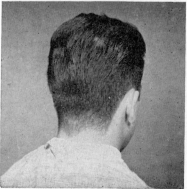

Fig. 105
Completed Neck-strip
Set-up

haircloth firmly over the neck-strip, over-lapping the left side over the right in back. Fasten the two parts of the haircloth with a non-pricking metal clip, and then turn the neck-strip down over the haircloth so as to form a cuff-like effect around the neck (Figs. 104, 105).

(2) **Small towel set-up:** Tuck the single thickness of a small towel across the back of the neck and under the shirt collar, apply about a three inch strip of the towel around the neck and over-lap it at the front of the neck. Arrange the haircloth over this strip, over-lap it at the left side of the neck, fasten the two ends of the haircloth, and then turn the towel down over the hair-cloth, forming a cuff-like effect (Figs. 106 to 109).

(3) **Paper towel set-up:** Arrange the towel in the same manner as prescribed for a "retouch."

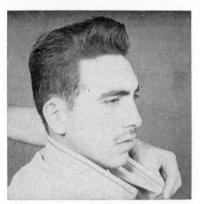

Fig. 106
Small Towel Set-up
Single Thickness

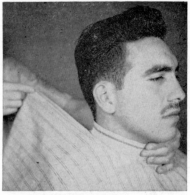

Fig. 107
Overlapping Towel in Front

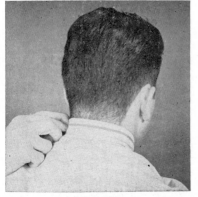

Fig. 108
Fastening Haircloth

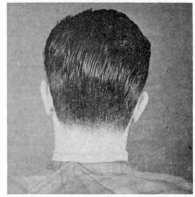

Fig. 109
Completed Set-up

Set-up for retouching hair cut: Retouching means a follow up cutting after outlining the cut with a razor. After outlining, there may be a few straggly ends that should be removed with the shears and comb. Then too, a final over-all look to discover any possible improvements is recommended. For retouching, the clothing and neck of the patron should be as meticulously protected as for the general hair cut. Fold the towel diagonally, place it over the collar in back and arrange it along the sides to the front of the neck where it is over-lapped. Bring up the ends of the haircloth, fasten it, and turn the towel down over the haircloth forming a cuff-like effect. Since the folding over of the towel is of double thickness, it may hold the haircloth in place without a clasp.

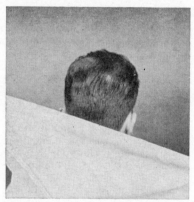

Fig. 110   Fig. 111

Diagonal Fold Retouch Set-up

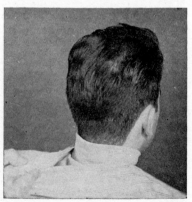
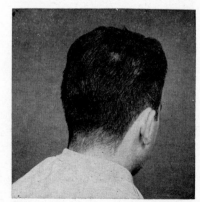

Fig. 112   Fig. 113

Diagonal Fold Retouch Set-up

Removing loose ends and dampness: Use smooth surface of towel to remove any loose ends or dampness. Pay particular attention to the forehead, nose, face, outlines, sides, and back of neck (Figs. 114 to 117).

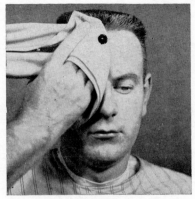

Fig. 114
Once Around Fold to Dry
Remove Loose Hair

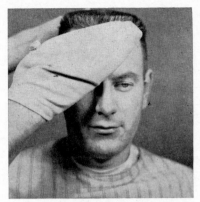

Fig. 115
Twice Around Fold to Dry
Remove Loose Hair

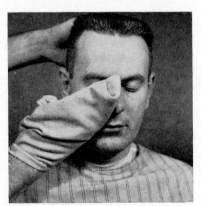

Fig. 116
Formal Fold to Dry
Remove Loose Hair

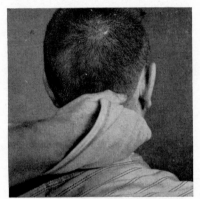

Fig. 117
Once Around Fold to Dry
Remove Loose Hair

POINTERS ON USE OF COMB

The comb should be held so that it can be manipulated easily and skillfully. If held properly the teeth can be turned either upward or downward, inward or outward, or changed from the fine to coarse part and reverse without the aid of the other hand.

1. Grasp the comb with the fingers and palm. The first finger is placed on the teeth about where the fine and coarse parts join, the thumb just below on the back of the comb, and the other three fingers are bent over the comb to assist in holding and manipulating it. Hold the comb firmly but not tightly.

2. While there is a scientific way to feed the comb into and through the hair, there is also a knack which one learns by concentrated

practice. With the teeth turned slightly towards the scalp at the edge, feed the comb into the hair until the hair rests firmly against the bar about an inch from the end of the comb and then turn the teeth upward. As the comb is pushed upward, pull the comb away from the scalp. **It is more important to move the comb itself away from the scalp gradually than to turn the teeth outward. The comb must be guided so as to keep it feeding into the hair until the desired amount is cut off. Turning the teeth outward may result in losing the hair to the shear and thus result in an abrupt blend. When hair is to be cut or blended, keep the comb feeding even though it may mean turning the teeth inward. The theory of turning the teeth**

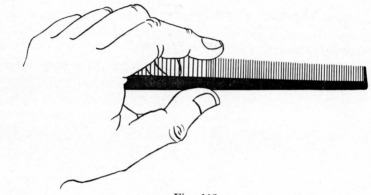

Fig. 118
Standard Method of Holding Comb

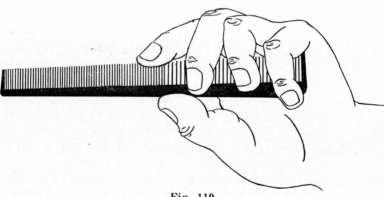

Fig. 119
Standard Method of Holding Comb

outward is applicable mainly to the extreme edge, especially when an extraordinarily full cut is to be given. To reiterate, emphasize moving the whole comb away from the scalp and keep the teeth feed-

ing until the follow through movement is completed. The comb should be manipulated so the hair to be cut is held approximately at right angle to the scalp. As a general rule the comb will continue to feed into the hair if it is held parallel to the contour of the head at the cutting point.

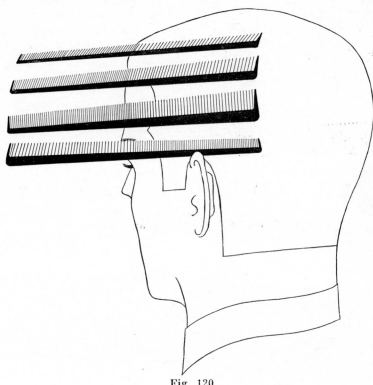

Fig. 120
Various Angles of Teeth of Comb

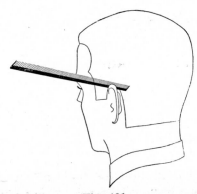

Fig. 121
Teeth Turned Inward

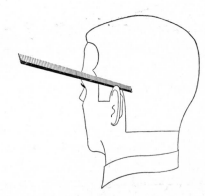

Fig. 122
Teeth Turned Outward

3. Use the coarse teeth of the comb wherever the hair is long enough to be picked up by them.

4. The fine teeth of the comb should be used only when the hair cannot be picked up with the coarse teeth. The fine teeth should be used to pick up hair at the extreme edge of the hair, to remove a clipper line, and to soften an arch or reduce sideburns.

5. In regular shingling, the shears and comb are held **parallel,** except at the sideburn and mastoid areas and wherever it would be awkward to hold them parallel.

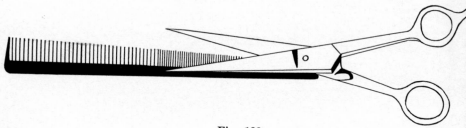

Fig. 123
Parallel Position of Shear and Comb

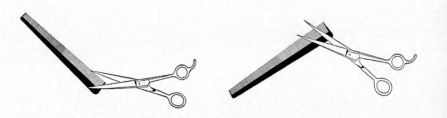

Fig. 124   **Fig. 125**
Diagonal Positions of Shear and Comb

POINTERS ON USE OF SHEARS

1. Hold the shears firmly but not tightly.

2. The thumb should not fit snugly in the thumb grip. Insert the thumb just far enough to be able to open and close the shears.

3. The third or ring finger should be inserted into the finger grip almost to the second joint.

4. The small finger should rest on the finger brace at all times.

5. The first and second fingers should be curved over the shank of the still blade to brace the shears.

6. For shingling, place the shank into the second crease of the first finger. In some instances, such as arching and fingerwork, place the shank into the first crease, because of the cutting position.

7. When the shears are held correctly, they can be slanted at any angle and even horizontally.

8. There should be a slight counter pressure applied to the blades.

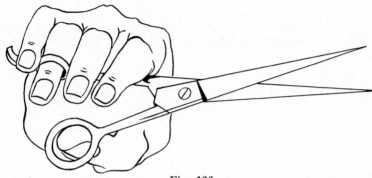

Fig. 126
Grasping Shears

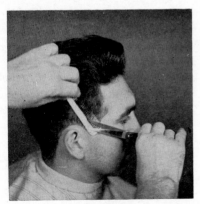
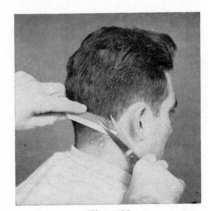

Fig. 127   Fig. 128
Diagonal Positions of the Shear and Comb

The finger grip is pulled toward the palm and the thumb grip is pushed from the palm.

9. **Do not over-use the points of the shears.** Save the points for the more delicate work such as arching over the ears. The over-use of the points dulls them, results in undue tediousness and inaccuracy.

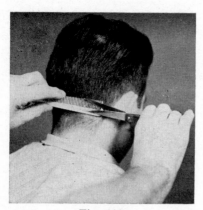

Fig. 129
Parallel Position
Shear and Comb

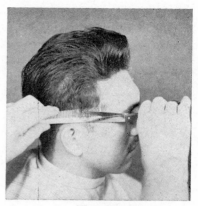

Fig. 130
Start Shear Work
Right Side

10. Make no unnecessary or superfluous movements; that is, open and close the shears only when cutting hair. Superfluous opening and closing of the blades wears the cutting edge down, sounds amateurish, and the resultant noise is undesirable.

11. Generally, close the shears just once on any single strand of hair. When the shears become so dull that this method cannot be used it is time have them sharpened.

12. Do not be noisy with the shears. Such noisiness may result from snapping the blades together too hard or from too loose blades. The blades should be so adjusted that either one of them can fall almost but not entirely closed on its own accord. (If the blades are too tight they tire the fingers and wrists.

13. **Start shear work on right side.** By proceeding from right to left, the points of the shears are directed into the next swath of hair to be cut, and thus, there is better visibility in the line of procedure. Conversely, proceeding from left to right, the shanks of the shears would be an obstruction to sight. When there is a problem area, it is often advisable to tackle it first wherever it is located. Left-handed persons should proceed from left to right.

SHEAR AND COMB EXERCISE

Shear and comb work can be practiced on any suitable object, such as a mounted bowling ball or manikin. One should develop **rhythm** in the use of the shears. Short, jerky, fretful, hesitant, and a mixture of fast and slow movements with the shears or any other implement characterize the amateur barber. For instance, in shingling make most strokes of about the same duration length and nature. The opposite of this would mean one or two quick, jerky strokes, followed by one or two slow, smooth strokes. Rhythm may even be developed to the place where the shears

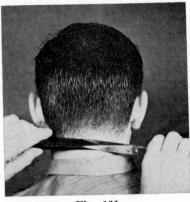 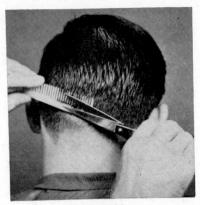

Fig. 131   Fig. 132
Edging with Shears and Comb

are opened and closed a certain number of times in the same length of
time on a given strand of hair.

One exercise to develop rhythm with the shears is to open and close
them four, six, and then eight times, starting at a given point and moving
upward in the air or on a wooden block. This is recommended as a preliminary to the first hair cut, but the exercise may be continued until
rhythm is developed.

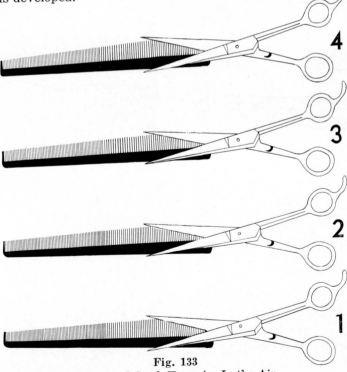

Fig. 133
Shear and Comb Excercise In the Air

POINTERS ON USE OF CLIPPERS

There are many good ways to use clippers. (Refer to the sections on Edging, Clipper-over-Comb Method, and Blade Attachments.)

1. Hold the clipper firmly but not tightly. Leave a small hollow space between the top part of the clipper, and the palm of the hand, irrespective of the make of clipper. (Gripping the clipper tightly stiffens the wrist.)

2. Feed the clipper slowly into the hair.

3. Gradually and slowly tilt the blades away from the head as they are moved upward.

4. Begin the clipper work at the base of the edge. Allow the still blade to become flattened on the surface of the scalp as it is moved upward; and at the place where you desire to start the actual taper, gradually tilt the blades outward, allowing the heel of the still blade to ride

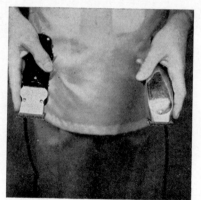

Fig. 134
Holding Clipper

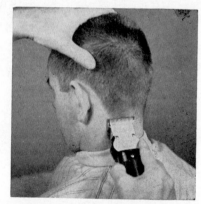

Fig. 135
Use Coarse Blade First

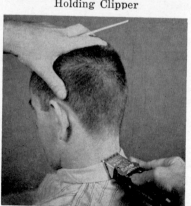

Fig. 136
Use Fine Blade Last

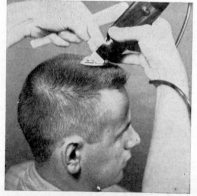

Fig. 137
Steadying Clipper

on the scalp to provide a support for guiding the clippers. Just how soon the taper is started, of course, depends upon the particular type of cut being given—sometimes the taper is begun at once.

5. When the clipper is used over the comb, the gauging of the degree of graduation is executed with the comb.

Where to start clipper work: In a **clipper all-around cut, start** the clipper work **on the left side.** The best reason for this procedure is that the clipper work is completed on the right side and at the exact place where the shear work is to begin. Another reason is that the hair part is usually on the left side. **When the clipper is to be used just in the back,** the general rule is to start on the left side of the neck, but if the edge appears indefinite it is preferable to **start at the middle of the neck.** By starting the clipper work at the middle of the neck, it is easier to get an accurate perspective of the back blend and thus assure not going too high. It is easier to visualize the correct neck-edge from the center cut strip than from the corner cut strip. Starting in the center, however, is optional with the barber. After completing the clipper work, step directly in back of the patron and view carefully all work done thus far. Check for balance and uniformity of shading. Notice the reflection in the mirror. The mirror sometimes reveals an otherwise unnoticed error.

MAJOR DIVISIONS OF HAIR CUT

Regardless of the type of a hair cut, it has three divisions.

1. Edges		1. Edging
2. Sides	or	2. Siding
3. Top		3. Topping

Sequence of cutting major divisions of hair cut: As a general rule, do the edges first, the sides second and the top last. When cutting a neglected head, the top may be tentatively cut to prevent the hair from riding the implements; a head of hair can be so voluminous as to make it impossible to determine the various divisions. It may be necessary to reduce the sides before edging. Shaping in these upper divisions first, however, is done only tentatively, the purpose being to clear the way for the edging. As soon as the clearance is completed, the haircut is begun and completed according to the standard procedure just outlined. In other words, this preliminary topping and shaping must be followed by finished topping and shaping after the edge is completed. There are other reasons for doing the upper divisions first. Such occasions arise (1) when the edge and middle consists of swirls, (2) when hair is matted, (3) when the hair is extremely dirty or greasy, and (4) when the head has bumps or eruptions.

Sequence of cutting three division is logical: The top cannot be merged or blended with something which does not exist. After the middle division has been completed, it is then possible to perform the topping with definite knowledge of its supporting division, the sides. Likewise, the middle section cannot be shaped to blend with something which does not exist; and so the logical step is to do the edge first. With the oundation laid, the hair cut can then be consructed by proceeding systematically from one phase of shaping to another. Conversely if the topping were done first, there would be loss of time resulting from the inevitable over-lapping of effort necessitated by the maximum element of guessing.

Merging three Divisions of hair cut: Each division merges into the division closest to it. The transition step between the edge and middle is so gradual that they become actually one. These divisions of course are strictly hypothetical, but they are more evident when the edging is done with the clipper. The edging may be extended into, and frequently through the middle section in a way so that it is all done as a general process. In this manner the edge is merged and blended with the middle section. Then, the top is blended to the middle division. This procedure is very logical—the edge is brought into blend with the middle, and the top into blend with the middle. While the topping is nearly always done as a separate process, the edging and siding are usually completed in one operation except for the clipper work. When the patron is bald or has only a scanty bit of top hair, all three divisions are cut as one general process.

Cutting top first theory: Although the standard cutting procedure of a hair cut is to follow the sequence just explained, the edge first, the sides second, and the top last, some barbers elect to do the top first. This method has been justified under certain conditions earlier in this chapter and even for general procedure it can hardly be deemed entirely wrong. The competent barber should be able to visualize the final result of his cutting and therefore whether the edge or top is done first makes no fundamental difference. It is true, however, that doing the top first often leads to over-lapping of movements, some re-doing, and thus more time. Perhaps architecture has the answer—first, the foundation, second, the sides or framework; and third, the roof.

METHODS OF EDGING

Edging is usually done with the clipper used alone or over the comb, when the hair is to be cut close at the base of the sides and back area. When the sides are to be left full, as in a Long Cut, the clipper is used to taper the edge in the back area only. Edging means tapering the hair so gradually that it fades out softly to the skin without a definite mark or line between the hair and the skin. In a hair cut in which the clipper is used just in the back, the edging on the sides is accomplished with the shears and comb, or with the clipper over the comb, depending on the style being given. While it is standard procedure to use the clipper wherever clipper-closeness is desired, practically the same effect can be achieved with the shears and comb, but this requires more time. There is no provable merit in the exclusive use of the shears and comb or the hand clipper to accomplish what can be done with the electric clipper to achieve a blended, tapered edge. If bumps or irregularities in the edge-area make the use of clippers impractical, use the shears and comb. However, if a customer is "touchy" in that he is afraid the barber will run the clipper too high, he may be pleased if the edging is done with either the hand clipper or the shears and comb.

To supplement the explanation here on edging, review the sections in this book on "Pointers on the Use of the Comb, the Shears, the Clipper, and the Clipper-Over-Comb Method."

Special Pointers on edging:

1. Start the clipper work on the left side in an all-around clipper cut; and in a cut in which the clipper is to be used just in the back, start either at the left side or at center of neck.

2. If just the clipper is to be used, place the coarse blade just below the edge and proceed upward vertically along a strip or swath of hair. Then switch to the fine blade to clip the extreme edge.

3. Finish each vertical strip as much as possible before moving to the next strip. The **finish-as-go** principle is applicable to each and every strip, and it saves time. It is incorrect to go "around and around" the head doing only a fraction of the edge on each round. The edging forms the foundation of the hair cut and so it should be done correctly and thoroughly. It is extremely difficult to build a good hair cut on a poor foundation.

4. When using either an adjustable or detachable blade clipper, use the coarse blade first and then follow-up with the fine blade at the extreme edge if greater closeness is desired. Do not run the fine blade high enough to destroy the blend made by the coarse blade. In brief, use the **Coarse-to-Fine** method whether the clipper is used alone or over the comb.

5. The head of the patron should be upright—natural position—during most of the edging.

6. The correct pattern of tapering with the clipper is illustrated in Fig. 141. It applies to the edge at the nape in a long hair cut. It is incorrect to proceed upward with the clipper and stop suddenly without tilting the blades outward and thus making a shelf effect. Instead, tilt the blades outward very gradually, making a taper.

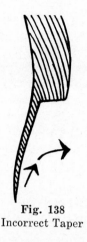

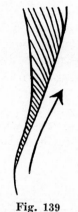

Fig. 138
Incorrect Taper

Fig. 139
Correct Taper

Methods of Edging Summarized: The methods of edging are largely a combination of the techniques already explained and illustrated, and they will not be reiterated here. All of these, along with the special pointers, should be borne in mind. Only four specific methods will be mentioned:

1. **Clipper edging.** Edging may be completed by clippers, using coarse and fine blades. Paramount in the use of the clipper for edging is to tilt it as it is advanced into the hair, and this can best be accomplished by riding the scalp with the heel of the still blade. Advance the clipper into the hair slowly to prevent the blades from jamming and pulling hair. This caution is particularly applicable to the use of hand clippers.

2. **Clipper-over-Comb method of edging:** The comb serves as a guard against lines and extreme closeness. The combination use of the clipper over the comb is simply another means of working from "coarse to fine" in edging. (Review the section on "Clipper-Over-Comb Method").

3. **The Line Method of Edging:** This method is still practiced by some barbers but it is not recommended. The fine clipper blade is advanced to the desired height without any graduation. A definite line is made and left to be removed with the shears and comb, or with the coarse clipper blade. The removal of this line entails unnecessary tediousness and time. Its remote merit is that it provides a definite and uniform point of demarcation between the edge and middle section; but the competent barber should be able to visualize this without a mechanically designated outline.

4. **Shear-Comb method of edging:** As stated earlier in this chapter, edging may be done with the shears and comb. This system is particularly fitting when the clipper cannot be used with advantage and

when clipper-closeness is not desired. Blades are being made so coarse, however, that almost any degree of closeness and of various short lengths can be accomplished with them. When the shears and comb are used for edging, the usual follow-up procedure is to use the clippers on the extreme lower edge to clip off the hairs, otherwise there would be too much tedious work with the shears.

CLIPPER-OVER-COMB METHOD

While the clipper-over-the-comb method is used in all divisions of some hair cuts, it is used primarily for edging. Learn the correct use and merits of this method. Do not overlook the fact that coarse blades as well as fine blades may be used successfully over the comb. The clipper-over-comb method is increasing rapidly in popularity. This method is simply a method of securing a coarse clipper effect. How can one be against

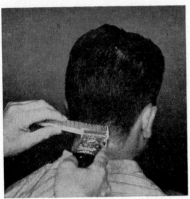 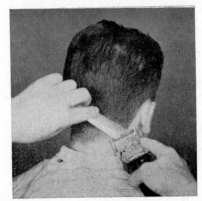

Fig. 140   Fig. 141
(Coarse Blade Over Coarse Part of Comb)

this method and still use coarse clipper blades. Some of the advantages of this method are:

1. It lends itself to greater versatility than coarse blades. Many degrees of closeness can be achieved simply by the proper manipulation of the clipper and the comb.

2. It is faster because different degrees of closeness can be secured without changing blades, changing clipper or pushing a lever.

3. Placing the clipper blade over the comb enables the barber to avoid undesired clipper closeness.

Pointers on use of clipper-over-comb:

1. The clipper blade teeth may be directed parallel, diagonal, or at right angles to the teeth of the comb.

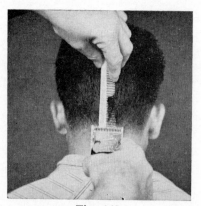

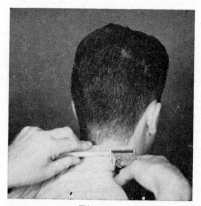

Fig. 142
Vertical Position of Comb
(Coarse Comb-Coarse Blade)

Fig. 143
Clipper over Comb Low Edge
(Fine Comb-Coarse or Fine Blade)

2. The **general rule is to use the coarse blade** over the coarse part of the comb first. The fine blade over the fine part of the comb may be used as a follow-up on the extreme edge in case it is not possible to clip that area close enough with the coarse blade over the coarse or fine part of the comb, or with just the coarse blade. If the non-detachable type of clipper is used, wherein the degrees of coarseness are obtained by a lever at the side of the clipper, it will be found that a little less than maximum coarseness feeds better for all purposes except on the extreme edge where the fine blade is preferred.

3. The coarse blade may be used over either the coarse or fine part of the comb, depending on the degree of closeness desired. As a general procedure, use the coarse blade over the coarse part of the comb in lower and middle areas of the edge, and the fine blade over the fine part of the comb on the extreme edge. For topping a butch, crew cut, short pomp, or flat-top, use the coarse blade over the coarse part of the comb.

4. At the extreme edge, ride the scalp firmly with the comb as the clipper is used over it.

5. Place the comb at the most advantageous position, horizontal, vertical, or at any angle.

6. Move the clipper and comb together in a coordinated manner if proceeding upward or moving across a given area. In some instances, such as flat-topping, the comb may be held momentarily still while the clipper cuts the hair projecting through the teeth of the comb.

7. When the edge is done with the clipper over the comb, in many instances there are advantages in doing the **upper area** of the **edge** first and finally the low area of the edge. This is not contradictory to the theory of sequence explained earlier, since the whole edge is

being done before the sides or middle section in forming the foundation of the hair cut.

8. Special combs may be used for the clipper-over-comb method. Such combs have longer teeth and they are usually coarser than the shingling comb.

Defense of clipper-over-comb method: Much of the prejudice formerly against this method has dwindled down to a negligible degree. Methods of working, of course, are typically controversial. It seems to be difficult for some draftsmen to change to new methods, and this has its virtue since it would be amateurish to adopt everything new that comes along. The test of a new method is simply this: Will it enable me to achieve good or better results? Will it lend itself to skillfullness? Will it lend itself to versatility? Will it lend itself to accuracy? Will it save time? Can one practice this method gracefully? This test in short should spell out quality, quantity and gracefulness.

In doing regular or standard hair cuts, the clipper-over-comb method should be restricted largely to the edging. This method has eliminated much of the tediousness of edging, and in fact, enables the barber to achieve a softer blended edge in less time. If it is used for shaping long hair in the upper middle and top sections of regular cuts, it will prove cumbersome and inaccurate. Some of the delicate touches of hair shaping in these upper sections of regular cuts can best be done with the shear-and-comb.

In doing **flat-tops, butches,** and **crew cuts,** however, the clipper-over-comb method is adaptable to the middle and top divisions also. The general rule then is to use this method wherever the hair is to be blended to a soft, natural feather-edge, wherever the hair is to be cut short or to a stubby length, and wherever the hair is to be levelled to a flat surface. Except for topping in the special kind of hair cuts, restrict the use of the clipper over the comb largely to the edge. In some instances it should be confined entirely to the edge, whereas in other instances where the hair is very obedient and where the customer has very little hair, or stubby short hair, or is partially bald, it may be used well into the middle section. Implements should have a reasonable correspondence in size to the kind of work for which they are used. A steam shovel should not be used to remove a pint of dirt. The shears has more versatility of use than the clipper; and the fine delicate touches of outlining, sizing, outline shading, and general shaping can best be achieved with the shears. The exclusive use of the clipper for the whole hair cut is not recommended. The use of the clipper-over-comb method to the exclusion of all other methods is not recommendable. Coarse blades and clipper-blade attachments often achieve the same results. The use of this method and of these implements do not lessen the emphasis that should be placed on the correct use of

the shears and comb in blending, tapering, and shaping. These two implements used together have their rightful place. Use them when it is proper
to do so; and use the clipper-over-comb method and the special implements
when it is proper to do so. It is advisable to use different methods to
achieve the same results, for the sake of making one's work more interesting.

METHODS OF SIDING

Siding refers to the back area as well as to the sides or to the section
between the edge and the top. As stated earlier, such a division is hypothetical and in some instances only theoretically existent. In siding, the
middle section is blended with the edge as well as with the top. The principles and pointers of cutting hair already explained in this chapter should
be kept firmly in mind. The correct manipulation of the comb is especially
important when cutting the middle section. Keep the comb feeding into
the hair. Depending somewhat on the contour of the head, keep the comb
feeding into the hair to be cut may mean pointing the teeth of the comb
straight up and often pointed slightly towards the scalp. The general
rule is to lift the whole comb away from the head rather than to point
the teeth outward from the head.

While in some cuts much, if not all, of the siding or middle section is
done with the clipper blade attachments or by the clipper-over-comb
method, the standard procedure in other hair cuts is to blend and cut
this section with the shears and comb. There are several **methods of
cutting the sides or middle section.**

1. **Shingling method of siding:** Shingling is a process of tapering,
   blending and shortening hair with the shears and comb. It is used
   for edging and for cutting the middle section. The comb is fed

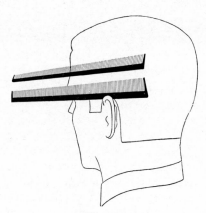

Fig. 144
Teeth of Comb Pointed Vertically Upward
And Inward Towards Scalp

through a whole vertical swath of hair in a continuous movement while the shears follow along cutting the hair projecting through the teeth of the comb. The comb serves as guage of how much hair to cut.

2. **Up-and-Over method of siding:** This method is used mainly to blend and cut the middle section; but it is also suitable for reducing moderately long top hair. In using this method, the hair is held up by the comb repeatedly without losing contact and is each time cut by the shears. Sweep a small batch of hair up and away from the scalp with the coarse part of the comb and hold it for cutting. Having cut the hair, place the blades astride the strand still held by the comb and immediately release the comb and bring it underneath the shears. Feed the comb upward through the hair into the next portion of the vertical strip to be cut. Repeat this process as many times as necessary. This method is identical with that of shingling except that it is a continuous process requiring the shear blades to hold a strand of hair until the comb is again inserted into the hair underneath the shears.

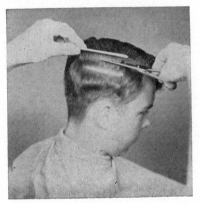
Fig. 145
Up-and-Over Method

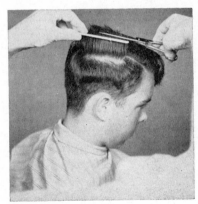
Fig. 146
Up-and-Over Method

3. **Siding by finger-work:** Finger-work is used primarily to shorten long hair, but it can also be used to shorten moderately long hair on the sides as well as on top. Since this method is used mainly for long hair, it will be explained under "topping."

4. **Siding by clipper-over-comb method:** This method can be used for siding in hair cuts where the sides are to be short. (See explanation of this method elsewhere in this chapter.)

5. **Blade-attachment method of siding:** (See explanation of this method elsewhere in this chapter.)

METHODS OF TOPPING

Topping is the most controversial areas of haircutting. There are several good methods of topping.

1. The most widely used method of topping is known as **Finger-work**. Finger-work is the process of picking up a strand of hair with the coarse part of the comb and holding it between the index and middle fingers of the left hand for cutting. These fingers follow the comb closely as it picks up the hair. While the hair is being picked up thusly, the shears are held firmly in the palm of the hand which is manipulating the comb. The thumb is released from the thumb grip, while the third finger remains inserted in the finger grip and the little finger remains on the finger rest. In this position the shears are closed. When the hair is in the proper position for cutting, and the fingers have a firm grasp on it, the comb is transferred between

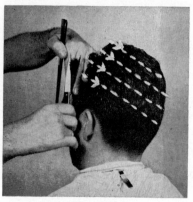

Fig. 147
Finger-work on Left Side

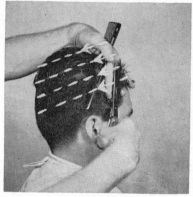

Fig. 148
Finger-work on Right Side

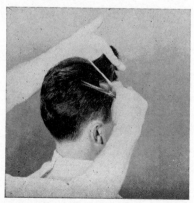

Fig. 149
Combing Through from Both Sides

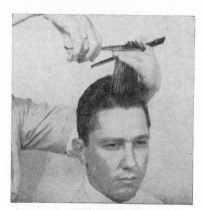

Fig. 150
Finger-work Across Top

the thumb and index finger of the left hand where it is held momentarily. Re-insert the thumb in the thumb grip and cut the hair at the desired place, above the fingers. Continue to hold the hair with the fingers until the comb is again inserted in the hair. Insert the comb beside the first finger and, as the fingers release the hair, comb through the upper portion of the strand held by the fingers and into another strand a little further—about an inch—along the swath. Repeat this whole process of cutting to the end of the swath, and then proceed to the next swath. Complete the left side first and then proceed to the right side. The following are some specifics on finger-work:

(1) Execute finger-work along strips or swaths from the front to back. While a single strand may be evened or shortened by finger-work, the "strip" procedure is more systematic for the whole area such as the upper middle section or the top. Direct the first strip low and move upward for the next strip. Make from three to five strips on each side of the head according to the size of the head. The final strip on each side should come to the center of the head.

(2) A given section may be combed through several times from either one or both sides before it is cut. Such combing assures that all hairs within the strand are in proper position. How many times it is combed through before it is cut depends on the texture and amount of hair, but two or three times usually suffices (Fig. 151).

(3) After the finger-work is completed on both sides of the head, check the center of the top for evenness by completing one or two more strips.

(4) In doing finger-work, apply the theory of "angles" as explained in this chapter. It is of paramount importance that the hair be cut at the proper angle to the scalp.

(5) The fingers holding the hair are pointed downward on the first strip on the sides and curved to conform with the contour of the head in the other strips.

(6) To do finger-work on the left side of the head, stand on the left side and to the front of the patron; for the right side and the center of the top, stand directly in back of the patron.

(7) The comb is passed to the left hand without turning it over. On the left side the teeth of the comb will point away from the hand and on the right side they will point towards the hand.

(8) On a patron who parts his hair, continue the finger-work from the long or full side over to the part.

(9) Finger-work is not recommended for cutting short hair, that is, for hair that can be successfully picked up with the comb.

(10) Exercise extreme caution when doing finger-work at the crown, and at the forelock, and in the back area, to avoid cutting the hair too short.

2. **Up-and-Over Method of Topping.** (Refer to previous explanation.)

3. **Topping by Shear-Lifting Method:** Stand forward at the right side. Comb all top hair forward. Insert the still blade of the shears under a strand of hair about two inches in front of the crown and follow-up with the coarse part of the comb to bring the strand to the proper angle for cutting. After cutting, release the strand from the comb and proceed as before. Direct the strips from left to right across the head (Figs. 151-154). Continue to cut such strips from the crown

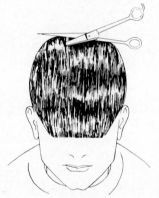

Fig. 151
Picking up Top Hair
With Shears

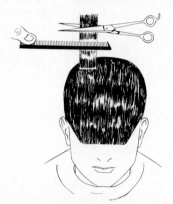

Fig. 152
Comb Holding Hair
Picked up With Shears

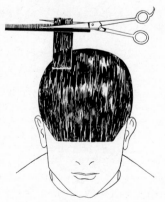

Fig. 153
Cuttting Position

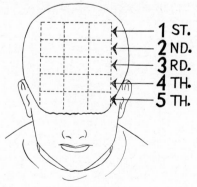

Fig. 154
Pattern of Strips

to the front hairline. This method is especially recommended for topping boys whose hair lies forward when not freshly combed or when the hair is combed straight back as a pompadour. It is much faster than the finger-work method. This shear-lifting method is the same in principle as the Up-and-Over Method except that each strand is managed independently in contrast to a continuous carry-through procedure in which the strips are directed from the side hairline upward or backward from the front hairline. The shear-lifting method is different in that the strips run crosswise the scalp, and each separate strand is completely released before proceeding to the next strand. **(The shear-lifting method can also be used for long hair on the sides and back area.)**

PRINCIPLES OF EDGING, SIDING, TOPPING IN A NUTSHELL

The essence of the principles of edging, siding, and topping is cutting the hair at the proper angle to the scalp. The essence of all the methods explained and illustrated for these major divisions of a hair cut rest upon the **theory of angles. The most important** principle of haircutting is the angle to the scalp at which the hair is cut. If the hair is cut at the proper angle to the scalp, the amount removed is comparatively immaterial as far as the smoothness and graduation of the ends of the hair are concerned. The proper angle ranges from forty-five to one hundred thirty-five degrees to the scalp. The degree of the angle depends upon the length of the hair, upon the section of the head being cut, and upon the extent of graduation desired. In brief, the theory of angles means lifting the hair upward and away from the scalp for cutting. For regular graduation, hold the hair to be cut at **right angle** to the scalp; for triple graduation, slant the hair slightly in the opposite direction or more than ninety degrees from which it is to be combed or is to lie. For example, take a strand of hair about one inch in diameter and hold it in a vertical position, cut straight through it making a flat surface. Now, hold the lower part of the strand secure and bend the top end over to forty-five degrees and then to higher degrees. Notice how the top ends seem to crawl upward and the lower ends seem to crawl downward. A neck duster or a roll of string will react in the same way. The inevitable result of cutting hair in this way is a sloped, graduated edge.

It is to be understood that the theory of angles is not to mean exactly forty-five or one hundred thirty-five degrees to the scalp—the angle may fall anywhere between these angles, such as sixty, seventy, or eighty. **The fundamental principle is to position the hair for cutting so that it slants in the opposite direction from which it is to be combed.** This principle applies to edging, siding, and topping.

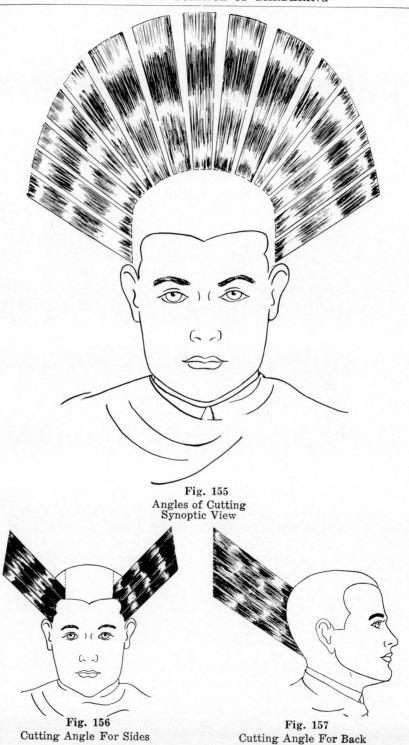

Fig. 155
Angles of Cutting
Synoptic View

Fig. 156
Cutting Angle For Sides

Fig. 157
Cutting Angle For Back

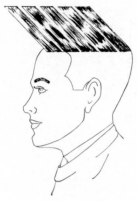

Fig. 158
Cutting Angle For Top

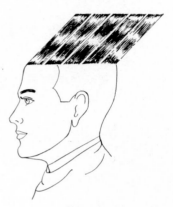

Fig. 159
Cutting Angle For Top

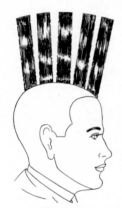

Fig. 160
Cutting Angle For Top

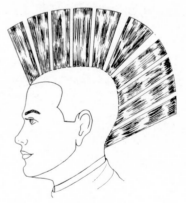

Fig. 161
Angles of Cutting
Synoptic View

POSITIONING HAIR WITH COMB FOR CUTTING

Hair can be positioned with the comb to the proper angle for cutting. Simply feed the comb into the hair and lift it to the proper angle. Start from any point above the hairline and move upward. This method is much faster than the finger method, and it is perhaps more accurate in that the amount being cut is clearly visible.

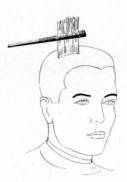

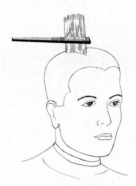

Fig. 162   Fig. 163

Positioning Hair With Comb

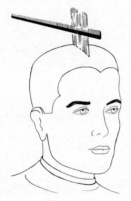

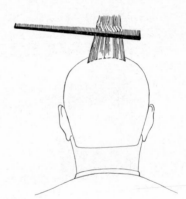

Fig. 164   Fig. 165

Positioning Hair With Comb

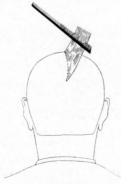

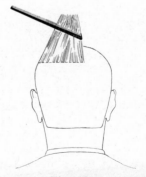

Fig. 166   Fig. 167

Positioning Hair With Comb

OUTLINING A HAIRCUT—ARCHING OVER EARS

Outlining a haircut or arching over the ears is usually accomplished with the points of the shears and the point of the razor. It is a good plan, except where the clippers are used all the way around, to mark the path of the outline with the points of the shears. Lay the moving blade almost flat against the scalp in front of the ear and, steadying it near the pivot with the cushion tip of the index finger of the left hand, make a continuous stroke over the ear and down the sides; then reverse the direction of the shears and in like manner return to the starting point.

Repeat until a decided path is made. Then bring the outline to a shingled edge, depending somewhat upon the style of hair cut. The line should either trail the natural hairline, or run into the hair just enough to form a distinct symmetrically shaped arch. Make the outline as straight down the side as possible.

Sharpness of outline at the mastoid region can be achieved with the fine blade of the clipper. This method is particularly applicable when a decisive line is desired. It is difficult to make a good line at this area where it is extended onto the neck. Clippers have been designed to make the whole arch and outline. The teeth of such a clipper are very fine and they cut very close. Some barbers like this method.

The perfect arch is comparatively low. It follows the natural hairline except when it is necessary to vary it to form a symmetrical and precise line. Observe that the outline behind the ear descends almost vertically— it does not lean noticeably towards the center of the neck.

Some recognition should be given to the school of thought that a razor should not be used over the ears to complete the arch, and that it should be completed with the shears and comb. Admittedly, except where the hair at the arch is too long, by reason of style, the hair should be tapered to a soft graduated edge, and the outline made as faint as reasonably possible, but it should be observable. Such an outline leans towards the casual and informal. A harsh, heavy outline is too mechanical looking to be artistic, but a perfect arch approaches a natural edge, although a properly made outline in all styles except the all-around close clipper cuts give "snap" and character to a style. The non-razor outline is called a natural edge, meaning that it is free from any noticeably artificial furrowing.

After an arch has been made with either the shears or clipper, apply lather along the path of the arch and down the sides of the neck. Do not use more lather than necessary and keep it out of the hair as much as possible.

Just before making the initial stroke with the razor use one of two methods to distribute the lather over the arch-way to straighten the hairs at the outline and distribute the lather evenly. Use the fine teeth of the

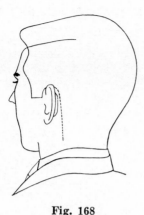

Fig. 168
Perfect Arch

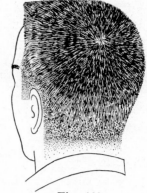

Fig. 169
Achieved with Shears and Comb
Natural Arch

comb or one finger of the left hand for the same purpose. The finger method usually suffices and it is much quicker. As the razor trails, the left hand should be placed open on the head so that the thumb may be placed firmly against the scalp just above the point of the razor. With the thumb in this position, pull up slightly with pressure against the scalp so as to hold the skin firm over which the razor is passing. Move the thumb along as the razor progresses.

Use the free hand stroke for the right side. Start at the sideburn and proceed over the ear from front to back, and then down the side of the neck. On the left side, start at the mastoid region with the free hand and proceed upward over the ear. Now switch to the back hand, outline the sideburn and then proceed from the mastoid down the side of the neck. As a general rule, wipe off the lather only when changing from free hand to back hand and upon finishing.

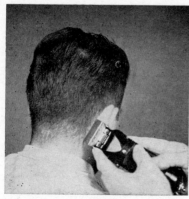

Fig. 170
Achieving Sharpness of Outline
Mastoid Area with Fine Blade

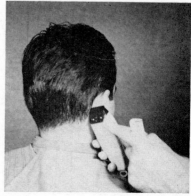

Fig. 171
Making Arch with Special Clipper

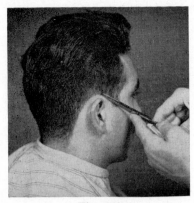

Fig. 172
Arching over Ear

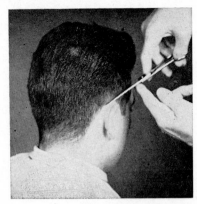

Fig. 173
Arching over Ear

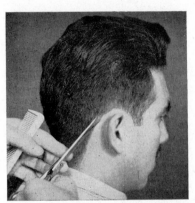

Fig. 174
Arching over Ear

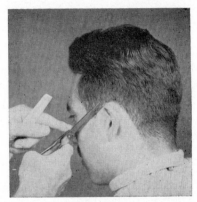

Fig. 175
Arching over Ear

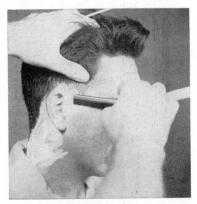

Fig. 176
Shaving Outline

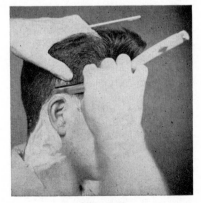

Fig. 177
Shaving Outline

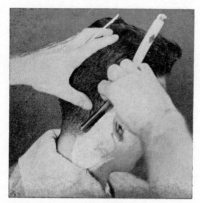

Fig. 178
Shaving Outline

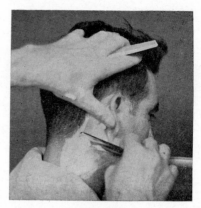

Fig. 179
Shaving Outline

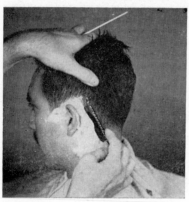

Fig. 180
Shaving Outline

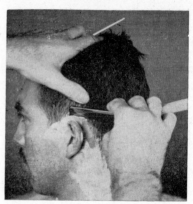

Fig. 181
Shaving Outline

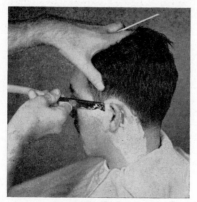

Fig. 182
Shaving Outline

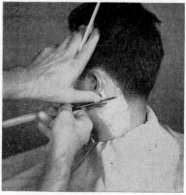

Fig. 183
Shaving Outline

Where to transfer lather from razor in arching:

1. To the palm of the left hand; or
2. To the base of the left thumb; or
3. To a strip of paper tucked over towel at center of neck.

Removing outline lather: After outlining a hair cut with the razor, the remaining lather may be removed as follows:

1. With the steam-towel as indicated in Figs. 184-185.
2. With a quick-end wrap of a steam-towel.
3. With a face-towel.
4. With a paper-towel or portion thereof.

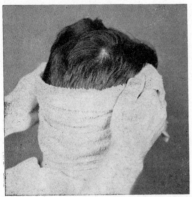 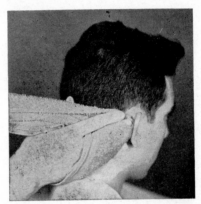

Fig. 184   Fig. 185

Two Ways To Remove Outline Lather With Steam Towel

Use a steam towel if it is already in use from some other service, such as a shave, facial, or shampoo.

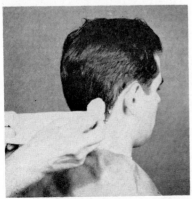 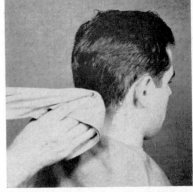

Removing Lather

Fig. 186 With Paper Towel   Fig. 187 With Linen Face Towel

POINTERS ON COMBING HAIR

1. Use the coarse part of the comb first and then follow up with the fine part. If the hair is coarse and voluminous, the coarse part of the comb may suffice.
2. Use a hairdressing comb for thick, coarse hair.
3. Hair on each side of a part is usually combed diagonally back or straight back.
4. The heavy side of a part may be roached in front to break the monotony of straightness.
5. Hair combed down perfectly flat gives lessened height effect.
6. Fluffy hair gives increased height effect.
7. To comb out tangles, use coarse part of comb. Hold comb perpendicular to the scalp, and comb through the **ends first.**
8. To add one final touch with the comb, lay it almost flat.
9. Seldom use the fine part of the comb for the final effect, unless the hair is fine and thin. It sort of cements the hair together and the hair separates easily.

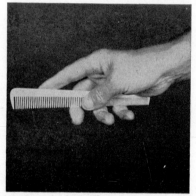 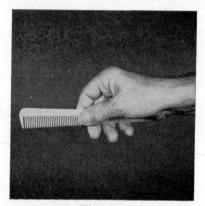

Fig. 190   Fig. 191

Holding Comb for Combing

10. After combing long hair through to the back of the head, push the ends of the hair upward and forward with the left hand just enough to break the tension of the hairs.
11. The left hand follows the comb except on short edges, to give a smoothing effect.
12. Comb clear through to the scalp, but do not scrape it.
13. Choose a big comb, such as a hairdressing comb, to hand to the patron who wishes to comb or part his own hair. A shingling comb is too fragile and too delicate for the layman to use.

14. In combing through the hair, either hold the index finger length-wise and along the back side of the comb to brace the part of the comb under strain, or hold it with the thumb and fingers astride the particular section being used. Otherwise, the comb will frequently break near the middle.

On some heads it is possible to do **camouflage combing** to cover top baldness. The hair on the sides and back may continue to grow normally. When this happens, the upper "rim" of one side and the back may be parted off and combed forward. In some instances, such hair grows long enough to cover the entire top area.

PARTING HAIR

A part may be made on any style in which the hair is long enough. Strive to make a precise straight part. A part usually runs **parallel with the sides of the head.** If it takes off at an angle it gives an unbalanced effect to the head. If it is not obvious where the patron parts his hair, ask him.

1. Hair may be parted on the left side, the right side, in the middle or at any other place. The conventional side for the man is the **left side.** Nature, however, usually sets a definite part and this has to be considered. The **natural part begins at the crown.**
2. Pompadour types may be parted if the hair is long enough.
3. Hair should be dampened before it is parted unless the patron objects.
4. A natural part is set by nature and is where two hair streams meet. (See p. 487).

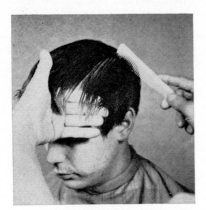

Fig. 192
Parting First Step

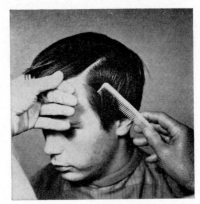

Fig. 193
Parting Second Step

5. Emphasize parting. An incorrect part is psychologically bad.
6. Step forward to the right side of the patron to do the preliminary combing. If it is to be a side part, step to the side on which the hair

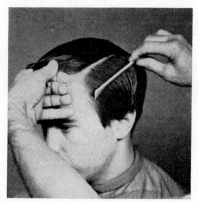

Fig. 194
Parting Third Step

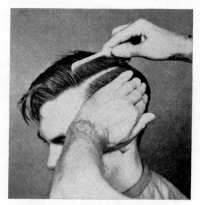

Fig. 195
Parting Fourth Step

is to be parted. With the coarse part of the comb, comb the hair forward. To make the line of part, start at the crown or crown area, and use the end tooth of the coarse section of he comb.

HAIR THINNING

Hair thinning is a scientific process; it not the removal of hair via a blind finesse. Two purposes of thinning are (1) to reduce thickness or volume, and (2) to shape the hair to conform to a certain style. The implements used to thin hair are the plain shears, thinning shears, and the razor.

Slithering is a method of thinning. Slithering actually strips the hair. This method of thinning is accomplished by sliding semi-opened plain shears towards the scalp astride a small strand of hair. Begin this procedure about one inch from the scalp. Hold the strand firmly between the index finger and thumb. The slithering may be facilitated by manipulating the movable blade. Slide over a given portion of the strand two or three times and then slide back about an inch and repeat. Continue in this manner along the strand. The blades should not be closed in slithering since they would cut off too much hair. The strand is held so that the palm of the hand holding the shears faces the barber. The hair should be lifted outward and upward to about a **ninety degree angle. While slithering** is a method of thinning, it may be used (1) to blend stubborn ends, (2) to shorten hair, (3) to encourage hair to wave, and (4) to do terminal blending (Fig. 196).

Hair should not be thinned from its top surface since this would cause certain hairs to isolate themselves and stand out and up wildly. It is a fundamental rule that hair should be thinned from an "imaginary" inner or underneath layer. In this way the slightly stubby shortened hairs will be kept under control by the surrounding hairs. This underneath layer may be considered the top side of the hair after all the hair is combed straight forward; but it is also any portion of hair over which other hair is to lie. Hair should not be thinned too closely to the scalp, because the short stubby hairs would tend to project through the hair over them and give the impression of a "field of spikes." A little thinning makes a great difference and, therefore, it should be done very cautiously and gradually.

Hair should be thinned first where it is thickest and then the remaining hair balanced with the desired thickness. This procedure enables the barber to determine more accurately the extent of hair to be removed elsewhere and to assure a symmetrical effect.

When a great deal of hair is to be thinned, it is preferable to **section off the hair,** and fasten each section. For incidental or slight thinning, sectioning is unnecessary.

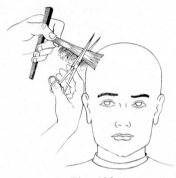

Fig. 196
Slithering Hair

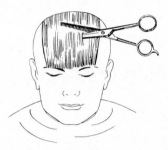

Fig. 197
Thinning Shear Thinning

Push-back Method of Thinning:

(1) The push-back method may be done with the plain shears and comb. With a strand of hair in position for thinning, push some of the hairs towards the scalp with the fine part of the comb and then execute slithering.

(2) The push-back method may be done with the thinning shears. Push some of the hairs of the strand towards the scalp with the notched blade of the thinning shears.

(3) The advantages of the push-back method are that the hairs thinned are left surrounded by neighbor hairs and thus they are prevented from sticking up, and it is easier to guard against thinning out too much.

Cutting Stubborn hair: It is a popular misconception that stubborn hair should be cut short to make it obedient. Cutting it short simply results in making it so short that even though it does stand up it will not be conspicuous. The chief way to control stubborn hair is to allow it to grow long; in this way, the weight of the long ends is sufficient to hold the other part of the strand in place, especially if it is helped with a few drops of hairdressing.

Attack the problem of stubborn hair as follows:

1. By slithering.
2. By making a part right in the middle of the difficulty and slithering or shaping the underneath hair; frequently it is the underneath section of the hair that is causing the trouble.
3. By cutting it very short, a last resort.
4. By letting it grow longer.
5. By thinning or end-thinning, with thinning shears.

Areas of hair to remove with caution: Remove with caution the hair at the crown and forehead. Leave the hair longer at these two places than anywhere else on the head, except when giving a short pompadour or some other short style.

Most common fault in haircutting: The most common fault is simply taking off too much hair. **The proper amount of hair to take off in some hair cuts can be put into a moderate sized thimble.**

This statement emphasizes the advisability of minimizing the cutting in many hair cuts. Hair cuts in this category might fittingly be classified as "retouch hair cuts." That is, cut off only the amount of hair that grew since the last hair cut in case no change of style is desired. The most common complaint of the public is that "the barber cut it too short." When styling a hair cut, becomingness along with the wishes of the customer should be paramount in the barber's mind. He should not feel that he must cut off a lot of hair to earn the charge.

Preferable kind of taper in back: The long taper is definitely preferable. By its longness, it gives the effect of naturalness. A taper should be so graduated that it appears to have neither a beginning nor an end. A long taper will reach a point about a half-inch below the lower tip of the ear, or as near that point as possible.

Wetting or dampening hair prior to cutting: As a general rule, the hair should not be dampened for cutting. When hair is wet and combed, it is in its unnatural position; if it is cut in such a position, when it is dry it will crawl back to a position impossible to estimate or determine and, therefore, irregularities will result. Shape it in its home-location. When side and top hair are extremely disorderly and defies any lying position, it may be dampened sufficiently to put it under control. It is correct to dampen a crew cut, short pomp or flat top for the final operation on the top. Hair should be wet for razor cutting, but this is only to keep from dulling the razor and to facilitate cutting.

Guessing factor in haircutting: The barber constantly makes snap decisions in haircutting as to where to minimize or maximize the quantity of hair and as to design. These decisions might be called "scientific guessing," at the basis of which is judgment, knowledge, and experience. The mechanics of cutting hair is a science, an act or process involving scientific methods, but not as an exact science as geometry. A set of definite measurements as to how much should be cut off, left on and where, applicable to each and every head would hardly be possible. At the discretion of the barber lies a large scope of decisions—"to cut or not to cut". His personal judgment plays an important role. Whatever his judgment is, he still necessarily relies on scientific methods. The barber's experience and special knowledge enable him to make his own mental photograph of the finished product to be. His judgment can hardly be perfect and so at this point the element of guessing seeps in, as he visualizes what he thinks should be done. He is going to make mistakes; and, since this is true, an element of guessing is almost inevitable. "To form an opinion" is the essence of what is meant by "guessing". The artistic yen and ability of an artist is impossible to spell out in its entirety. This brings us to the border of guessing. When guessing becomes perfected it is "scientific guessing". At its foundation are the art and science of haircutting.

Use of mirror reflection: The back section of a hair cut is vividly reflected in the mirror. The mirror reveals any defects in shading and balance. While the barber should be able to detect these without a mirror, many barbers find the mirror helpful.

Cut hair before shampooing: The general rule is to cut the hair before shampooing it. An exception comes when the hair is excessively dirty or has sand in it. Right after a shampoo it is hardly possible to determine the natural lying position of the hair since it is inclined to be fluffy and disorderly. It is easier, however, to cut clean rather than dirty hair. Hair does respond differently, and in some instances giving a shampoo first would not be wrong.

Choice of implements for cutting hair:

The barber should use good implements, but whether he gets results with the shears and comb or clippers with or without the comb, or uses some improvised gadget, is unimportant. It is how he uses the implements that counts. There is no merit in the exclusive use of the shears and comb in haircutting. Hair can be butchered or nicely shaped with any cutting implement. All any of such implements are designed to do is to **cut hair.** The results are entirely dependent upon how they are used. This holds true also with clippers. One can do anything with an electric clipper that can be done with a hand clipper—it is just that the electric requires less effort and that it cuts faster. In fact, for flat tops and for many delicate touches, the electric clipper is much more versatile. The barber should guard against prejudice toward the different kinds of any implement. He should experiment with the various kinds.

Standing position with respect to cutting point: The cutting point should be to the barber's right, approximately in line with his right shoulder. The reasons for this are:

1. For ease of movement. This reason is immediately self-evident, once the position is taken. If the management of either the shears or clipper is carried on directly in front of the body, the hands, arms and body will be cramped.
2. For gracefulness. The ease consequent from this position makes possible a greater degree of gracefulness.
3. To avoid becoming round shouldered.
4. For systematic procedure.

Turning customer's head in upright position: Use **both hands** opened with fingers curved to turn customer's head as desired in doing any phase of a hair cut. Place the left hand on the left side and the right hand on the right side of the head. Move the head gently and gracefully to the position desired and come to a definite stop and then remove the hands. This may be done while holding the shears and comb or clipper and comb.

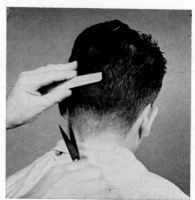

Fig. 198
Wrong Way to Move Head

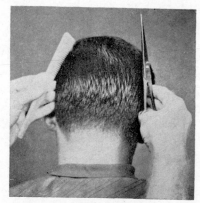

Fig. 199
Right Way to Move Head

Cutting hair below hair-piece or toupee: Do not cut off any of the hair-piece. Do the middle section first and blend the edge in with it. If you elect to do the edge first, keep it very low.

Cutting Dyed Hair: Proceed with extreme caution to prevent cutting off too much hair. The treacherous area is the middle section at the points where it is merged with the edge and top.

How to trim eyebrows and nostril hairs:

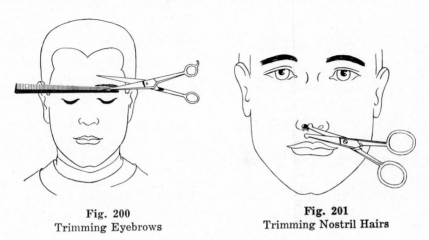

Fig. 200
Trimming Eyebrows

Fig. 201
Trimming Nostril Hairs

SIDEBURNS

The term "sideburn" refers to the narrow strip of hair grown on the region just in front of the ear. The term may also be interpreted to mean side whiskers. The term originates from General A. E. Burnside (1824-1881) who popularized the wearing of sideburns. Sideburns also bear a relation to the length of the neck, and, of course, to the height of the neck-edge. A normal or medium length sideburn goes with a normal height neck-edge; and a long sideburn goes with a low neck-edge. As a general rule, the medium length sideburn goes well with all hair cuts except where there are conspicuous irregularities of features.

A sideburn is necessary to give balance to a hair cut.

1. All men's hair cuts should have some kind of sideburns. To shave straight forward from the arch is inartistic.
2. Short sideburn means one-half inch drop.
3. Medium sideburn means one inch drop. This length is most popular.
4. Long sideburn means from one-and-a-half to two inches in length.
5. Extra long sideburns are usually not recommended but they may be worn by persons with abnormally long chins and, of course, for fiestas or a lark.
6. The length and thickness of a sideburn should have a reasonable correspondence to the style of hair cut it accompanies. For instance, the short, medium, and long ones look best with the hair cuts described by these terms. The extra long cut takes longer and thicker sideburns.
7. Sideburns may be used to fill out sunken temples.
8. The bottom edge of the standard sideburn should be horizontal.

9. The width of sideburns is usually set by nature. From three quarters of an inch to one inch is regular.

10. Where the sideburns are to be distinctive, the coarse part of the comb is suitable for gauging the desired thickness. The term "coarse comb thickness" might be used. All straggling hairs should be removed.

11. Sideburns usually should come to a shingled, graduated edge.

12. Give **special attention** to the **sideburn.** It is a conspicuous part of a hair cut.

Four basic lengths of sideburns: The guide line to the length of sideburns is the corner of the eyes, since they are in a straight line. The ears are often unbalanced in that one is lower than the other.

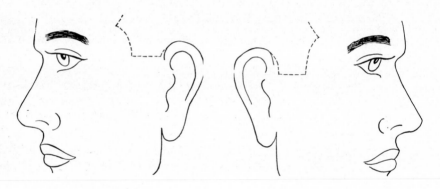

Fig. 202
Short Sideburns

Fig. 203
Medium Sideburns

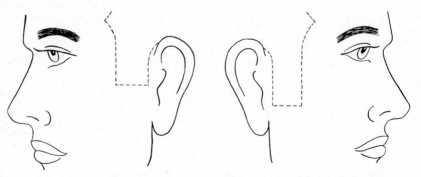

Fig. 204
Long Sideburns

Fig. 205
Extra-Long Sideburns

PSYCHOLOGY IN HAIRCUTTING

A great deal of **psychology** is **involved** in **haircutting,** especially in the styling area. Putting the customer at ease and leading him to believe that he is getting competent service and a well-designed style are very important. The barber should be aware of the fact that it is not entirely **what** he does, but **how** he does it that most influences the customer and that induces him to tell his friends about him and to continue patronizing his shop.

1. Put the customer at ease as quickly as possible. The methods of doing this are numerous. One right word spoken to the adult often suffices, even if it is about the trite old subject, the weather. The intonation in speaking to him may be enough. The tone of the voice is very important; it may give the impression of confidence in your skill or the lack of it. Usually, face your customer when discussing an important point in designing the hair. If the patron is a child, especially a first timer, the barber should spend a moment or two getting acquainted with him before attempting to cut his hair.

2. Indicate that you are very glad to serve. Come to attention immediately, standing erect.

3. Consistently wear a cheerful countenance.

4. Put a good ring in your voice.

5. Speak distinctly, but guard against speaking too low or too loudly.

6. Have a ready smile.

7. Maintain a good posture.

8. Manifest an eagerness to give the kind of hair cut the customer wants.

9. Be immaculately clean.

10. Converse according to the suggestion in the chapter on conversation.

11. Stick to pleasant remarks.

12. Do not be argumentative.

13. Heartily thank him for his patronage.

14. Don't be "touchy."

15. Be willing to accept criticism gracefully.

One of the most important phases of psychology in haircutting is the **willingness** to **make changes** or **corrections.** Most of these acts take only a moment and your willingness to make them cheerfully greatly impresses the customer. Some things you may have an occasion to do or say are:

1. Admit the oversight if it is a matter of correction.

2. You may say that perhaps you misunderstood.

3. Appear glad to do any alteration.
4. Tell the patron you are sorry.
5. Typical major mistakes in cutting hair are taking off too much, not taking off enough, and not giving the style desired by the customer.
   (1) If you have taken off too much, you may say, "I am sorry but it will grow back to the length you desire in a short time. You have a healthy scalp." Or you may say, "After a shampoo, your hair will not look so short."
   (2) If you did not take off enough, simply take off more.
   (3) If your failure to understand was serious, the best thing to do is apologize and to assure the customer that you now understand and that you will keep firmly in mind the style he desires, and guard against making the error again.
6. Never explode. When you lose your temper, you place obstacles in the road to success. Everyone wants to be a success in whatever he is doing.
7. Use a lower tone of voice than usual when discussing any correction to be made.

The amount of hair a customer instructs the barber to cut off is a psychological problem. The instructions have to be carefully analyzed. Discount about sixty percent of what the customer requests in this regard, and the final result will generally be satisfactory with him. The customer does not understand how to instruct the barber nor how to guage the amount of hair that should be cut off. Just a little experience teaches the barber that "a little makes a great deal of difference" in removing hair. As to the amount to cut off, the barber should use his own judgement. This advice is not contradictory to the idea that a customer should feel that he is getting what he wants. For instance, should a patron tell you to cut off about two inches from the top, cut off about three-quarters of an inch and this will usually meet with his full approval.

Suggesting a change of style likewise involves psychology. It is quite fitting to suggest a desirable change of style. But this is seldom appropriate the first time you serve a patron. After you have come to know him well, such a suggestion will be more readily accepted. If he, however, asks for your opinion, willingly and quickly suggest the style he should wear. But never get into the habit of trying to make everyone change his hair cut.

Coping with an irregularity of the customer's head or hair is also a psychological procedure. Any irregularity should not be pounced on the first time you serve a patron. The patron may have become bored from listening to every barber refer to the defect. Either give him a "break" by not mentioning it, or, if you deem it advisable, quietly and politely offer a brief suggestion as to how the condition can be minimized.

It is even a **psychological approach to honor the customer's idio-syncrasies about his hair cut.** Some customers have just one and perhaps two points by which they judge a **hair cut.** Some customers give special attention to the sideburns, to the arches, to the height on the sides, to the height of the neck edge, to the way the hair is parted or combed, or to whether the hair has been clipped low at the back of the neck. The patron may volunteer to tell you about his "touchy" points, but if not, discover them as soon as possible and give them ready consideration. When you have become acquainted with him, he will appreciate your reiterating these points as a preliminary to cutting his hair.

Handing the customer a hand mirror so that he may view the back of his head is psychologically good. The fact that you are willing to let him see what you have done favorably impresses the customer.

It is **psychologically bad to finish a hair cut too quickly or to take too long.** If you finish too quickly, he may feel you have slighted him and that he has not got his money's worth; conversely, if you take too long, he may feel that you are amateurish and that his cut is inferior.

It is also **psychologically bad to talk too much or too little.** The skill of the blabber-mouth is usually discredited; and the reticent barber may convey the impression that he dose not know what he is doing. Whatever you say should be on the positive side and in a pleasant vein.

HOW TO DETERMINE STYLE TO BE GIVEN

Ideally, the decision of style should result from a study of the shape of the man's head, the kind and amount of hair he has, and his occupation. But a more direct method is imperative, though, in view of the fact that an immediate decision must be made with the least possible annoyance to the customer. The keynote pointer is to tell or suggest to the patron rather than ask him. It is extremely difficult for the average patron to explain the style he wishes; the barber, on the other hand, who is familiar with the styles and the words and phrases that quickly and clearly "paint the picture" should rise to the occasion and attempt to phrase for the customer just the style he wishes. This is really possible most of the time. **The proper time to find out what sort of cut is desired is while combing the hair prior to any cutting.** But the barber should be analyzing the head while putting on the neck strip or towel. Note the following pointers:

1. Quickly look the head over at the earliest opportunity, and judging from the type of hair cut he last had, come to a tentative or temporary conclusion as to what is probably desired. Explain this conclusion briefly and simply to the patron and either gain his approval or listen to any change or revision that he may make. If he is firm in

what he says, accept it without hesitation, assure him that you understand, and proceed with the cut at once. The best guide to what style of cut the patron wishes is his last hair cut.

2. Ask only the **major questions first;** that is, do not take up all the necessary minor questions, such as those that pertain to the length of the sideburns, to the length or thickness of top. Instead, after finding out in general terms what is desired, start cutting, and **wait until the appropriate time in the process of the cut to ask further questions.** By so doing, the patron will be more at ease. The customer would be annoyed by a "cross examination" in detail of every step to be taken throughout the cut. Exception: an extraordinarily particular person may wish several points settled at the beginning especially if it is the first time that you have cut his hair and more especially if his last hair cut was not what he wanted.

3. The following is a list of suitable **questions for ascertaining what kind of hair cut is to be given.** Ask the patron only enough questions to ascertain; often just the answer to one question will suffice. Do not ask all these questions. The questions you ask should reflect your tentative decision as to the style desired. For instance, if the patron's hair is full at the sides, and obviously for his last hair cut the clippers were used just in the back, do not ask him if he wishes an all-around clipper cut. Instead ask if he would like the sides left full. An affirmative answer should give you sufficient knowledge to start the hair cut. Ask the question which will anticipate his saying "yes" and which will make it unnecessary for him to do any explaining. The questions may be classified as General Preliminary and Later Detail questions.

4. Questions to ask customer.
    (1) Would you like your hair cut the same as it was the last time?
    (2) Would you like a clipper edge all around? If so, ascertain what height he wishes—low, medium, high.
    (3) Would you like an extra low edge in back?
    (4) Would you like the sideburns shortened a little?
    (5) Would you like your sideburns the same length?
    (6) Would you like a little off the top? (If not, suggest that you check it for evenness.)

Brief description of a good haircut:
    (1) Becomingness. The cut should do something for the person. The style should "fit" the person to whom it is given.
    (2) Creativeness. Does the style have originality? Is it an interesting variation in style—something different?

(3) Balance. The shading in the corresponding areas of a haircut should be identical in effect. The sideburns should be of even length; and the arches should be the same height.

(4) Smoothness. This means it must be free from nicks.

(5) The outline should come to a soft, gradual edge. In an all-around clipper edge this is correct, but in styles with enough side hair for definite arches, the rule applies just to the neck edge.

ROUTINE STEPS OF HAIR CUT

Except for the actual cutting and shaving, all the routine steps of a hair cut can be rehearsed. By such an exercise, the student will gain a mental vision of the procedure and mechanics in a hair cut. This preliminary knowledge will enable him to relate various aspects of the subject to procedure. Even at this point it is important that the student learn to socialize a split moment with the customer to put him at ease before the hair cut is begun. The customer should be made to feel that he is in willing and competent hands. Even a cheerful "good morning" and "Como esta Ud?" or "Comment allez-vous?" along with pleasing manners may suffice. The following is a resume of the routine steps:

1. Recognize customer.

2. Seat customer (in locked chair).

3. Spread haircloth.

4. Wash hands with soap and water and dry them.

5. Place implements in sterilizer.

6. Place neck-strip or face towel around neck.

7. Adjust chair to proper height.

8. Comb hair tentatively. Observe texture and quantity of hair, any irregularities of hair and shape of head.

9. Find out what style of cut patron wishes. This may be ascertained while combing his hair or right after set-up for hair cut.

10. Do clipper work.

11. Do shear and comb work. (This will include preliminary arching.)

12. Complete edging and siding.

13. Do topping, working from left to right side.

14. Comb through hair thoroughly and check details.

15. By cutting remove hairs from ears and any projecting nostril hairs. You may trim eyebrows but only with consent of patron.

16. Drum out loose hair-ends with finger tips of both hands and re-comb.

17. Dust off loose hair-ends from forehead, ears, and neck with duster or towel, or by some mechanical device such as hair "vacuum," und(haircloth, remove neck-strip or towel and finish dusting off.

18. Remove haircloth and shake it free from loose hair. Do this noise-lessly.

19. Replace haircloth.

20. Arrange towel for outlining.

21. Clip any remaining hair on neck. Dust off.

22. Lather outline area.

23. Trace outline with point of razor.

24. Remove remaining lather with a damp towel and dry area.

25. Dress customer for retouching. (Refer to section on "Set-up for Retouching Hair Cut.)

26. Do retouching, especially checking arches.

27. Massage scalp just a moment. (This is psychological time to sug-gest a shampoo, scalp treatment, or tonic.)

28. If no tonic is given, find out if patron wishes his hair dry or damp.

29. Comb hair neatly.

30. Remove the retouch set-up.

31. Remove loose hair or dampness. Pay particular attention to fore-head, outline area, nose, and face. Use smooth surface of towel.

32. See that chair is locked before patron steps out.

33. Make out check and hand it to customer as you remove haircloth, or immediately afterwards.

34. Thank patron when you give him check.

NAMES OF STYLES OF MEN'S AND BOYS' HAIR CUTS

Standard styles of men's and boys' hair cuts:

1. There are six standard styles:

    (1) Short Hair Cut   (4) Short Pompadour
    (2) Medium Hair Cut   (5) Medium Pompadour
    (3) Long Hair Cut or Trim   (6) Long Pompadour

2. The variations of these representative styles are **innumerable**. Every head is different, and this fact means that each hair cut has some degree of variation from any established style.

Terminology of Styles: There is very little standardization of terminology of styles. Many names of styles are originated and popularized locally and have no national acceptance. Among the current styles nationally recognized are the crew cut, butch and flat top, and even these are differently interpreted in the various sections of the country. What is an appropriate name for a hair style? An appropriate name should be descriptive of the style either by definitive terms or self-explanatory words. Such terms as "short", "medium", and "long", however, are relative in their connotation in that the degree of shortness or longness varies according to the individual barber's interpretation, but these terms suggest the general category of the length desired. Such terms as the following are apropos: very short, slightly shorter or longer than medium, and extra long or extra full. Occasionally a style of local origin receives national recognition, such as the Ivy League or Princeton. These names are not descriptive and require explanation. Among the names that are ideally descriptive is "Flat Top". Whatever the variations of this style are in length of the top and sides, the top is flat. Such names as "professional cut", "business-man cut" are improper because they are neither descriptive nor self-explanatory. They mean one thing to a particular barber and something very different to another barber. The most that can be said for these terms is that they connote a conservative design, but this design can be of any category.

The term "Two Line Hair Cut" does not indicate a particular style but simply means continuing the outline straight down the sides of the neck. This method is in contrast to the outmoded way of shaving across the back of the neck, thus continuing the outline over one ear to connect with the outline over the other ear—a "One Line Hair Cut".

Do not pay much attention to **local fashion names.** Lean more on descriptive terms readily understood by customers than upon non-descriptive names of styles. Recognize that there are multiple variations of the basic styles or of any other established styles. Place emphasis upon stylistic adaptation and creative hair styling. Aside from a definite demand by the customer, strive for the cut that will be the most becoming to him, disregarding adherence to established patterns or styles. Remember that the customer wants "individuality" of design, although he usually does not want a design that is conspicuously different from the prevailing style and neither does he want to wear an obsolete style.

Pompadours: This term originated with the name of the person who first popularized combing the hair away from the face and directly back. He was Marquis de Pompadour. Besides meaning the combing of hair away and back from the front hairline, it also means cutting the hair so short that it will stand erect on top of the head, resembling the surface of the bristles of an oval-shaped hair brush held horizontally.

Names of current hair styles: These names are used nationally and in most instances are fairly descriptive:

1. Crew Cut
2. Flat Top, Regular
3. Flat Top with Long Sides
4. Flat Top Ducktail
5. Flat Top Boogie
6. Boogie
7. Butch
8. Ducktail
9. Brush Cut
10. Convertible

Convertible Hair Cut: It is possible to cut a head of hair in such a way that it can be combed to more than one style. Such a hair cut may be referred to as "convertible." It is not possible to cut some individual styles, such as the Butch or Flat Top so that they are convertible, but cuts in the medium and long category can be so cut. The variations of such a cut would range from Medium Cut to Medium Pompadour, Long Cut or Trim to Long Pompadour, Semi-forward Boogie to Short Medium Cut, and from any of these styles or from any other to any different style wherein the length of hair is suitable. Cut the hair in such a way that it can be combed all natural directions from the crown and still be of even length.

MEN'S HAIR STYLES

The following illustrations and photographs consist of standard and special hair styles along with several variations. Two views of the six standard styles will be illustrated first. Some of the standard styles will also be illustrated along with the other styles.

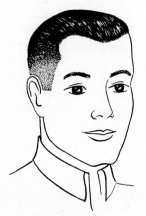

Fig. 206
Regular Short Cut

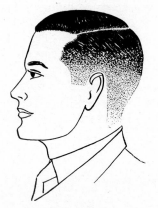

Fig. 207
Regular Short Cut

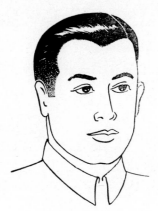

Fig. 208
Regular Medium Cut

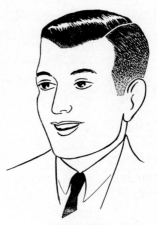

Fig. 209
Regular Medium Cut

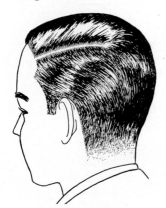

Fig. 210
Medium Long Cut

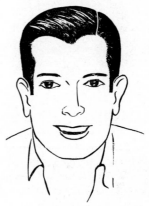

Fig. 211
Regular Long Cut

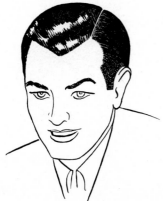

Fig. 212
Regular Long Cut

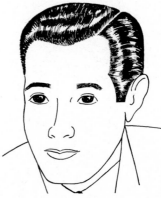

Fig. 213
Extra Long Cut

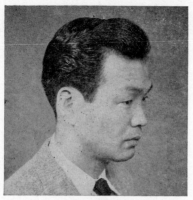

Fig. 214
Regular Long Cut

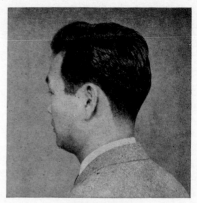

Fig. 215
Regular Long Cut

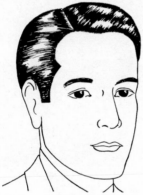

Fig. 216
Extra Long Cut

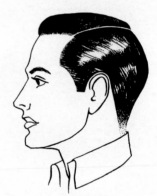

Fig. 217
Extra Long Cut

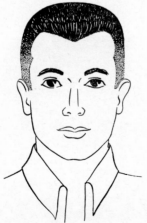

Fig. 218
Short Pompadour

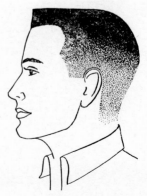

Fig. 219
Short Pompadour

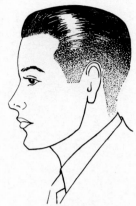

Fig. 220
Medium Pompadour

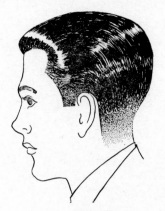

Fig. 221
Medium Long Pompadour

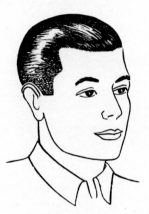

Fig. 222
Long Pompadour

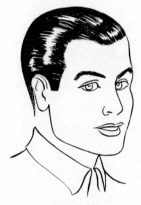

Fig. 223
Extra Long Pompadour

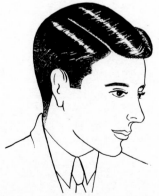

Fig. 224
Casual Roach
Top Hair To Side

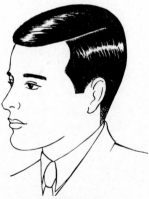

Fig. 225
Casual
Top Hair Forward

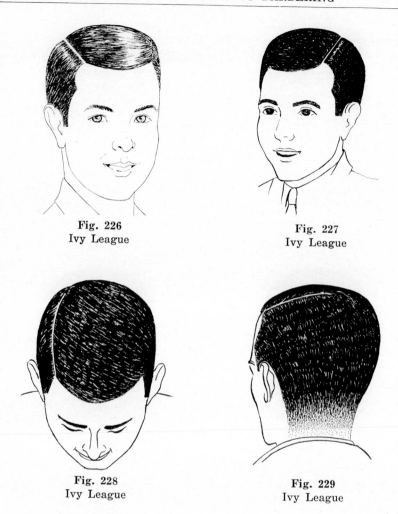

Fig. 226
Ivy League

Fig. 227
Ivy League

Fig. 228
Ivy League

Fig. 229
Ivy League

BOYS' HAIRCUTTING

The general principles and methods of cutting hair apply equally to boys' and men's haircutting, and the styles are nearly all identical. In boys' haircutting, however, the cuts tend to run shorter and less shear and razor outlining is done. The edges on smaller boys are typically casual and are usually soft clipper edges. The discussion here pertains largely to **boys under twelve years of age.**

The principles of cutting hair will not be reiterated in this section. The pointers to be enumerated are outside of those principles. They should be helpful for cutting the hair of boys in the age category just mentioned.

Special pointers on boys' haircutting and styles:

1. Put the boy at ease. This can be done in many ways. Two ways are:
   (1) Speak to him gently and nicely.
   (2) Ask him something about himself, but fitting to his age. Such questions as "do you have a kitty", "do you like trains", or "where do you go to school" are fitting.

2. Determining the hair style:
   (1) Judge from the last hair cut.
   (2) If he is a very small boy, ask his escort.
   (3) If he is old enough to know, ask him.
   (4) Use good judgment.

3. Except in long cuts, the clipper edge should be a little higher than on a man. This is particularly advisable in the back because of the vertical groove in the middle of the neck. It is very difficult to make a good taper in this groove. A high neck edge permits the blending to start above this groove and the final appearance will look smooth and neater.

4. Cut the hair a little shorter than on adults.

5. If the electric clipper frightens the child, try the hand clipper. Sometimes, shawing the child the clipper drives fear away. Letting him see you run it across the back of your hand also helps.

6. Be on your guard and ever-ready to remove implements from the child's head. He is likely to move or turn his head quickly and unexpectedly.

7. Do not try to give a perfect cut to a very small child, since this would keep him too long, and, consequently he would become fretful and restless.

8. Do as careful a job as possible in a reasonable length of time. Never slight a child's cut. Any defects will likely be noticed by the escort or parents and meet with instant disapproval.

9. Generally, a boy's hair may be dampened without asking the escort. But it is always fitting to ask.

10. Leave haircloth intact until the haircut is finished—until the hair is dampened and combed. (Exception: It might sometimes be necessary to clip extreme lower part of neck after the haircloth is removed from the neck.)

11. Be sure to dust off loose hair from ears and neck before dampening the hair, else these loose ends when wet will cling to the skin and be very hard to remove.

12. Dampen the hair before final combing unless requested not to do so.

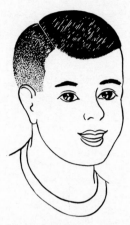

Fig. 240
Regular Short Cut

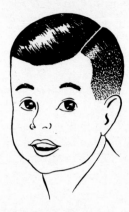

Fig. 241
Regular Medium Cut

13. Emphasize the final combing and parting.

14. Topping in boys' haircutting. The regular finger-work is often cumbersome because the top hair does not yield itself to being combed directly upward or backward, and holding the hair thusly between the fingers may be uncomfortable to the boy. The-Up-and-Over and Shear-Lifting methods are recommended.

Styles of Boys' Hair Cuts: As stated earlier, boys' styles are of the same general pattern as men's styles. The usual variations were presented uder "Special Pointers on Boys' Haircutting and Styles."

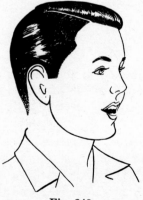

Fig. 242
Regular Long Cut

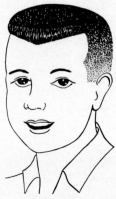

Fig. 243
Short Pompadour

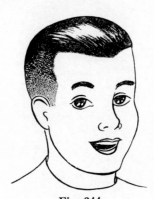

Fig. 244
Medium Pompadour

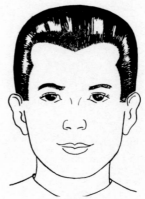

Fig. 245
Long Pompadour

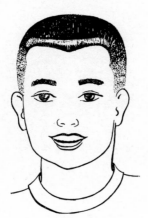

Fig. 246
Short Crew Cut

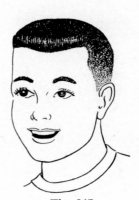

Fig. 247
Medium Crew Cut

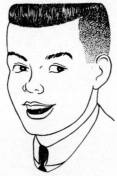

Fig. 248
Flat Top

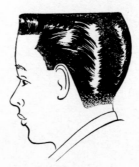

Fig. 249
Flat Top Ducktail

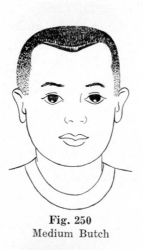

Fig. 250
Medium Butch

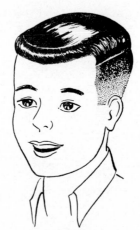

Fig. 251
Forward Boogie

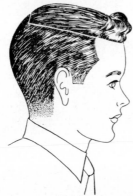

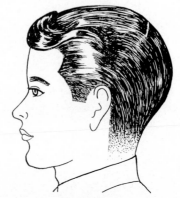

Fig. 252   Fig. 253
Medium Long Cut with Top Hair Combed Forward or a Forward Flip Style

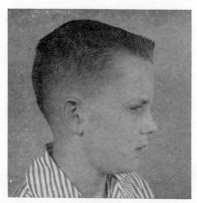

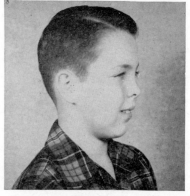

Fig. 254   Fig. 255
Butch   Medium Long Hair Cut

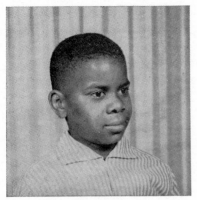

Fig. 256
Short Brush Cut

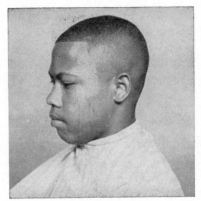

Fig. 257
Quo-Vadis

HOW TO DO CREW CUTS

The three essential features of a crew cut are: (1) a short, smooth surface on top, (2) a slightly round effect at the point where the top merges with the sides, and (3) the side and back hair is comparatively short and has a continuing, **elongated taper.** The top hair should be graduated in length from front to back so that it is almost horizontal when the head is in its normal position. The surface of the top hair should form a slight curve and conform with the general contour of the head. If an arch effect is made across the top from side to side, it should be so slight that it is barely observable; a perfect rounding effect across the top following the natural shape of the head is not as artistic as the **brush** top or short pomp top.

The "crew" cut has outgrown a definite singular design. Until a few years ago, the term crew cut was used synonymously with "short pomp" or "brush" cut. In some areas, however, a crew cut simply means a very short hair cut with a low all-around clipper edge. There are several designs of crew cuts, but in all of them the top hair is cut largely the same. The descriptions run something like this:

1. Crew cut with a low all-around clipper edge.

2. Crew cut with medium long sides that reach to the hairline where there is a definite outline over the ears. The back hair is correspondingly medium long, but it comes to a blended, soft edge usually achieved with the clipper. Sideburns are suitable and correct with medium long cuts. When the **sides** are medium long and the taper is elongated to the hairline, the edges are formed by either a very coarse clipper or by the shears-and-comb.

3. A **short** crew cut is simply a short pomp with a low clipper edge.

4. A **medium** crew cut is a short pomp with side and back hair that runs to the hairline at a length graduated from about one to one-eighth of an inch with a blended clipper edge in back and a definite outline over the ears.

5. A **long** crew cut means that the hair on the sides and back area is longer than medium.

The difference between a short or regular crew cut and a medium or long crew cut is the amount of hair on the sides and back. The length of the top runs almost uniform. Typically, the length of hair in a crew cut is short—it may be short, medium, or medium long. The length varies in the realm of shortness; long hair and the crew cut are opposites.

The standard sequence of cutting the edges, sides, and top may be followed. Some barbers prefer to do the crown area first, or the sides and crown area as one process, then the edging, and then the topping either with the clipper over the comb or with blade attachments. The finishing touches, especially of the siding and topping are done with the shears and comb.

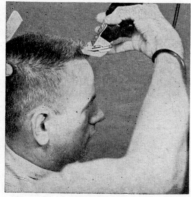 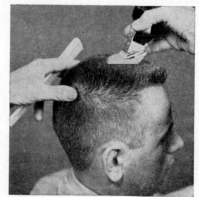

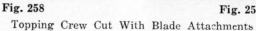

Fig. 258   Fig. 259
Topping Crew Cut With Blade Attachments

The preliminary procedure of giving a patron his first crew cut is to "box" it in (Fig. 260). Where the previous cut was a crew cut, simply employ the general principles of edging, siding, and topping, following the pattern observable or a mental picture.

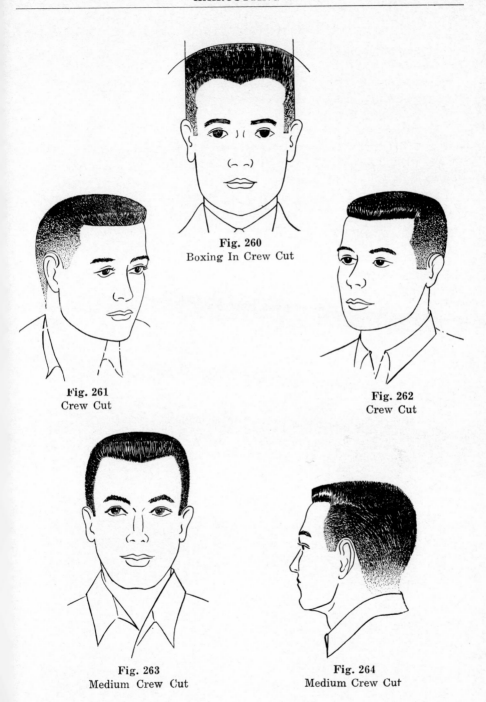

Fig. 260
Boxing In Crew Cut

Fig. 261
Crew Cut

Fig. 262
Crew Cut

Fig. 263
Medium Crew Cut

Fig. 264
Medium Crew Cut

HOW TO DO A FLAT TOP

The procedure of giving a crew cut is practically identical with that for the flat top. In the flat top, there is emphasis on flatness and there is a decided squarish effect where the sides meet the top. The top of a flat top is generally cut shorter on top than in a crew cut, but this difference is not a major point of differentiation.

The initial time a patron has a flat top, do the "boxing in" as illustrated in Fig. 265. Otherwise, merely follow the pattern already set. The "boxing in", however, is usuable when the sides are to be left medium full, or full enough to be called fenders.

Flat tops may be classified in four categories—the regular or short flat top, medium flat top, long flat top, and flat top with ducktail. As in the case of the crew cut, the difference between short, medium, and long is a matter of hair length on the sides and back area. The length of the top runs fairly uniform. The top hair should not be short enough to expose the scalp.

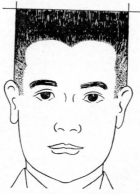

Fig. 265
Boxing in Flat Top

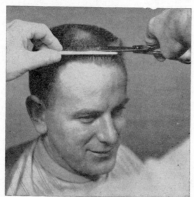
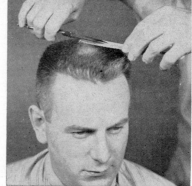

Fig. 266   Fig. 267
Flat Topping with Shears and Comb

The **general procedure and methods** used in cutting crew cuts are applicable to cutting flat tops. The theory, though, of doing the crown area and top first often has more advantages, except when there are to be "fender" sides or a ducktail. Since the top is the paramount feature of a flat top, its flatness and design must not be jeopardized by doing any other part of the cut first unless it is the extreme edge. Blade attachments are especially helpful in achieving flatness on top. Such attachments come in various sizes. Some barbers prefer special combs, usually large ones, if they use the clipper-over-comb method of topping a flat top. This method lends itself to more versatility in arriving at the desired length. For instance, the length is graduated downward from the front hairline to the crown. With blade attachments the result would be hair of the same length unless the attachments are changed or guided through some areas without contact with the scalp, and this is possible.

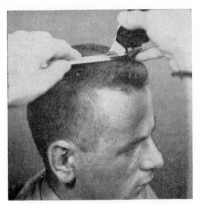

Fig. 268
Flat Topping with Coarse
Clipper Blade over Comb

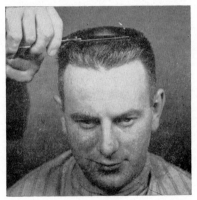

Fig. 269
Smoothing Flat Top
With Shears

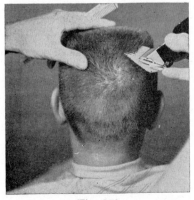

Fig. 270

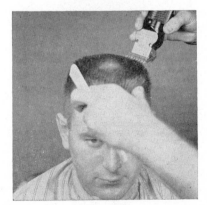

Fig. 271

Flat Topping With Blade Attachments

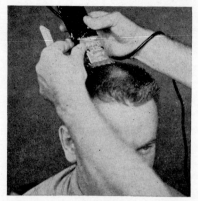

Fig. 272   Fig. 273
Smoothing Top with Coarse Clipper Blade

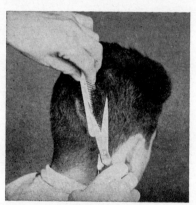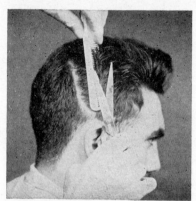

Fig. 274   Fig. 275
Trimming Sides of Flat Top with Long Sides

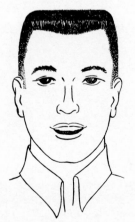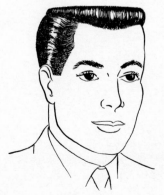

Fig. 276   Fig. 277
Flat Top with Short Sides   Flat Top with Long Sides

HOW TO DO BUTCH CUTS

A **Butch** is the simplest style to cut. Essentially it means short hair in all three dimensions of a hair cut. The only variation is that the sides and back area should be coarse clipper shortness or of such medium length as can be achieved by clipper blade attachments. The top ranges from three-quarters to one-quarter of an inch in length. The upper portion of the middle section and the top are made the same length. A fitting variation is to graduate slightly the length of top hair from front to back. The same clipper blade attachment may be used for both of these areas.

The top hair and the hair at the curvature is rounded to conform with the contour of the head. A little "flip" or a quickly graduated bit of hair across the top at the front hairline appropriately breaks the monotony of sameness of length.

In nearly every respect, the same procedure and techniques of giving a crew cut are followed to give a butch, except there are only two types of butches—the short and the medium, and these terms apply to the sides and back area. The hair is characteristically and uniformly short on top. The butch may be called a **short brush cut**. Refer to the techniques of cutting explained for crew cuts and flat tops.

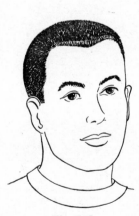

Fig. 278
Regular Butch

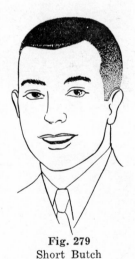

Fig. 279
Short Butch

HOW TO CUT DUCKTAILS

The principal feature of a ducktail hair cut is the "dove tailing"—fitting together in the back. For hair to be made to do this it must necessarily be long on the sides and in back. The top hair is typically long, but it may be just medium long or flat as in a flat top. The only instruction needed

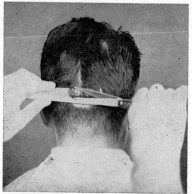
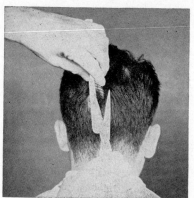

Fig. 280
Fig. 281
Furrowing Center for Sides of Ducktail

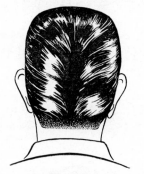

Fig. 282
Regular Ducktail

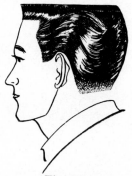

Fig. 283
Ducktail with Flat Top

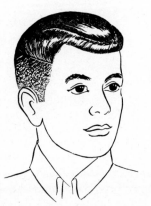

Fig. 284
Forward Boogie with Short Sides

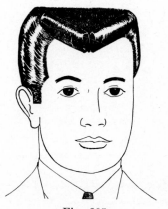

Fig. 285
Flat Top Boogie
(Long Sides)

in addition to that given for the flat top pertains to the back area where the ends of both sides are cut so as to cling together. A slight vertical furrow is made in the center of the back area. The long ends of the sides are cut and **slithered.** Slithering the ends makes them obedient and cooperative, and only a little hair wax is needed to get them to form a ducktail effect. Properly tapered and slithered ends create an interlocking of the multiplicity of the terminal hairs. This is true in all hair cuts, but it is especially needful in ducktails.

A ducktail cut is on the feminine side, and can indicate affectation. They look well on comparatively few persons.

BOOGIE HAIR CUTS

A **Boogie** hair cut is combed forward on top and has a scroll effect at the front hairline. It is usually referred to as the Forward Boogie. This scroll may be rounding or sort of "V" shaped. This style is designed to be florid and different. It is worn almost exclusively by the younger set. The only special pointers necessary to give this cut are (1) make a high side part on each side if it is a Regular Forward Boogie, (2) make no part on the Long Boogie, and (3) **slither** the ends to form the scroll.

NEGRO HAIRCUTTING

Negro hair is characteristically very curly and kinky. It can be described as "nappy". Many of the principles of cutting straight hair are applicable to the cutting of nappy hair; however, it is noteworthy that some different techniques and additional clipper blades or blade attachments are necessary to do a good job in a reasonable length of time. Clipper blades ranging in sizes from 0000 to number 2 are recommended. The sizes most used are 000, 0, 0A, 1 and 1½. The coarse blade sizes are so designated on detachable blade clippers. Much the same effects can be accomplished by an adjustable blade type of clipper by the use of blade attachments.

Styles of Negro hair cuts: Many of the styles for straight hair are worn appropriately by those whose hair is very curly or kinky. The standard styles are especially adaptable to both kinds of hair. Such a style as the flat top, though, would be extremely difficult to give in soft, kinky hair, unless it was varied to minimize the stubby uprightness on top. Because Negro hair is inherently curly, it is possible to achieve many nice effects in styling not possible with straight hair. Two of the hair styles very common among Negros are Front Shingle and English Brush Back. The English Brush Back may be designated as low, medium, or high brush cut. Styles designed to keep the hair fairly close to the scalp are popular with the Negro. This is accomplished either by cutting the hair short or cutting it in such a manner that it responds readily to hair wax or hairdressing.

The **Front Shingle** is designed by shingling the top hair so that it slopes towards the front. The shingling begins at the posterior portion of the vertex, but it is graduated so as to leave the hair heavier in front. The hair is usually clipped very close and high all around the head. This is a very practical type of hair cut, especially for those whose occupation exposes them to dust and dirt. If the hair is nappy, this cut can be almost completed with the clipper. Begin with the 000 blades and run them up high all around, and then, with a coarse blade or blade attachment, continue upward to the top portion of the middle section. With the clipper set for coarseness, or with a coarse blade, start at the posterior portion of the vertex and proceed forward to the front hairline. With the most appropriate size blade, blend the hair of the top, middle and edge by directing the clipper from the top area downward with the **teeth of the blade pointing downward**. A razor outline is optional.

The **English Brush Cut** is a very popular style with the Negro—to him it is also known as the Pompadour. The texture of Negro hair is such that it lends itself easily to straight back combing on almost any shaped head. As stated earlier, there are three standard variations of the brush cut—low, medium and high.

The **Low Brush Cut** has a very low all-around clipper edge. Typically, the top is left long. A frequent variation is to cut the top short and blend it with equally short hair on the sides and back.

The **Medium Brush Cut** is designed with slightly less hair in the middle and top areas than the Low Brush Cut. The Medium Brush Cut also has an all-around clipper edge. The 000 blades are used just in back across the neck. The No. 1 blades are used to continue up into the hair in back and also to make the clipper-edge on the sides. These coarse blades are moved upward about one and a half inches, but not higher than a point which corresponds to the eye-brow. Then a very important procedure is followed. Continue with the No. 1 blades, but turn the clipper upside down so that the teeth of the blades point downward. With the clipper in this position work from the top downward in narrow strips. It is in this way that the graduation or blend is mainly accomplished.

The **High Brush Cut** has a close and high all-around clipper edge. The top is left long enough to be combed straight back. The siding is done with both the coarse and fine clipper blades. In this style a razor outline is optional. The High Brush Cut was very popular with Negroes in the Armed Forces during World War II.

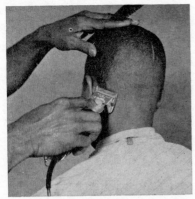

Fig. 286
Styling Quo-Vadis

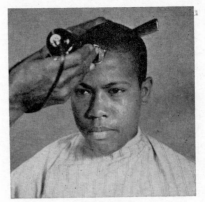

Fig. 287
Styling Quo-Vadis

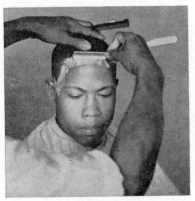

Fig. 288
Styling Quo-Vadis

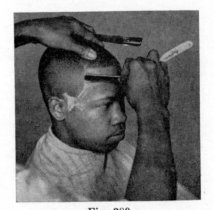

Fig. 289
Styling Quo-Vadis

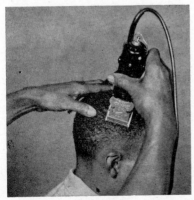

Fig. 290

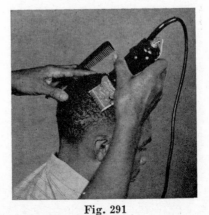

Fig. 291

Techniques of Cutting Negro Hair

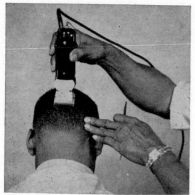 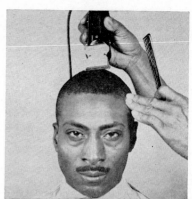

Fig. 292   Fig. 293

Techniques of Cutting Negro Hair

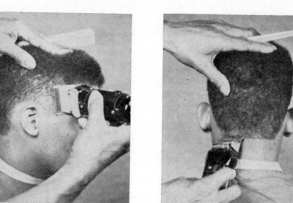

Fig. 293A   Fig. 293B

Techniques of Cutting Negro Hair

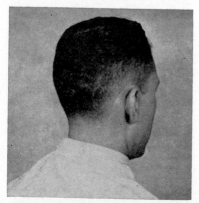 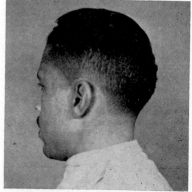

Fig. 294
Short Cut—Front Shingle

Fig. 295
Medium Brush Cut or
Medium Pompadour

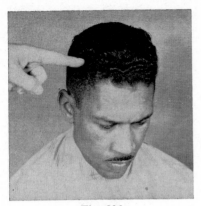

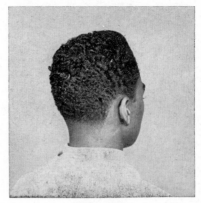

Fig. 296
Medium Brush Cut

Fig. 297
Full Brush Cut or Long Pomp.

The **Long Pompadour** is also a Negro type of cut. This style is not of the "Brush" variety since the hair is left long on top. Typically all the hair is combed back, without a part.

The **Medium Pompadour** is the same general design as the Long Pompadour except that the hair is shorter on the sides and top. It is a very popular cut and it is often parted.

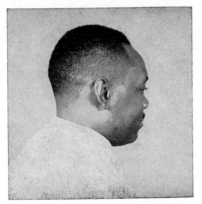

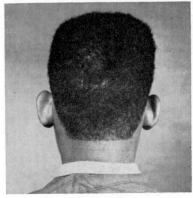

Fig. 298
Medium Brush Cut

Fig. 299
Medium Pomp Square Back

WOMEN'S HAIRCUTTING

The fundamental principles of men's haircutting are applicable to women's haircutting. The end products, of course, are entirely different. That is, the designs, styles, and final effects are different. To do women's hair cuts, the barber should have a mental storehouse of the standard and popular styles. The pointers to be enumerated on women's haircutting also apply to girl's haircutting.

Review the scientific and artistic principles set forth earlier in this chapter. The various techniques of cutting, shaping, thinning, tapering and blending apply to both men's and women's haircutting. Many of the artistic principles are also equally applicable. Review various shapes of faces, sizes of nose, sizes of ears, lengths of chin, and lengths of neck.

To do women's haircutting, one needs to know (1) the fundamental principles of cutting hair in all its phases, such as tapering, thinning, and slithering, (2) an understanding of the artistic principles of balance and symmetry, (3) a mental storehouse of styles, and (4) imagination or creative ability. (These are the same requirements for men's haircutting.) In general, styles of women's hair cuts tend to be easy, loose, and casual and free from the crisp or static lines in men's styles.

The woman is inclined to favor such terms as "style" and "shape" to "cut". Hair-shaping appeals to her more than "haircutting".

Acquire a mental storehouse of styles: Acquire a large variety of mental pictures of styles. Detail instructions on how to develop these pictures or images are given in this chapter. Study the styles you see on women, in newspapers, and in cosmetology magazines.

Seeing is doing: What the artisan sees, he can reproduce. Some people who play the piano can play a piece of music after hearing it just once. While they may do this by only hearing, you may reproduce a style by just seeing.

Shingle Category: A shingle means a comparatively short hair cut with the back area of the head tapered to a soft blended edge. A shingle on a woman differs from that on a man in that it is left much fuller and the blend is quick or steep, to the point of being somewhat abrupt.

Identical elements in men's and women's haircutting:

(1) The same implements used are—the shears, combs, clipper, and razor.
(2) The shears and comb are used in the same way.
(3) Slithering is done in the same manner.
(4) Shingling is done in the same manner.
(5) Feathering is done in the same manner.
(6) Thinning is done in the same manner.
(7) The haircloth is used in the same manner.

(8) For edging or making a feathered neck-edge the clipper is used in the same manner.

(9) The principles of balance, symmetry, and proportion are the same.

(10) The same general artistic principles are applicable.

(11) The same emphasis is placed on sanitation and sterilization.

Neck-edge styles on women: Neck-edges are usually informal or casual. There are many variations of the standard patterns. The four standard patterns are Feather Edge, Rounding Line Edge, Semi-Circular "V" Edge and the Regular "V" Edge. The "V" shaped patterns may come either to a definite line or feathered edge. Neck-edges may be blunt, swirled, turned under or upward, rolled, or clubbed. A very casual or informal neck-edge is also known as "jungle" edge. Such an edge does not conform to an established pattern—it is a rambling edge that harmonizes with an informal or casual design. It is usually done by slithering or end thinning.

NECK EDGES

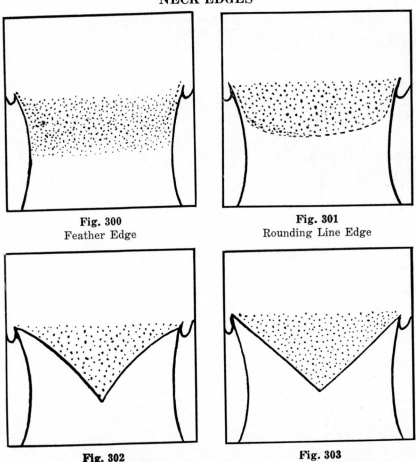

Fig. 300
Feather Edge

Fig. 301
Rounding Line Edge

Fig. 302
Semi-Circular "V" Edge

Fig. 303
Square "V" Edge

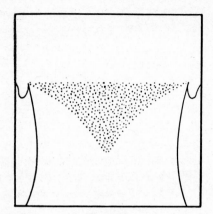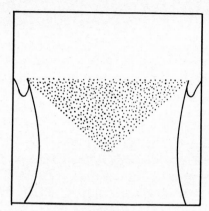

Fig. 304   Fig. 305
Featheredge "V" Patterns of Neck-Edges

CUTTING AND SHAPING LADIES' HAIR

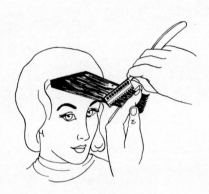

Fig. 306

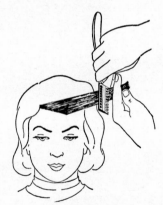

Fig. 307

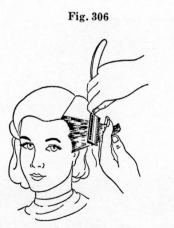

Fig. 308

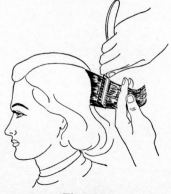

Fig. 309

Resume of effects achievable in ladies' haircutting:

1. To achieve a **pompadour effect** softer than the classic pomp, strands are parted parallel to the hairline and positioned off the face for cutting. In this way, underneath hair is cut at ends.

2. To achieve a **toplock or side angled bang,** position the strands parallel to the forehead, and shorten hair to a point that is about level with the outer fringe of the eyebrow.

3. To achieve an **off-the-face styling effect,** make vertical partings on the side and position strands back from the hairline. Begin cutting about three inches from the face hairline and shorten as designed.

4. To achieve a **blended taper** for a **lifted nape effect,** section the hair vertically across the back from the crown downward, and graduate the lengths from about three to two inches at the nape.

One purpose in styling is to draw attention away from the less attractive features. This can be accomplished in two general ways:

1. Partially conceal such a feature. For example, design bangs on a broad forehead. Sometimes an abnormality such as large ears and extra long neck can be made to appear almost normal by optical illusion; otherwise, concealment can be achieved through good hair designing.

2. **Counteract** such a feature by arranging an effect in the opposite direction. That is, a receding chin would be emphasized by sweeping hair back, and if the nose is prominent, don't design bangs to hang low over the forehead, since they would point to the nose like an arrow.

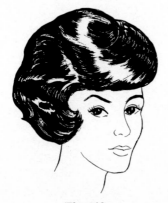

Fig. 310
Casual Fluff

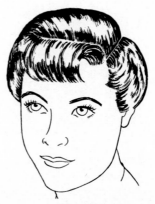

Fig. 311
Forward Scroll

Women's and girls' hair styles: There are innumerable styles of women's and girls' hair cuts. The term "hair style" is more widely used than "hair cut" when it applies to women. Outside of a handful of names, there is no standardization of name terminology of women's hair styles. In general use are such terms as shingle, bangs, short, medium, long, feather edge, line edge, Dutch Bob, "touch-up," etc.

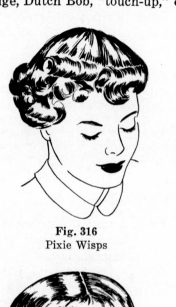

Fig. 316
Pixie Wisps

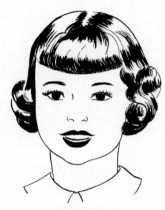

Fig. 317
Dutch Bangs Casual Sides

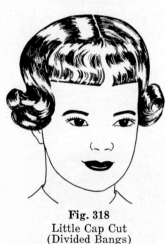

Fig. 318
Little Cap Cut
(Divided Bangs)

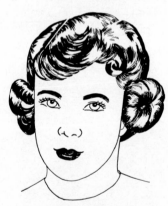

Fig. 319
Twinkle Bang
(With Ear Puffs)

Bangs: Bangs are the hair that lie over a portion of the forehead. They may be worn by both women and girls. A bang will do a lot to cover an unusually large forehead. If a woman has a prominent nose, the bang should not cover more than one-third of her forehead. Properly designed bangs add smartness to a hair style. A bang is that portion of the front hair that is cut so as to cover a given part of the forehead. There are styles and individual variations of bangs.

1. The range of lengths of bangs is from the eyebrows to two inches above the eyebrows. A long bang falls about a half inch above the eyebrows; a medium bang falls about one inch above; and a short bang falls about one and one-half inch above. Bangs tend to run shorter on girls.

2. Stubborn bangs cut too short will be uncontrolable.

3. Bangs may be cut back into the sides as far as the hairline; and in cases in which the hair grows well forward on the forehead, they may be cut beyond this line. In this latter case, clip the short hair that is left just underneath the back part of the bangs.

4. To cut bangs, steady the shears with the index finger of the left hand; start in the middle and work back to one side and then to the other. In this way, it is easier to judge the cutting. On the left

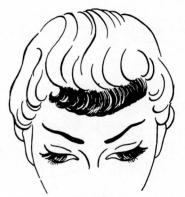

Fig. 320
Wisp Bang

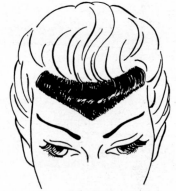

Fig. 321
Chevron Bang

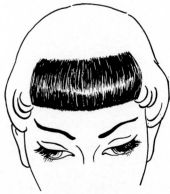

Fig. 322
Dutch Bang

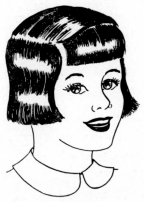

Fig. 323
Dutch Cut

side work with the palm of the hand down; on the right with the palm up. Both sides of the bang may be cut from one standing position. Make big carefully directed swaths and bring the blades of the shears together very quickly. The portion of hair within a single stroke will be straight; and it is easier to stop and start evenly three or four times than seventy-five times. And, by closing the shears quickly, better control of the hair is gained.

5. After the first outline is made, dampen the bang and retouch. Do a great deal of combing and checking.

6. Gauge the straightness of bangs by looking at them from about two feet directly in front of the customer and by looking at them in the mirror.

7. Make the final touch a cutting stroke. The result will be a smoother edge to present for approval.

8. A great deal of combing through the bangs is necessary. It is really difficult to make a perfect bang. A good eye and steady nerves are required. Just before the final touch just mention, again dampen the bangs slightly, re-comb, and do the final edging.

9. Bangs may be partial or all the way across the forehead.

10. Bangs may have either a formal or casual edge.

11. Bangs may be horizontal, diagonal, or slanted at any angle.

SELECTED TERMS IN HAIRCUTTING

1. The **base** means the foundation of a hair cut.

2. **Blending** means cutting the hair so that there is no line of demarcation within or between sections—graduating or tapering.

3. **Blunting** means blunt cutting. This is done by cutting the hair square off while holding the hair at right angles to the scalp or straight downward.

4. **Bobbing** means cutting the hair square off, making no taper.

5. **Chevron** means "V" shaped.

6. **Clubbing** is synonmous with bobbing. It produces a stubby effect.

7. A **coiffure** is a hairdo. It is a completed style of dressing the hair.

8. A **coiffeur** is a male hairdresser; and a **coiffeuse** is a female hairdresser.

9. **Cutting** is the process of severing hair—shortening and tapering.

10. **English thinning** means thinning the hair from an imaginary underneath section, leaving it longer on the outside.

11. **Feathered** means a soft, beveled edge.

12. **Layer cut** means cutting the hair so as to produce layers that resemble shingles on a roof.

13. **Shingling** means graduating or blending, usually producing a featheredge.

14. **Shredding** means cutting in long, narrow vertical strips, usually from the base upward.

15. **Slithering** means cutting in long, narrow vertical strips, usually from the base upward.

16. **Teasing** means back-combing to produce a hat—ratting.

17. **Thinning** means reducing the weight or bulk of hair near the scalp, through a strand, or at the extreme ends.

18. **Trimming** means partial cutting, that is, the removal of the ends—just taking off a little.

19. **Blending, graduating, tapering, sloping, and feathering** are used to mean the same thing. "Feathering" originates from the arrangement of the feathers of the wing of a fowl which came gradually to a soft natural edge. (The edge of a hair cut should be made so as to fade out so gradually that it is almost impossible to tell where the edge actually begins.)

Possible Faults in Haircutting

1. Cutting off to much hair.
2. Not cutting off enough hair.
3. Giving an incorrect style.
4. Unbalance.
5. Cold lather for arching.
6. Pulling from dull razor.
7. Pulling from the shears.
8. Nicks in the hair.

HAIRSTYLING
(Basic Principles)

Hairstyling means designing and doing individualized hair styles for particular persons.

This chapter is only an **introduction** to men's hairstyling. It is not necessarily a part of a regular beginner's course in barbering.

The **avenues to this artistry** are studying, thinking, experimenting, and observing artisans. Fundamentally, when one understands the scientific and artistic principles of haircutting, he can create a style of his own, or duplicate any style which he sees even if it is just an illustration or picture. Just as an architect knows how to draw blueprints for many kinds of buildings, the barber knows how to blueprint in his mind many kinds of hair styles. After the barber has mastered the fundamentals of cutting and styling, he needs only to see or to have either an actual or mental picture of the style to be given. The same general principles of edging, blending, cutting and visualization apply to all hair cuts. Many pianists can play a new piece of music after having heard it played once. Just so, the competent barber can duplicate any style he observes. The section on "mental images" will be studied later in this chapter.

There is no mystery in designing hair styles. Some barbers are, however, capable of developing individual knacks which can be learned by others. These knacks are often referred to as "tricks-of-the-trade." They are not actually tricks but rather some ways, approaches, and methods discovered and perfected by an individual barber or artisan. Every barber who works thinkingly and creatively develops knacks which supplement the fundamental principles of hairstyling.

MEN'S AND BOYS' HAIRSTYLING

Types of heads and faces: A study of the types of heads as to contour, outline, general shape, and the most becoming style is one of the major considerations of this chapter. All the artistic principles explained and illustrated in this chapter are applicable to those considerations. The present discussion, however, will be confined to "parts" and indications as to where to minimize or maximize the amount of hair.

It is important to know where to part the hair on a given shape of head and where to have the hair short or long, thin or thick. In brief, how can the most becomingness in a hair cut be achieved. The answer is in the composite of the artistic principles of hairstyling. In this section, then, the question will be only partially answered. The barber should be thoroughly familiar with the different types of heads as a starting point to hairstyling. The following illustrations are presented for this purpose, to designate where to part the hair, and, to some extent, the proper amount of hair at the proper areas.

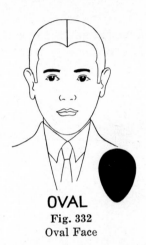

OVAL

Fig. 332
Oval Face

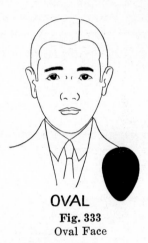

OVAL

Fig. 333
Oval Face

The **oval face** is the ideal shape. It is designated as the "egg" shape. It is wider at the forehead and tapers to a well-rounded chin. This type of face looks equally becoming with hair worn low or high on the head; and likewise, either a center or side part or no part at all is becoming, depending somewhat on other facial characteristics (Figs. 332, 333).

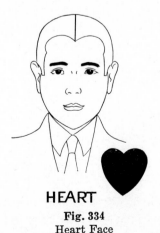

HEART

Fig. 334
Heart Face

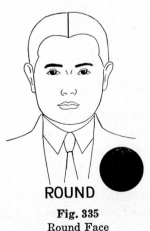

ROUND

Fig. 335
Round Face

The **heart-shaped** face is broadest across the cheek bones and has a wide, broad forehead. It is narrow at the jawline and wide at the eyes. The jawbones curve either to an oval or pointed chin that completes the heart shape. Almost any style is becoming on this normal type of face. The hair may be either short or long, but preferably a little fuller on the top than on the sides. A center part is recommended, or one made fairly close to the center of the head (Fig. 334).

The **round face** is short with a wide forehead, a rounded hairline, curved jawbones that slope either to an oval or rounded chin. The forehead, cheeks, and jawbones are of equal width. Try to break down the round look. Maximize the top hair to balance the jawbones and thus lengthen the face. A part directly in the center to divide the face in half is recommended (Fig. 335).

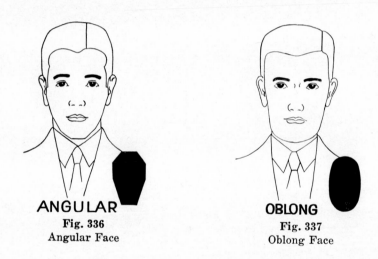

ANGULAR

Fig. 336
Angular Face

OBLONG

Fig. 337
Oblong Face

The **angular face** is broadest across the cheek bones, but has a wide forehead. It has sunken temples, hollow cheeks, and prominent cheek bones. The jawbones are curved so as to form a squarish chin. The hair should be kept close to the head, especially at the sides. A side part is most suitable (Fig. 336).

The **oblong face** is a long, slightly oval face with a rounded chin. The width from the forehead to where the jawbone curves to the chin is frequently the same. Minimize the top hair and maximize the hair at the sides. A low side part is most appropriate (Fig. 337).

The **inverted triangle face** is widest across the forehead. From the cheeks downward it tapers sharply to a pointed chin. The temples, fore-

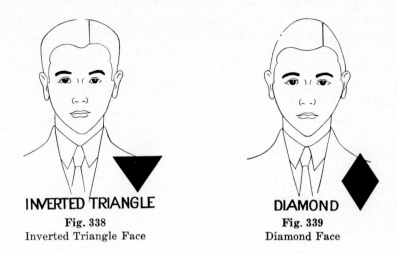

INVERTED TRIANGLE
Fig. 338
Inverted Triangle Face

DIAMOND
Fig. 339
Diamond Face

head, and cheek bones are about the same width, although the temples may be slightly recessed and the cheek bone area may be narrower than the forehead. Keep the hair close to the head. An off-center side part is most becoming (Fig. 338).

The **diamond face** is wide at the eyes and cheek bones and narrow at the forehead and chin. It's oblique jawbones taper sharply to a pointed chin. Minimize the top hair and maximize the hair at the sides. A low side part is recommended (Fig. 339),

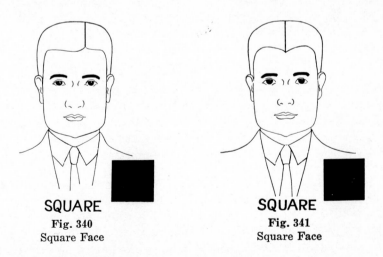

SQUARE
Fig. 340
Square Face

SQUARE
Fig. 341
Square Face

The **square face** has a wide, squarish forehead, and squarish jawbones and chin. The width of the forehead, cheek bones, and jawbones is practically the same. This is a difficult shape of face to style. Maximize hair at the sides to subjugate the squareness of the jaws. The top hair should be reasonably full. A center part is suitable if the nose is fairly normal in size and shape (Fig. 341).

A **square face** may also be parted off-center, if the nose is prominent. (Fig. 340).

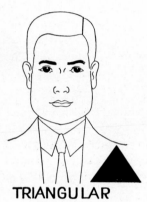

TRIANGULAR

Fig. 342

Triangular Face

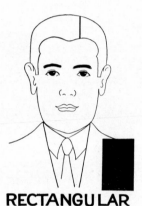

RECTANGULAR

Fig. 343

Rectangular Face

In the **triangular face** the upper half is narrower than the lower. It has a narrow, tapering forehead and the width through the square jawbones is emphatic. The chin may be slightly squarish or pointed. An attempt should be made to make the upper portion of the head seem wider to balance the wide jawline. Maximize the hair at the narrow portions of the head and minimize, or keep close to the head the hair at the wide portions of the head. A low side part is most suitable (Fig. 342).

The **rectangular face** is long and squarish. It is longer than it is wide. The forehead, cheek bones and jawbones are of identical width. The squarish jawbones slope to a slightly oval or squarish chin. The hair should be minimized on top and maximized at the sides to give a rounding contour effect. An off-center part is recommended (Fig. 343).

Heights of Neck-edges: The height of neck-edges at the nape of the neck is very important, especially with respect to the length of the neck. The length of the chin should also be considered. There are four standard heights, namely, high, standard, low, and extra low. A high neck-edge runs about one-half inch above the lower tip of the ear. A normal or standard neck-edge runs about even with the lower tip of the ear; a low neck-edge about one-half inch below, and an extra low neck-edge about one inch below.

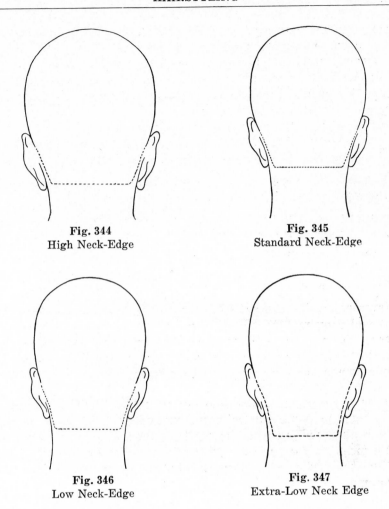

Fig. 344
High Neck-Edge

Fig. 345
Standard Neck-Edge

Fig. 346
Low Neck-Edge

Fig. 347
Extra-Low Neck Edge

The height of a neck-edge may be determined by the way the hair grows. Where the barber has the choice, he should make a normal height neck-edge in the absence of irregularities. If the patron's neck is short, recommend a high neck-edge; if the patron's neck is long, recommend either a low or extra-low neck-edge, depending on the length of the neck. The length of the face and the drop of the chin also should be considered when deciding upon the height of the neck-edge. Make the neck-edge as low as possible on a person with a long pointed chin. Conversely, while the normal edge is usually preferable, a higher than normal is recommended for a person with a short chin.

Designs of neck edges: The designs of neck edges, as well as the heights of them, are important in hairstyling. Heights of neck-edges will be further discussed and illustrated in the following pages, showing that they relate to the length of the chin, the length of the sideburns, and in fact to all the prominent physical features of the face, head, and neck In the current trend of hairstyling, the major emphasis is on the top sides, and back. Even though the public observes mostly these divisions the fact still remains that the artisan gives particular attention to the neck-edge — its design, height, precision, finish, and relation to the other parts of the style. A vague, unbalanced, improper height, unfin ished neck-edge, to the artisan, detracts from the whole effect of the style. The following are some imperfections to avoid:

1. A horse-shoe design. This means rounded corners. Instead taper the edge so that it reaches the side outlines of the style.

2. Abruptness. A properly blended neck-edge fades out gradually to a soft edge, giving a natural edge effect.

3. Improper height. Relate the height to the physical features dis cussed in this section of hairstyling, such as the chin, sideburns ears, and neck.

4. Improper width. An extra-wide neck can be somewhat normalized in width by making the width of the neck-edge a little narrower than the neck; and likewise, an extra narrow neck can be made to look slightly wider by the maximum width of neck-edge. This is a camouflage but respected by artisans.

Kind of outline over ears: One school of thought is that the outline over the ear should be precise, definite and symmetrical. The other school of thought is that the outline over the ears should be just the opposite; and this means a feather edge without a definite line. Which type of an outline the stylist gives is at his option, except for the choice of the customer.

Neck-edges in relation to chin: The height of the neck-edge should be made, as far as possible, according to the length of the chin. If the length of the chin is normal, the height of the neck-edge should be normal—about even with the lower tip of the ear. If the chin is short, the height of the neck-edge may be made of normal height, or a little above the lower tip of the ear. If the chin is long, the height of the neck-edge should be low— from one-half to one inch below the lower tip of the ear. If the chin is abnormally long, the height of the neck-edge should be as low as possible. The illustrations immediately following present the four standard heights of neck-edges in relation to four different lengths of chins. (Figs. 348-351.)

Sideburns in relation to chins: Sideburns are a major factor in the illusion to normalize the distance between the outward corner of the eye and the point of the chin. For a normal chin, recommend a normal or medium

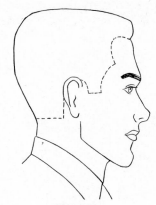

Fig. 348
Neck-Edge for Normal Chin

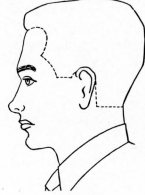

Fig. 349
Neck-Edge for Short Chin

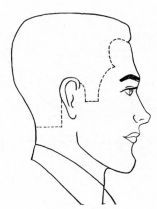

Fig. 350
Neck-Edge for Long Chin

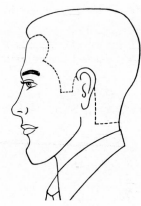

Fig. 351
Neck-Edge for Extra-Long Chin

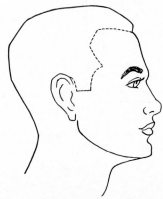

Fig. 356
Normal Chin and Normal
Length Sideburn

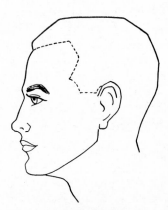

Fig. 357
Short Chin and Short
Sideburn

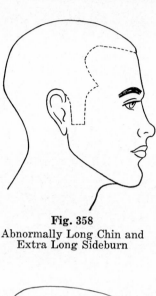

Fig. 358
Abnormally Long Chin and
Extra Long Sideburn

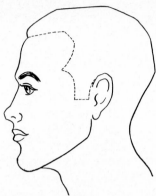

Fig. 359
Long Chin and Long
Sideburn

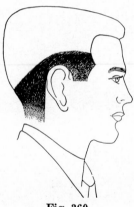

Fig. 360
Normal Size Ears
Normal Height Arch

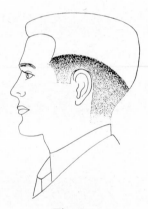

Fig. 361
Small Ears and Higher Than
Normal Arch

length sideburn; for a short chin, recommend a high sideburn; for a long chin, recommend a long sideburn; and for an abnormally long chin, recommend an extra long sideburn. The following illustrations present these principles:

Arches and amount of hair behind ears in relation to size of ears: The general attempt is to form an arch that will tend to make small or large ears look reasonably normal. If a small ear is isolated by a higher than normal arch, it will appear larger; and if a large ear is crowded by an arch lower than normal, it will appear smaller. The illustrations to follow also show that the amount of hair immediately behind the ear helps to give

the illusion of smallness or largeness. Isolate the small ear with comparatively little hair; and crowd the big ear with more than the average amount
of hair. Study the following illustrations: Figs. 360-363

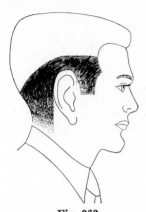

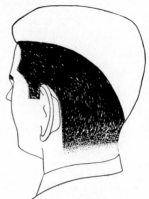

Fig. 362
Large Ears and Lower Than
Normal Arch

Fig. 363
Projecting Ears and Lowest
Possible Arch

Mental storehouse of styles: The barber should have a mental storehouse
of styles. Such a storehouse provides blueprints of styles and enables him
to select and adapt a style to a given person. The barber should have a
clear mental picture of the final product before he starts cutting. Some
of the details may not be decided upon at the starting point, but the
general style and shape should be. That is, a blueprint of the cut should
be drawn in his mind before he cuts a single hair. There are many ways
to acquire or develop mental pictures of styles for a mental storehouse.
Here are some of the ways:

1. By studying pictures of styles in books and in magazines.
2. By reading explanations of styles.
3. By studying hair cuts on people through observation.
4. By listening to the patron's requests.
5. By using one's own imagination.
6. By reasoning from knowledge of the theories of artistic haircutting.
7. By an understanding of balance, symmetry, harmony, and proportion.
8. By observing and listening to other barbers and artisans.
9. By studying the principles of artistic haircutting.
10. By creative thinking. This means originating your own variations
    and styles.

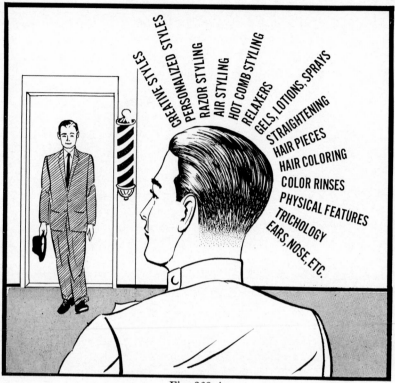

Fig. 363-A
A Mental Storehouse of Styles

RAZOR SHAPING AND STYLING

Shaping hair with the razor has been practiced for many years. Such practice is presently very popular in Europe and in some parts of the United States. Razor haircutting is a somewhat controversial subject. There are pros and cons. Some artisans say they can achieve certain styling effects by the razor that cannot be realized by any other implement, while others say they can achieve the same results with shears and with less probability of damage to the hair. The razor can be used (1) to thin hair, (2) to shorten hair, (3) to taper and blend hair, and (4) to break the resistance of stubborn hair by stripping it and thus making it more obedient. The structure of hair can be damaged by excessive stripping. Stripping means slicing. Excessively stripped hair becomes dry, frizzy, and lifeless. Moderate stripping along a strand of hair is not necessarily damaging. Terminal or end stripping does little or no damage, since the ends will soon be replaced by growing hair. It might be established that razor stripping is faster, more accurate and more graceful than shear stripping. One advantage of the razor stripping over shear stripping is that the razor strips and blends the very ends of hair.

Types of razors used for cutting hair: The straight open-blade razor is widely used, especially by barbers. The **wedge** is preferred, size 9/16 to 3/8. The guarded blade is also used. The argument is that a guarded blade is (1) inexpensively replaceable and (2) prevents the blade from cutting too deeply; whereas the unguarded straight razor (1) does not gather cut hair at its edge and (2) the cutting edge can be suited to the artisan's liking by honing and stropping. Some barbers prefer a coarse honed edge unstropped or stropped only on a canvas; others prefer a smooth stropped edge close to a shaving edge, and still others use a special wedge razor, a special hone, and a short European-type strop (a combination of wood and leather).

Basic fundamentals of razor cutting and shaping:

1. Tentatively complete the basic edging with the shears and comb and clippers. This includes outlining over the ears and blending at the nape. If the hair is excessively long by neglect or as is often true in virgin styling with a razor, the shears may be used to "rough in" the general desired shape or volume. Basic edging is done prior to dampening or shampooing.

2. The hair should be damp. Dampness facilitates cutting by softening the hair. Soft hair is less dulling.

3. **Freshly** shampooed hair is best for razor cutting, since the hair must be free from grease, oil and dirt. Towel dry the hair and leave it slightly damp. Freshly shampooed hair lends itself more readily to new positions and moulding and its natural flow is more evident.. Dirty hair does not respond to different styling positions and effects. Shampooing follows basic edging and outlining.

4. Do the basic edging prior to dampening or shampooing.

5. Tilt the blade to about 45 degrees to cut hair off.

6. Tilt the blade very little to strip the hair, whether along a strand or at the ends.

7. As a general rule keep the razor within about one inch of the comb, but this is a flexible rule. Keep it closer for terminal cutting and blending and on short hair. The comb arranges the hair for proper directional cutting. Cut the hair in the direction it is combed. Whether the razor precedes or follows the comb is at the discretion of the artisan, but much depends on the length and texture of hair. For terminal cutting and blending, the razor usually precedes the comb. In the **revolving** or **windmill** movement the razor and comb alternate positions repeatedly.

8. **Underneath** and **surface** cutting and shaping:

   (1) **Underneath cutting:** To diminish the general volume of hair do underneath cutting. Comb a section of hair in the opposite

direction from the final position to be combed; that is, if the top hair is to be combed back, comb it forward for cutting. A **right angle** cutting position away from its final combing is correct for the back area. The strokes for diminishing volume are comparatively long, and the blade is only slightly tilted.

(2) **Surface cutting:**

(a) For terminal blending (end tapering), use comparatively short strokes, with the blade tilted about 45 degrees.

(b) For surface blending, the length of the strokes runs from short to moderate, with the blade tilted according to the amount of stripping or terminal blending to be done.

(c) For surface blending, use the razor after the hair is combed into its final position.

(d) When tapering surface hair, direct the comb and razor in the direction the hair is to be combed. Good meshes are sometimes best achieved by the razor following the comb.

9. **Sectioning the hair:** Sectioning is usually not done for surface or terminal blending, and it has little merit in the back area, depending on the length of the hair. Hair that is cut every ten days or two weeks can usually be **re-cut or re-touched without formal** sectioning. It is necessary to section the hair for a virgin styling job or hair that has grown long. There are various good ways to section the hair.

(1) **Bi-sectioning.** Divide the hair into two sections. This is done by parting the hair from ear-to-ear, passing through the crown, combing forward all hair in front of the part, and combing downward all hair behind or below the part.

(2) **Tri-sectioning.** This means dividing the hair into three sections. Part the hair widthwise, running from ear to ear and through the crown to the hairline. Comb top and side hair all forward. Make a vertical part from the crown to the nape, dividing the back area in halves, and comb the hair in each section forward which would be at about right angle to the sectioned line. Fig. 364. Tri-sectioning when there is to be no part and sides and top are to be combed back.

(3) **Quartering.** This means four sections. Simply add one section to tri-sections. Make a top center part and comb the hair on each side downward. Do mainly terminal blending, beginning from one and a half to two inches from the sectional line. **Fig. 366.**

(4) **Umbrella sectioning.** Comb the hair all natural directions from the crown, similar to each rib of an open umbrella. Cut along the top and sides and then do mainly terminal blending in the back area. This is a very flexible method and the most practical approach to underneath cutting of the sides and top. (Fig. 367.)

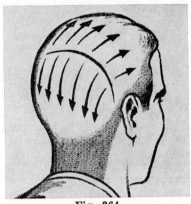

Fig. 364
Bi-Sectioning

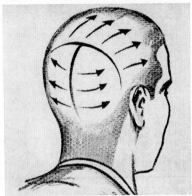

Fig. 365
Tri-Sectioning

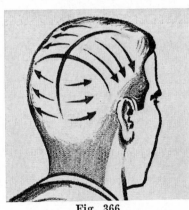

Fig. 366
Quartering

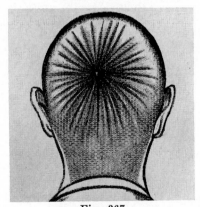

Fig. 367
Umbrella-Sectioning

10. When cutting to diminish hair, whether by underneath or surface cutting, start about 1½ inches from the frontal hairline, part, sectional line, or crown; but from a stubborn crown, start about 2 inches. The cutting may start closer to the frontal hairline at the sides.

11. Razor cutting can be done in all hair cuts except the short cuts, such as the Butch and Short Pompadour.

12. Contour designs give a full long effect, but the hair is only about two inches long in the upper middle and top areas. Contour designs are moulded to conform to the shape of the head, but the length is varied to allow for irregularities of the scalp, the size of the ears, and the length of the neck. (Refer to chapter on Hairstyling.)

13. When approaching the ear, place the comb against the ear at right angle to the scalp to protect the ear. (Fig. 387)

14. Razor cutting can be continued to within one half to one inch of the outline or edge.

15. Blow waving often follows razor cutting. (Refer to chapter on Hairstyling.)

16. Hold the razor firmly, placing the thumb on the heel of the razor, but the wrist should be flexible.

17. To guard against cutting too deeply, the straight razor should ride the hair lightly.

18. In non-parted styles, the hair may be combed on the bias across the top from either the left or right side. In bias combing, follow the hair streams—the direction in which the hair naturally slants.

19. The length of the razor stroke is short to moderate.

20. Razor cutting may be used to supplement shear cutting. When so used, usually only terminal shaping and blending are done.

21. Anyone interested in learning razor cutting should not only know the basic principles set forth in this chapter, he should have individual lessons. Some barbers have developed their own system and it is recommended that you contact them. They often advertise in barber magazines.

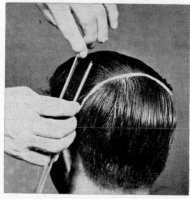 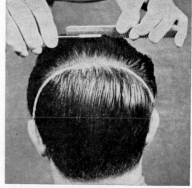

Fig. 368   Fig. 369
Underneath Cutting of Bi-Sectioned Head

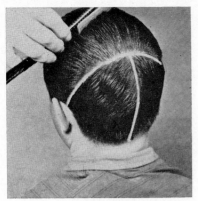

| Fig. 370 | Fig. 371 |

Underneath Cutting of Tri-Sectioned Head

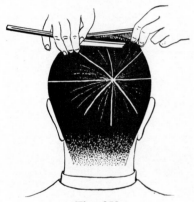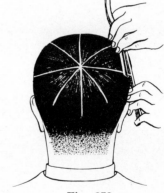

| Fig. 372 | Fig. 373 |

Underneath Cutting of Umbrella Sectioning

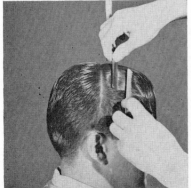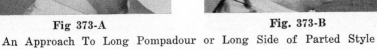

| Fig 373-A | Fig. 373-B |

An Approach To Long Pompadour or Long Side of Parted Style

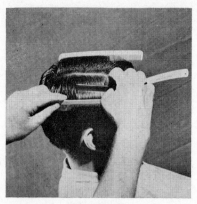

Fig. 373-C

An Approach to Long Side
of Parted Style

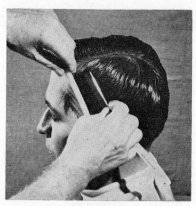

Fig. 373-D

An Approach to Short Side
of Parted Style

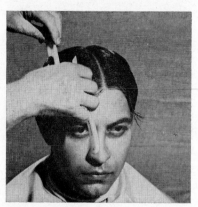

Fig. 373-E

An Approach to Long Pompadour

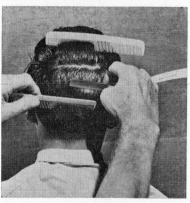

Fig. 373-F

An Approach to Stubborn Crown

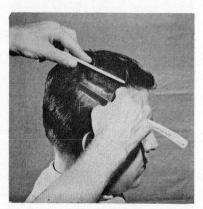

Fig. 373-G

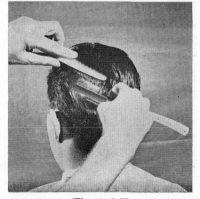

Fig. 373-H

Informal Spot Shaping With Razor

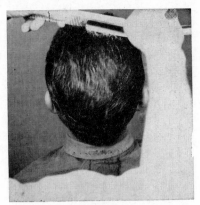

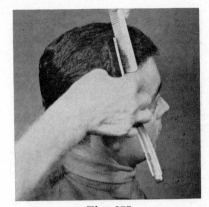

Fig. 374   **Fig. 375**

Surface and Terminal Cutting and Blending

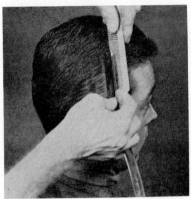

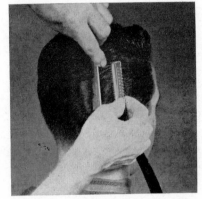

Fig. 376   **Fig. 377**

Surface and Terminal Cutting and Blending

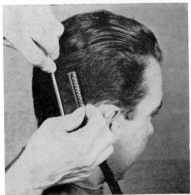

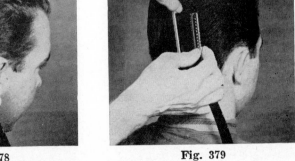

Fig. 378   **Fig. 379**

Surface and Terminal Cutting and Blending

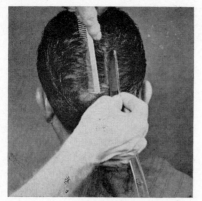 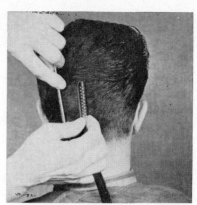

Fig. 380   Fig. 381
Surface and Terminal Cutting and Blending

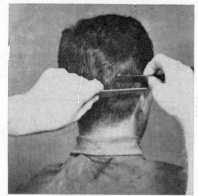 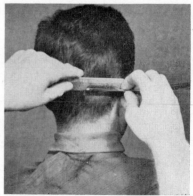

Fig. 382   Fig. 383
Surface and Terminal Cutting and Blending
Windmill Movement

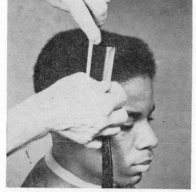 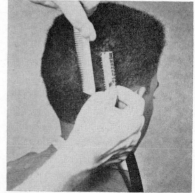

Fig. 384   Fig. 385
Surface and Terminal Cutting and Blending

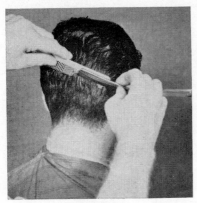

Fig. 386

Cutting Hair Over Comb

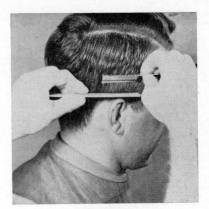

Fig. 387

Protecting Ear

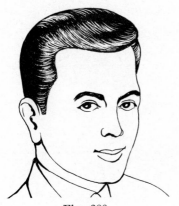

Fig. 388

Two Inch Contour Pomp

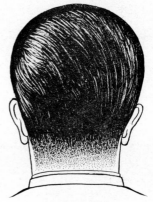

Fig. 389

Two Inch Contour Swirl

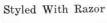

Styled With Razor

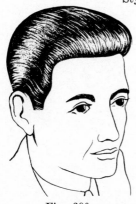

Fig. 390

Two Inch Contour with Part

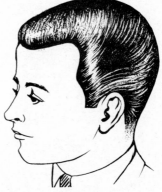

Fig. 391

Two Inch Contour Swirl

Styled With Razor

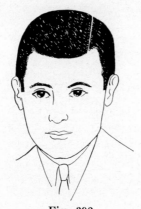

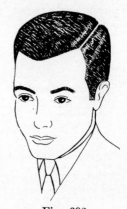

Fig. 392
Short Parted Contour

Fig. 393
Medium Parted Contour

Styled With Razor

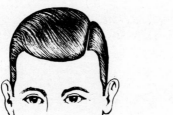

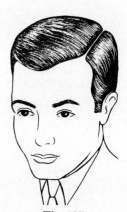

Fig. 394
Short Parted Contour

Fig. 395
Medium Parted Contour

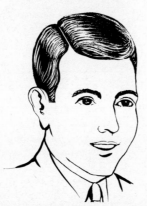

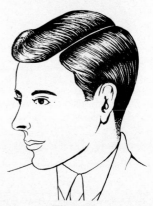

Fig. 396

Fig. 397

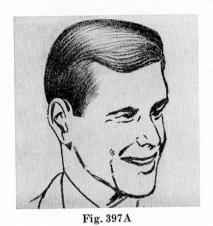

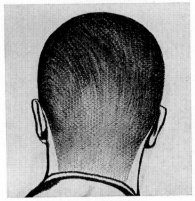

Fig. 397A   Fig. 397B

AIR STYLING

(Also Known as Blow Waving)

Air styling embraces two major phases of hairstyling, air shaping and air waving. **Air Shaping** means redirecting and controlling of hair, and is also known as air contouring, air arranging and blow shaping. Air waving is also known as **blow waving.**

The size and kind of combs or brushes used are partly a matter of individual preference. Much also depends on the volume of hair. There is a variety of brushes, ranging from three to fourteen rows of bristles, with a surface that is flat, oval, curved or contour.

AIR SHAPING

The procedure of air shaping will be illustrated and outlined. Hair can be redirected to a general swirl from left to right or right to left depending on the natural flow of hair. By such redirecting the monotony of plain straight back pompadour can be avoided and a natural variation of shape can be achieved and hair that clings too snugly to the head may be lifted to give it a slight bombage effect and better contour. Slightly lift the hair and dry it in that position. Lift the hair about 1½ inches across areas to be lifted, but a single lift may suffice. Often hair has to be directed against the styling direction.

Stubborn crowns, undesired swirls, tight curls, obstinate cowlicks, or stubborn hair difficult to manage can often be controlled and redirected by a blow waver. The blower usually follows or precedes the brush or comb closely. Repeatedly pass through the trouble spot, directing the hair to the position desired. Either press the hair down or lift it, depending on what is desired to blend with the coiffure. The extreme ends of the side and top hair may be turned under with the comb and blow waver.

Procedure of air shaping:

1. Complete basic edging and size head by regular methods.
2. Shampoo and towel dry hair, but leave it damp.
3. Razor style hair.
4. Follow with plain shears on extreme ends of hair wherever needed
5. Apply styling gel, lotion or warm water.
6. Following the redirecting comb or brush with a blow waver.
7. Finish with sparing amount of hair creme, oil or/and spray.

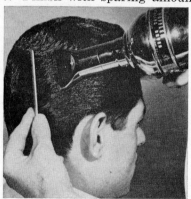 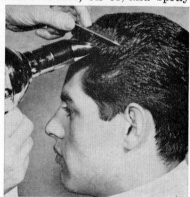

Fig. 398   Fig. 399
Redirecting and Controlling Hair with Blow Waver

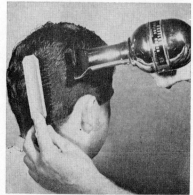 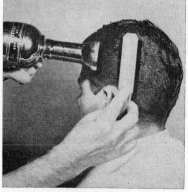

Fig. 400   Fig. 401
Controlling Stubborn Hair   Controlling Stubborn Hair
At Vertical Curvature   At Temples

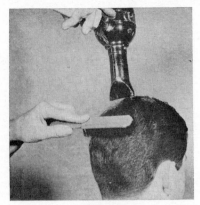

Fig. 402
Controlling Stubborn Crown

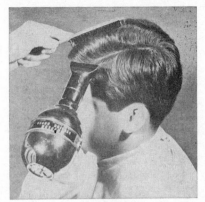

Fig. 403
Achieving Bombage
Lifting Hair Without Waving

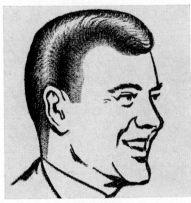

Fig. 404

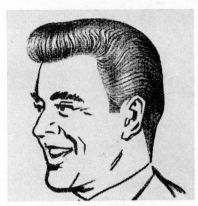

Fig. 405

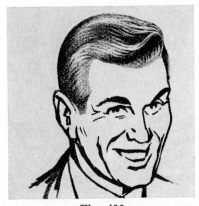

Fig. 406

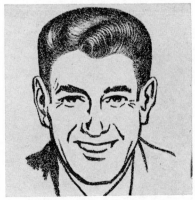

Fig. 407

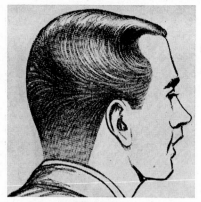

Fig. 407-A

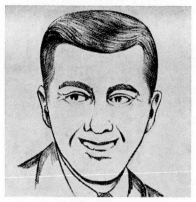

Fig. 407-B

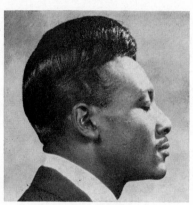

Fig. 407-C

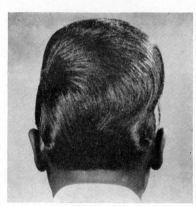

Fig. 407-D

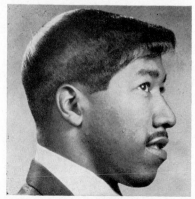

Fig. 407-E

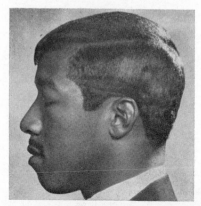

Fig. 407-F

NOTES

BASIC PRINCIPLES OF AIR WAVING
(Also known as Blow Waving

Air waving is a process of waving hair with a hand man dryer and a comb or brush. Air waving takes only a few minutes to do and lasts longer than a finger wave. It will often survive dampening or swimming. Besides setting waves, blow waving can be used to improve an unbecoming hairline. Air waves are made according to an **S-shaped pattern.** Air waving is also known as blow waving.

Pointers on Air Waving

1. The hair should be from two to three inches long, but it can be done on longer hair. Such waving is less successful in long hair.

2. The hair must be clean, but freshly shampooed hair responds most successfully. Oily or dirty hair does not respond to new positions.

3. The hair must be slightly wet. If freshly shampooed, towel dry only. If the hair is too damp after towel drying, remove the excessive dampness by trailing a coarse comb with blower.

4. Adjust the portable blower to moderately hot. Just warm air will have no effect and air too hot will damage the hair.

5. Direct the hot air away from the scalp.

6. The number of waves given depends on the patron's choice. Just one wave at the forelock often suffices, but two waves are also in good taste. More than three waves border on femininity.

7. The waves should be soft and natural looking. Avoid bouffant or large puffed out waves.

8. Use the fine part of a medium sized hairdressing comb or a small hair brush to arrange and position the hair. **A brush works better on short hair.**

9. As a general rule, if the hair is naturally wavy follow the pattern of the natural waves.

10. A non-oily tonic may precede air waving; however, some artisans prefer a styling gel, styling lotion or very warm water. Such styling agents are applied before and sometimes during the **air styling. They may feel silky to the fingertips, but leave** no trace of stickiness, oil or grease.

11. Make each ridge of a wave secure before forming the next one.

12. Sufficient drying is often accomplished by continuing to comb through the waves with a coarse comb with the blower trailing. But to dry the hair thoroughly place a hair **net over the hair,** press the first and second fingers astride each ridge to further secure the wave while directing the blow waver on each wave.

13. **To form the ridge** of a wave, push the comb or brush through the hair from the hairline or part to a place just beyond where

the ridge is to be formed. Simply stop and back up the comb or brush, pushing the hair slightly upward from the scalp until a tentative ridge is formed. When backing up the comb or brush, it sometimes helps to slide it slightly to the left or right depending on the disposition of the hair and the beginning direction of the wave and of the next wave. Hold the hair in this manner until the wave is formed. When forming the next ridge, comb or brush the preceding wave and to the stopping point all in one stroke to make sure you are following the direction of the wave and directing all hairs belonging in the next ridge. When forming waves, the comb or brush should penetrate through the hair to the scalp to make sure that every hair is included.

14. The final effect should be personalized and moulded to the general contour of the head. A sculptured effect is best achieved in hair from two or three inches long in which the ends of the hair run inside the waves. Waves made in this way are soft, smooth and natural looking.

Summary of procedure of Air Waving:

1. Shampoo and towel dry hair. (If hair has been just shampooed for razor cutting, it will only be necessary to dampen the hair slightly with warm water.)

2. Comb hair as desired, noting direction of any natural waves.

3. If hair is still too wet, comb through several times with blower trailing.

4. Leave hair slightly damp. Apply very warm water, or a styling gel or lotion.

5. Form a ridge.

6. Direct the stream of air along the wave to be formed until the ridge and wave are fairly secure.

7. After waves are formed, further secure each wave by complete drying.

8. Brush or comb through hair several times.

9. Apply a little hairdressing with spray on finger tips to the surface of the hair. Hair spray is also recommended.

10. Comb or brush hair neatly.

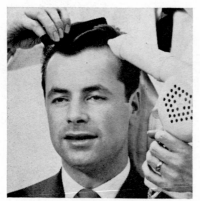

Fig. 408
Forming First Wave

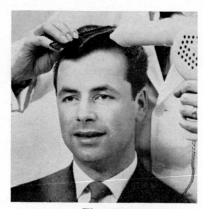

Fig. 409
Blow Wave Completed

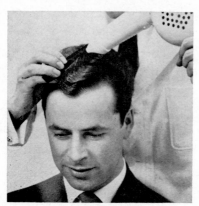

Fig. 410
Forming Second Wave

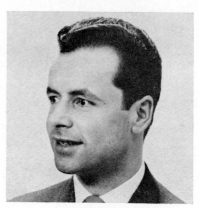

Fig. 411
Wave Completed

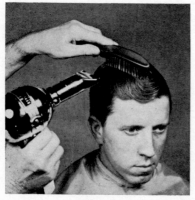

Fig. 412

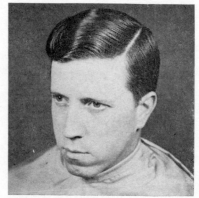

Fig. 413

Casual Top Swirl
Making Fly-away Hair Into Soft, Casual Wave

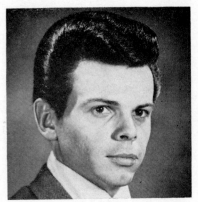

Fig. 414

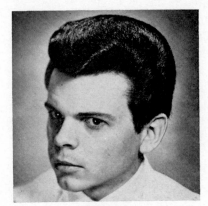

Fig. 415

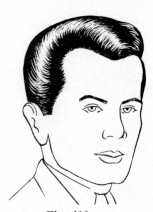

Fig. 416

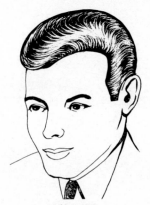

Fig. 417

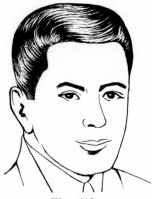

Fig. 418

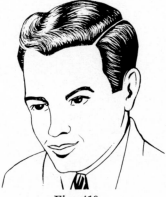

Fig. 419

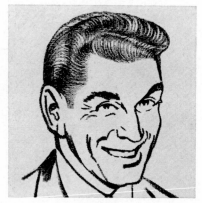

Fig. 420

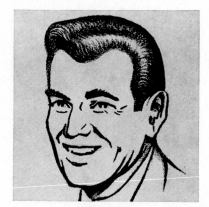

Fig. 421

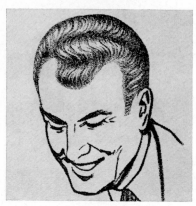

Fig. 422

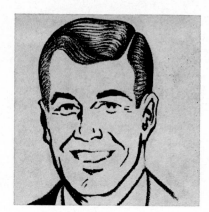

Fig. 423

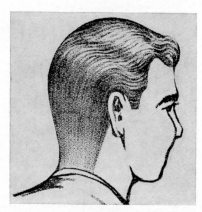

Fig. 424

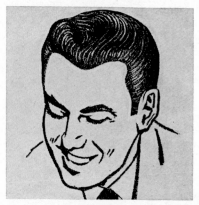

Fig. 425

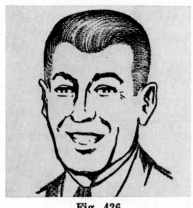

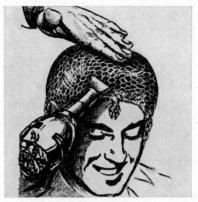

Fig. 426   Fig. 427

SOME HAIRSTYLING POINTS SUMMARIZED

The type of the face is determined largely by the bone structure and general outline of the face. The chin, jawbones, cheekbones, temples, forehead, and skull, form the outline of the face. The immediately foregoing discussion is in the most difficult and controversial areas of hairstyling. A hair style parted or non-parted, and in which the minimizing and maximizing of the amount of hair might be just the opposite of that recommended in some instances and still be a great success. The artist must have the stamina of his own convictions in his creative hairstyling and be tolerant.

STRAIGHTENING OF HAIR

Introduction

The beginner's course may be too short, in some states, to teach this subject and also it may not be required.

Hair that is excessively curly or kinky can be straightened. The straightening is permanent or more properly semi-permanent in a qualified sense; that is, it generally lasts from 60 to 90 days if accomplished by chemicals; however, some manufacturers contend that when their product is used the hair straightened will not "go back" and only touch-ups are needed on new growth in 4 to 6 weeks. Hair straightened by hot irons is temporary and usually lasts only to the next shampoo.

PURPOSES OF STRAIGTENING HAIR

1. To make hair more manageable.
2. To make hair more stylable.
3. To make hair easier to take care of.
4. To satisfy one's taste.

METHODS OF STRAIGHTENING HAIR

There are two general methods:

1. **By chemical compounds.**

    (1) Sodium Hydroxide. This kind of relaxer penetrates into the hair as it straightens. Sodium Hydroxide relaxer is the **more commonly used.** These are the most effective chemicals for relaxing the hair. A sodium relaxer is the best because it takes less time to relax the hair.

    (2) Thio compound. (Technically, it is Ammonium Thioglycollate). This kind of relaxer merely softens and straightens by altering the sulphur and amino acid content of the hair. This relaxer requires much longer time to straighten the hair and is therefore less popular or practical, especially for men. It has a tendency to shrink the hair and cause frizziness; whereas the sodium relaxer expands the hair, making it more manageable. Read manufacturer's instructions carefully.

2. **By electric straightening combs.** This method will be explained a n d illustrated elsewhere in this chapter. The **most popular method of straightening hair** i s b y chemicals, because of time saving and longer lasting than with hot combs.

DIVISIONS OF CHAPTER

This chapter will be divided into two parts, namely, chemical hair relaxers and electric comb straighteners.

PART I — CHEMICAL HAIR RELAXERS

As before mentioned, there are two kinds of chemical hair relaxers, known as Sodium Hydroxide Relaxer and Thio Relaxer. The following discussion pertains to the sodium hydroxide relaxer except where otherwise indicated. Some of the discussion applies to the Thio Relaxer also; and its procedure will be outlined separately. The sodium hydroxide relaxer is the kind most used.

Hair processing: This term means straightening hair by chemical preparations.

Hair relaxer: This term means a hair straightening product.

POINTERS ON CHEMICAL HAIR RELAXERS

A thorough and repeated study of Pointers is essential and imperative. Do not give a hair relaxer treatment without having all these pointers firmly in mind.

1. Follow manufacturer's instruction.

2. Examine scalp carefully.

3. Do not apply over eruptions, abrasions or open sores. Dermatitis would result.

4. **Protect** ears, forehead, neck, scalp and hairline skin with manufacturer's special product or with pomade, vaseline, mineral oil petroleum jelly or a pre-straightener cream base (this is a form of petroleum jelly.) This specially prepared scalp and skin protector is easier to wash out and is preferred over other agents.

5. Cover entire scalp with the skin protector before applying relaxer, unless manufacturer instructs differently.

6. Keep relaxing creme away from scalp — about 1/8 to 1/16 of an inch.

7. Hair must be dry for a sodium hydroxide relaxer, but for a Thio relaxer the hair should be slightly damp.

8. If hair is damaged, use the manufacturer's hair conditioner prior to applying relaxer, but follow manufacturer's instruction. The conditioner is used to **prevent** breakage of hair. Hair may be damaged by over-exposure to the sun, hot irons or combs, bleaching, or coloring.

9. Apply hair relaxer with the bar of a large comb or a special paddle. **Simply lay the creme on the hair.** With a coarse toothed comb spread the creme through the hair. **Direct the comb upward** and

in various directions and try not to touch the scalp. But at the edge comb the creme downward very gently. You may proceed in a **horseshoe pattern starting at the front** and working around. Finally comb the hair in the direction that it is to be styled. Follow the illustrations of application given in this chapter.

10. Avoid getting relaxer into eyes. Be mindful of the fact that the relaxer is a potent chemical.

11. If the relaxer burns to a degree uncomfortable, remove it immediately.

12. Full "take" time is from 5 to 25 minutes, depending on the condition and texture of hair. If the hair is straightened it will look straight and shiny and it will not spring back to curly. Free a small strand or section of relaxer to test. Simply presing hair down with back of the comb may suffice to determine straightness.

13. **Before rinsing relaxer out of hair remove the bulk of it with a fine or medium tooth comb rapidly.**

14. When shampoo is recommended use a **neutral shampoo.** This is a soapless and high quality non-alkaline shampoo; it is soothing and unperturbing. A neutral shampoo is also known as **bland** shampoo. Manufacturers of hair relaxers may have such a shampoo. **Creme shampoos** are examples. Soap would cause excessive tangling and give a gummy effect.

15. Relaxing creme must be applied rapidly and removed rapidly, since its action is fast.

16. A tepid water rinse should always be used, because hot water can cause tangles, matting, scalp irritation and possibly weaken the relaxer. Cold water does not remove relaxer sufficiently.

17. **A Neutralizer Rinse** is very important. It further stops the action of the relaxer, helps prevent a reddish cast, and helps to keep the hair straight. If a shampoo is given, apply a neutralizer immediately afterwards; if a shampoo is not given, apply it after the water rinse. Read the manufacturer's instructions carefully, for some require that the neutralizer be **rinsed out** and others require it to be **left in the hair.** When a neutralizer is to be rinsed out **leave it in the hair from 3 to 5 minutes or as instructed.** Saturate all sections of the hair thoroughly. The comb may be used to separate the hair to assure thorough saturation of the neutralizer in all portions of the hair. Catch the drippings in

a plastic pan or bowl and pour it on the hair several times. Continue to distribute this rinse into the hair with the finger tips and coarse comb. Comb in the general direction hair is to have its styled position.

18. Do not use heated waving or straightening combs or irons over freshly relaxed hair. Breakage could result.

19. A hair **conditioner** applied after the shampoo adds luster, helps to prevent breakage, eliminates tangles and gives manageability to hair.

20. **Do not distribute the relaxing creme with a wet comb, since water drops could reach the scalp and cause smarting and possibly burning and streaking of the relaxer.**

21. **Do not mix sodium hydroxide with a thio relaxer.** That is, do not apply one on top of the other, since hair breakage could result.

22. **Hair is not shampooed before a relaxer is applied.** However, if the hair is excessively greasy, remove the excess grease with a neutral shampoo. The relaxer is also a cleansing agent.

23. Over-relaxing and straightening can **cause breakage.** The timing should be very exacting. Never leave a customer with a relaxer on his hair.

24. **Symptoms of allergy to relaxers** are inflammation, irritation, burning and itching, headaches a n d sometimes nausea.

25. **Application of color rinses and reconditioners:** A color rinse may follow a neutralizer, or a shampoo. Some manufacturers have a combination neutralizer and color rinse in the same bottle, called **neutralizer color rinse.** Such a combination is applied and distributed through the hair with a large tooth comb and the finger tips. **After about 5 to 10 minutes rinse out** with warm water. The rinse removes the neutralizer but not the color. A hair conditioner may follow a neutralizer or color rinse or both.

26. USES OF PRE-STRAIGHT CREMES. There are two general uses of these cremes.

(1) They are used to protect the scalp, skin at the hair line, forehead, temples, top and back of ears and neck. This use especially applies when the manufacturer states that no scalp protector is needed. This c r e m e should remain on about five minutes before applying relaxer. Not all manufacturers r e c o m - mend a pre - straight creme.

(2) They are used not only to protect the scalp, skin at hair line, forehead,

temples, back and top of ears and neck, but also to pre-condition the entire hair for the relaxer.

When so used it should remain on about five minutes before applying straightener.

BRIEF SUMMARY OF PROCEDURE FOR SOME RELAXERS

Read Manufacturer's Directions Carefully.

1. Scalp examination.

2. Skin or patch test 24 hours before applying relaxer, if required by manufacturer.

3. Protector to forehead, ears, nape of neck and entire hairline.

4. Relaxer (on dry hair).

5. Rinse (tepid water).

6. Shampoo, if required by manufacturer. Use neutral shampoo such as creme shampoo. It must be soapless to prevent excessive tangling.

7. N e u t r a l i z e r (stabilizer). Leave on 3 to 5 minutes. Rinse out thoroughly.

8. Give color rinse if desired.

9. Dress hair as desired.

STANDARD PROCEDURE FOR SODIUM HYDROXIDE RELAXER

Standard procedure is meant to be an outline of the steps common to most chemical relaxers with a sodium hydroxide base. These steps should be adapted to the particular manufacturer's product and instructions. This procedure assumes that the stylist or barber has read the section on **Pointers on Chemical Hair Relaxers.** THIS IS VERY IMPORTANT. It also assumes that the scalp has been examined and found free from eruptions and open sores, that the hair is in proper condition. The **most important advice** is to follow the manufacturer's instructions. **Before application** select the relaxer and review the manufacturer's instructions. If the hair is overly porous or has been damaged by overexposure to the sun, by hot irons or combs, or by bleaching or

tinting, a condtioner should be used prior to the relaxer. A conditioner may be applied with finger tips.

1. Linen set-up same as for shampoo. A plastic shampoo cape is recommended.

2. The mixture is cleansing and so the hair does not need to be freshly shampooed. But it should not be applied on excessively oily or greasy hair. Follow manufacturer's directions.

3. Comb hair free from tangles.

4. Protect forehead, ears, skin at hairline and scalp with a petroleum base creme or the manufacturer's product. Do not rub the base into scalp. The purpose of this base is

to protect the skin and scalp from irritation by the relaxer.Some protectors are made to cover the hair also. Some manufacturers say no protector is needed for their relaxer.

5. **Put on rubber gloves** if you give relaxers continuously or have any scratches or openings on the skin of your hands. However, gloves are not needed for an occasional job. The fingers need not touch the relaxer. It is applied with the bar of a comb or paddle, and may be distributed with a comb. But for the occasional job, the finger tips may be used with or without gloves, if there is no breakage in the hand-skin.

6. Apply mixture quickly on hair from front to back. Use special spreader or back of large comb. Apply on sideburns and long hair first. Completely cover hair before combing through. Guard against touching scalp with teeth of the comb and against getting relaxer on scalp. Distribute the relaxer through the hair. Do not rub in. Simply lay the relaxer onto the hair gently with a paddle or bar of a large comb. Longer hair is parted for the application. Distribute it through the hair with wide tooth combs and the finger tips.

7. After the hair is completely covered, comb preparation through hair until it is straight. Use coarse comb, and place it almost flat. Comb hair mostly upward and in various directions. After five minutes, **test development** by freeing a small section from relaxer, and pressing hair down with bar of comb to determine s t r a i g h t n e s s. Straightened hair looks a little shiny and does not spring back to curly when combed. If straight, quickly **remove most of relaxer with fine or medium tooth comb before rinsing with tepid water.** IT IS VERY IMPORTANT TO REMOVE AS MUCH OF THE RELAXER AS POSSIBLE BEFORE RINSING WITH WATER, AND MORE ESPECIALLY WHEN THE MANUFACTURER D O E S N O T RECOMMEND A SCALP PROTECTOR. THE REASON IS THAT WATER AND THE RELAXER TOGETHER CAN C A U S E SMARTING, IRRITATION AND HAIR BREAKAGE.

8. Time on head averages about 5 to 25 minutes, but less for fine texture and more for coarse, resistant hair.

9. Rinse with tepid water. Be sure to use only warm water. Cold water does not release the substance from the hair and too hot water, along with the relaxer, might irritate scalp and cause excessive tangles. Touch scalp gently.

10. Some manufacturers say no shampoo is needed, but some

do. When instructed, use a **neutral shampoo** (it is soapless). Some manufacturers make a special relaxer shampoo (see Pointers on Relaxers). Shampoo movements should be given gently.

11. Apply a neutralizer rinse (also known as stabilizer). Saturate the scalp and hair thoroughly. This rinse helps prevent reddening, gives manageability to hair and helps remove tangles. Distribute with finger tips and wide tooth comb. Lay comb almost flat and comb hair straight. Comb neutralizer slowly and gently through the hair. Leave the neutralizer on about five minutes. Remove with tepid water; however some neutralizers are designed to remain on the hair. Follow manufacturer's instructions. A neutralizer rinse is not required by some manufacturers. Color rinse may follow neutralizer, and so may a hair reconditioner or both.

12. Finish as desired. If waves or contour shaping is desired, either finger waving or air waving may be done. If blower is used, the air should be only warm, not hot. Do not use hot irons.

13. A seasoning of hair creme before the final combing and hair spray afterwards may be applied. A conditioner may also be recommended or a series of conditioner treatments when conditions of the scalp and hair warrant them.

HAIR RELAXER PROCEDURE OF ONE MANUFACTURER
SODIUM HYDROXIDE RELAXER

CAUTION: For safe results, cover the scalp with Pre-Strate petroleum jelly before applying relaxer. **Do not use soap shampoo** to remove relaxer.

1. Apply our special pre-strate to the forehead, temples, back and top of ears, nape of neck, hairline, **scalp** and **hair.**

2. Allow the pre-relaxing skin protector to remain on the areas covered for 2 or 3 minutes before applying straightener.

3. Now apply straightener to thick part of hair first, leaving thin parts and temples to the last. **Lift hair while applying, hold comb flat, making** certain that neither the creme nor comb touch scalp.

4. Taking time 10 to 15 minutes.

5. Rinse out thoroughly with lukewarm water.

6. Give black rinse on black hair for black, glossy well-groomed appearance. This rinse will also tone down gray streaks.

7. Dress hair as desired.

METHODS OF APPLYING RELAXERS

Follow the manufacturer's instructions, but the following illustrations should be helpful. Refer to **pointer No. 10 on Pointers On Chemical Hair Relaxers.** (page 159)

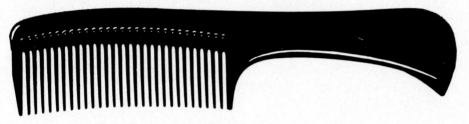

Fig. 427-A
Type of Comb For Spreading And Distributing Relaxer

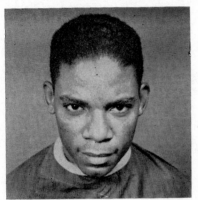

Fig. 427-B
Before

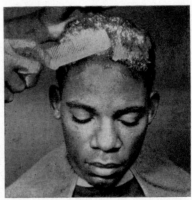

Fig. 427-C
Laying Relaxer On With Back
Of Large Comb

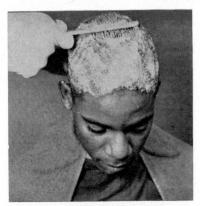

Fig. 427-D

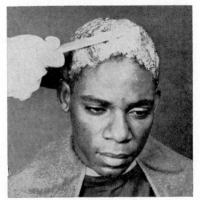

Fig. 427-E

Combing Relaxer Through Hair

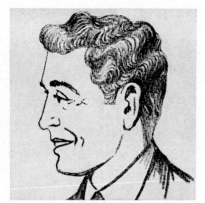

Fig. 427-F
Hair Before Relaxed

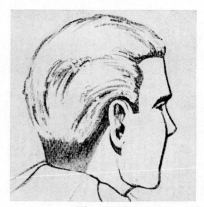

Fig. 427-G
Relaxer on Hair

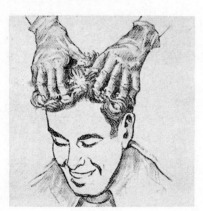

Fig. 427-H

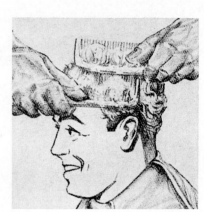

Fig. 427-I

Distributing Relaxer

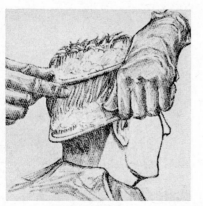

Fig. 427-J

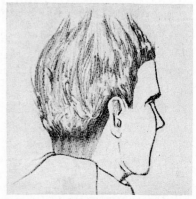

Fig. 427-K

Distributing Relaxer

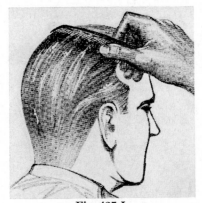

Fig. 427-L
Removing Relaxer with Comb
Before Water Rinse

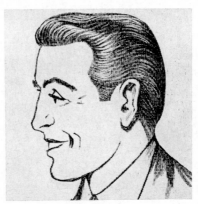

Fig. 427-M
Hair Relaxed and Styled

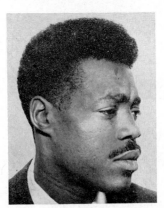

Fig. 427-N
Before

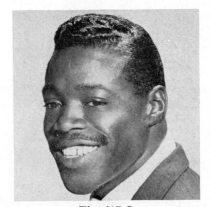

Fig. 427-O
After

Straightened with Casual Wave

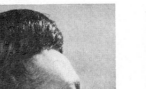

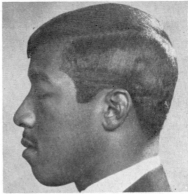

Fig. 427-P

Fig. 427-Q
From Curliness to Straightness

HAIR STRAIGHTENING BY COMBS

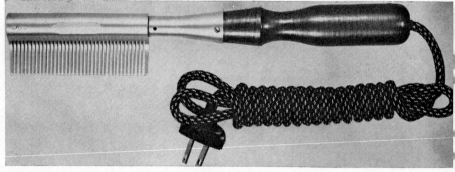

Fig. 428

Electric Hair Straightener

Procedure of Straightening Hair by Electric Comb

1. Linen set-up.

2. Shampoo hair if needed. Hair must be free from oil or grease.

3. Dry hair thoroughly.

4. Apply a special **pressing oil** and comb through hair.

5. Section top hair, from side to side, into strips about one inch wide, starting at front hairline. Do not make the second strip until the first strip is straightened. Comb each strip forward and hold it taut between the first two fingers.

6. Feed hot comb through each strip of hair until straight.

7. Proceed all across the top from front hairline to crown.

8. Comb and dress hair, but do not use aqueous solutions.

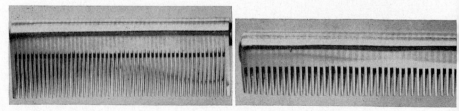

Fig. 429

Non-Electric Hair Straightening Combs

Non-electric hair straightening combs may be used to straighten short hairs at the forehead, temples and nape. These combs have to be heated.

Mustaches

Mustaches, more so than beards, are worn throughout the world, and they frequently accompany beards. There are innumerable designs of mustaches, and they often reflect a great deal of individuality of customers. Mustache services consist of designing, trimming, shaping, and waxing. It is a safe assumption that the person who wears a mustache is particular as to how it is shaped and trimmed, since his purpose is personal adornment. This purpose still holds true irrespective of whether it is worn to cover a scar, to minimize the effect of a wide upper lip, to call attention from an extremely large nose, or break down extreme flatness of profiles. There is, of course, also a sort of professional reason for wearing a mustache—to add that something which says "here is a professional man." Then, too, this means of adornment is sometimes used simply as a change or rest from one's appearance—to break the monotony of sameness.

The shaping requires the use of several implements. The outline is best made with the points of the shears. The finishing touches are most successfully done with the barber's most delicate implement, the razor. Cold cream allows for a greater visibility and thus makes for a higher degree of accuracy. The length is conveniently reduced with the shears over the comb. Use the part of the comb that corresponds to the size of the

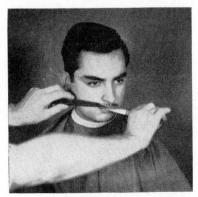

Fig. 436
Trimming Mustache

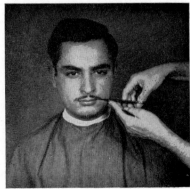

Fig. 437
Outlining Mustache

mustache. The use of the clippers over the comb to outline and reduce a mustache is somewhat crude as the cutting implement is much out of proportion to the specimen. In shaping extremely large mustaches, however, the clipper may be used.

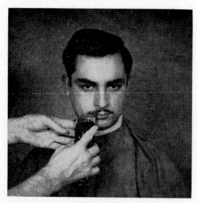

Fig. 438
Outlining Mustache

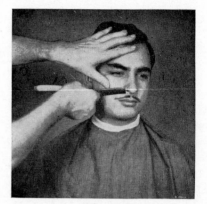

Fig. 439
Outlining Mustache

POINTERS ON DESIGNING MUSTACHES

It is not enough to know the procedure of trimming and shaping mustaches. The barber should be familiar with the artistic principles, such as the following:

(1) Turned down corners give a droopy effect.

(2) Turned up corners give the effect of cheerfulness.

(3) Straight lines are almost neutral as to sadness or cheerfulness of impression, but they convey honesty, reliability, conservative judgement and neatness.

(4) A very small "eyebrow" mustache has a laughable proportion to an exceptionally large face; likewise, a large mustache is unproportional to a small face. Therefore, the size of such adornment must have some correspondence to the size of the face.

(5) A mustache should not project over the edge of the upper lip. Such over-lapping conveys unneatness and uncleanness.

(6) The length of a mustache that greatly exceeds the length of the lip may look clownish.

(7) A mustache should not be allowed to grow free as to outline, else it will look unkempt and unbalanced.

(8) Generally, a mustache that covers the full bearded portion of the upper lip is too large to look artistic but there are exceptions to this rule.

(9) The lower edge of the mustache should not always follow the edge of the lip—the edge may be made above the edge of the lip at both ends or all the way across, depending on the design.

(10) Radically turned up corners are clownish.

(11) Twisted turned up or down corners are strictly sheikish and are worn mainly by the Beau Brummel type of men.

(12) The corners should be slightly rounding on a squarelike face.

(13) The corners should be somewhat squarish on a round face.

(14) A mustache on a bald-headed man should be as large as his face will admit. It's size draws attention away from the baldness above, but a dainty little mustache in such a case would seem ridiculous because it would accentuate the baldness

(15) A mustache should contain the elements of balance, symmetry, and character.

(16) A person with a conspicuously large or scarred upper lip may advisedly wear a mustache.

DESIGNS OF MUSTACHES

Designs according to physical features: While individual taste must be considered, some designs are more becoming for certain physical features. Basically, the size of the mustache should correspond to the features and size of the face—a larger design for coarse, heavy facial features, and a smaller design for fine, small, smooth, facial features.

1. When there are coarse facial features and a large area between the lip line and nose, a heavy chevron mustache is becoming.

2. A prominent nose calls for a larger mustache.

3. For a long, narrow face, design a narrow, thin mustache.

4. For an extra large mouth, design a pyramidal shaped mustache, heavy and about mouth length.

5. For an extra small mouth, design a narrow, short, thin mustache.

6. For smallish regular features, a small mustache, triangularly shaped or separated at the nose ridge is becoming.

7. For a wide mouth and prominent upper lip, a heavy handlebar or large divided mustache is becoming.

8. For a round face with regular features, a semi-squarish mustache is becoming.

9. For a square face with prominent features, design a heavy linear mustache with ends curving slightly downward.

10 The length of the mouth, the size of the nose, and the upper lip area are the most important factors

DESIGNS OF MUSTACHES

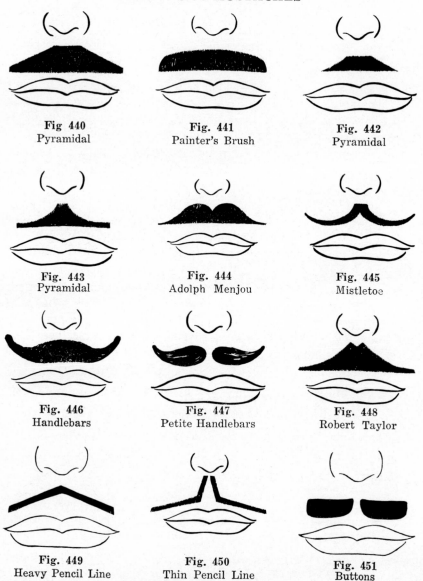

Fig 440
Pyramidal

Fig. 441
Painter's Brush

Fig. 442
Pyramidal

Fig. 443
Pyramidal

Fig. 444
Adolph Menjou

Fig. 445
Mistletoe

Fig. 446
Handlebars

Fig. 447
Petite Handlebars

Fig. 448
Robert Taylor

Fig. 449
Heavy Pencil Line

Fig. 450
Thin Pencil Line

Fig. 451
Buttons

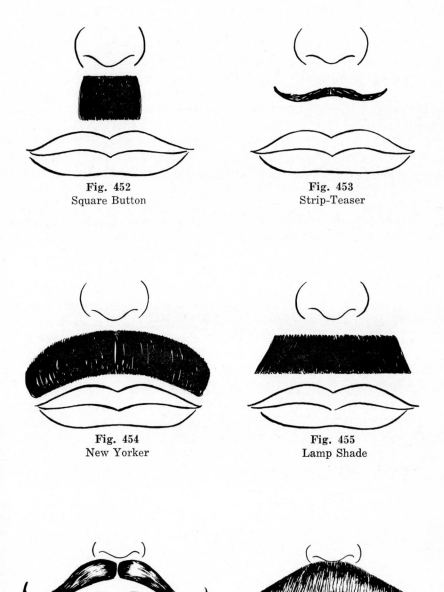

Fig. 452
Square Button

Fig. 453
Strip-Teaser

Fig. 454
New Yorker

Fig. 455
Lamp Shade

Fig. 456
Handlebars

Fig. 457
Chevron

Beards

Beards have been worn from time immemorial. In ancient times, they were worn as signs of manhood, strength, wisdom, and dignity. Poets, philosophers, and the dignitaries wore beards to indicate their distinction. Even Lincoln was clean shaven until he became president of the United States. Shortly after his election he grew a beard to lend dignity to his office in correspondence to the nobility in many other countries of the world at that time. Powerful tribal gods wore beards, and the kings of Persia plaited their sacred brambles with golden thread. Even today we associate beards with such notables as Santa Claus, Samson, and Socrates. Even at the end of the nineteenth century, a book entitled "Notable New Yorkers" listed 2337 men of whom almost fifty per cent are pictured with some kind of beard. Prior to the invention of some cutting implement, of course, all men wore beards. The Mosaic beard best typifies the earliest beards. Moses, however, commanded certain people to shave off their beards. In honor of the Pharoah before whom he was summoned to appear, Joseph had his bearded face shaved. For the sake of strategy, Alexander the Great required his soldiers to be clean-shaven so that the enemy warriors could not throw his soldiers to the ground by their beards.

The reasons for beards run from necessity to custom, although cognizance should be given to racial and religious reasons. After Hadrian grew a beard to cover his warts and scars, beards became the fashion among his Roman subjects. In contrast, William, Archbishop of Roven, France, prohibited the wearing of beards. Beard trimming, the major work of early barbers, became a prevailing vogue after 500 B.C.; before this time beards were allowed to grow at will.

The cult of pognotrophists (beard growers) is more ancient and medieval than modern. Pognotrophy gains and dwindles. The cult of the beard is peculiar to Oriental people. In Punjab the Sikhs wear full beards rolled up and pinned under their chin as "one essential requirement to a man." Akin to this trend of thinking is a quotation from Shakespeare: "He that hath a beard is no more than a youth, and he that hath no beard is less than a man." Beards have different meanings in different countries. While the Egyptians shaved them off, the Jews traditionally wore full beards and were forbidden to stoop to trimming them artistically like neighbor tribes. And still another view was taken towards beards in ancient Peru where the Incas made laws against the wearing of beards. Interesting too is the fact that Chinese are typically beardless, but Confusius is always represented wearing one.

In the 15th century the big whisker was unfashionable in Europe. But it made a return in the 16th century with Henry VIII of England, the possessor of a beauty. Out went the beard in the 18th century, only to make another comeback in the 19th. Following a lot of pro-beard propaganda in the latter half of the 19th century in America, beards flowered in a profusion of sizes and styles. But led by the aesthetes of 1890, men gave up this kind of personal adornment often referred to as a "badge of masculinity" and as a "symbol of strength," and they have been shaving their faces ever since.

While shaving the face was practiced to some extent in ancient and medieval times, it is primarily a modern custom and it is almost universally practiced. There are still a few professional men today, as well as some farmers, who wear beards. The beards these men wear are largely the Van Dyke type popularized by the great painter, Van Dyke, during the sixteenth century.

Beards are frequently worn in Western America in seasonal festivities, especially to reproduce the pioneer customs. Of course, in fraternal ceremonies, on the screen and stage, beards, real or false, are worn for characterization.

There is tremendous versatility in the designs of beards and their sporadic appearance, along with the fact that they have survived the caveman's clamshells, the primitive razors, is a fact that should not be overlooked. While there are various differing opinions as to smartness of beards, it can scarcely be denied that a clean shaven face is easier to care for as well as far more sanitary.

In the United States, except for religious reasons, many beards are grown for a lark At state centennials beards are worn for historical purposes. But since the days when men used clamshells and sharpened artifacts of flint to shave, shaving has grown increasingly popular. And now with the modern means and conveniences of shaving, beards seem to be largely a thing of the past. Wherever beards have staged a faltering temporary comeback, the styles mostly worn were Van Dykes and full mutton chops. A study of the face of contemporary man reveals a high preference for the apple-cheeked over the stubbled chin.

TRIMMING BEARDS

Beard trimming is done largely with the shears and comb. It is also correct to use the clipper-over-comb method, except for the preliminary shortening of a long beard. The detail shaping, however, is best accomplished by the shears and comb. A systematic starting place is advised. Work from the chin to the ear or from the ear to the chin. Honor to the full extent the customer's preference as to length and design. Beards are very personal to those who wear them. Check frequently during the trimming, allowing the customer to view the beard in a mirror. For some of the finishing touches, it may be necessary to use a razor. In the Goatee type of beard, as well as in partial beards, do the general shaping first, and then shave the portions or sides of the face as desired. While it is proper to view the beard from a front position of the customer, do the trimming by standing at a side position.

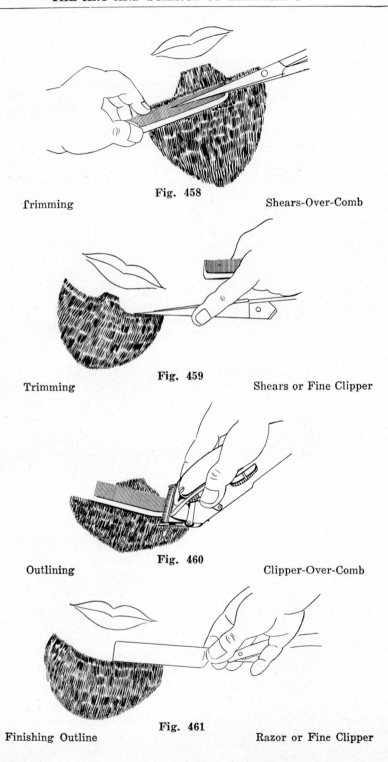

Fig. 458

Trimming   Shears-Over-Comb

Fig. 459

Trimming   Shears or Fine Clipper

Fig. 460

Outlining   Clipper-Over-Comb

Fig. 461

Finishing Outline   Razor or Fine Clipper

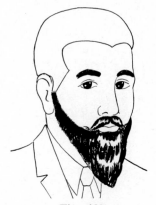

Fig. 462
Van Dyke

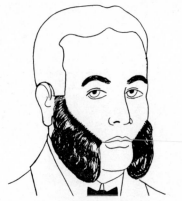

Fig. 463
Mutton Chops

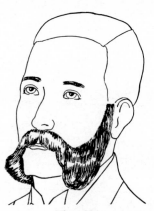

Fig. 464
Friendly Mutton Chops

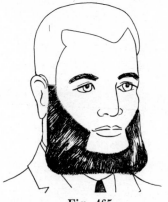

Fig. 465
Old Dutch

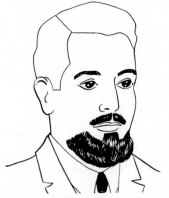

Fig. 466
Balbo

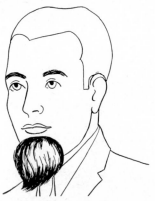

Fig. 467
Norris Skipper

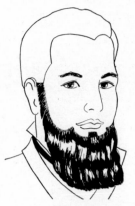

Fig. 468
Spade or Shenandoah

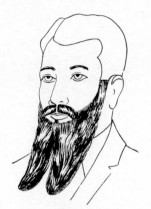

Fig. 469
French Fork

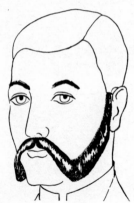

Fig. 470
Franz-Josef

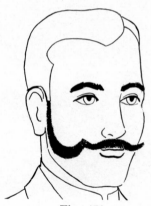

Fig. 471
A la Souvarov

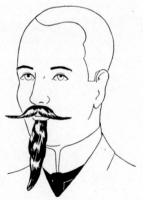

Fig. 472
Napoleon III Imperial

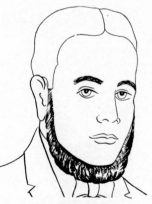

Fig. 473
Chin Curtain

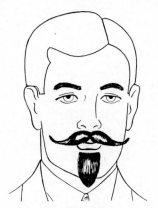

Fig. 474
Handlebar and Chin Puff

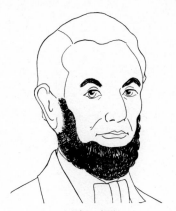

Fig. 475
Lincolnic

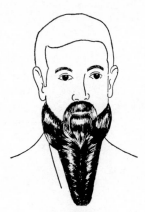

Fig. 476
Ducktail

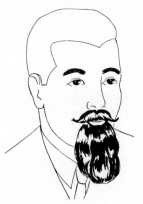

Fig. 477
Goatee

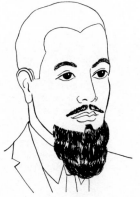

Fig. 478
Modified Goatee

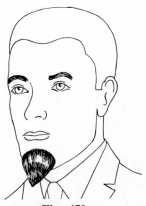

Fig. 479
Petit Goatee

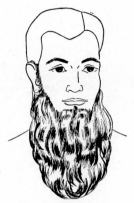

Fig. 480
Jumbo Junior

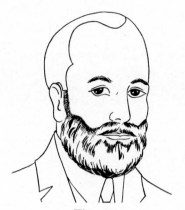

Fig. 481
Medium Full Beard

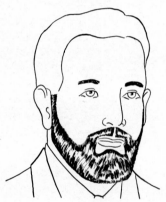

Fig. 482
Short Boxed Beard

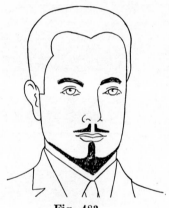

Fig. 483
Hulihee
(After Hawaiian King)

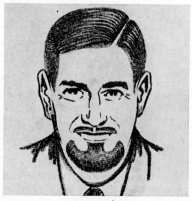

Fig. 484

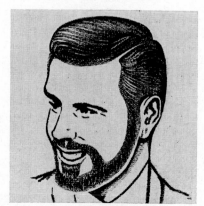

Fig. 485

Hairpieces

Custom-made hairpieces, formerly known as toupees, now meet with universay acceptance. The clumsiness and artificiality of the grease painted hairlines of early toupees were as conspicuous as a wheelbarrow in a plate of spumoni. The nondetectable hairpieces of today are created and styled to individual requirements, and thus replace "stock" hairpieces. Hairpieces can be designed for heads of any size or shape, and for baldness of any degree or type, with complete assurance of a perfect fit, and a completely natural life-like appearance, with the hair seeming to grow upon the head. Hairpiece designers take into consideration the characteristics of the face and of each individual feature.

Barbers, who were renowned as wig-makers in the eighteenth century, have had an emphatic place in the development of contemporary hairpieces. Today the barber can derive commissions serving as the middleman between the manufacturer and the customer, either by promoting sales through recommendations or by selling the hairpiece direct to the customer. Informational and promotional kits are available for both of these procedures. It is comparatively easy to make accurate head measurements. With these measurements, along with a sample of hair and a simple picture of the head, it is possible to obtain a hairpiece by mail order. Additional hairpieces are still simpler to obtain since the customer's head measurements, hair sample, and picture are kept on file in the wigshop or hair department of the manufacturer.

Wearers of hairpieces do not only include those character players and comedians, such as Edgar Bergen, but also many well known persons in private and picture life. The most pretentious wig-making job on record was that of Max Factor, Hollywood, for "Marie Antoinette," with 22 elaborate natural white hair coiffures for Norma Shearer, and hundreds of not so elaborate ones of revolutionaries and their opponents. The weirdest job was one which called for a carefully crafted and fitted toupee and goatee for a large land turtle, for a film comedy scene. Wigshops now supply beautifully crafted coiffures for actresses in their picture scenes or social appearance, hairpieces for men in pictures or private life, and all of the false beards, mustaches and even chest hair. In these wigshops are conditioners of human hair which goes into the various hairgoods; expert hairlace seamstresses who fashion the lace "scalps" of toupees and wigs; "ventilators" who knot the hairs into the hairlace scalps, one by one, and who are masters of the unique technique by which undetectable toupee and wig hairlines are created; hairdressers who dress and trim the toupees and wigs into their final coiffure pattern.

The "scalps" of toupees, wigs, beards, mustaches, and eyebrows are a[l] made on hair lace foundations. After this lace net has been stitched t[o] form a close fitting cap over the real human scalp, the wig hairs are knot ted into it one by one. The "scalp" is placed over a wooden hairpiece bloc[k] shaped and contoured according to the subject's measurements. When hairpiece is completed it is made secure by the lace edge with spirit gum and the lace, which is of spider web transparency and of a flesh tone, is un[-] detectable.

Some important details about hairpieces:

(1) Hairpieces are made from actual human hair. Such hair i[s] from women. Some of the countries from which hair is bough[t] are Spain, France, Italy, Korea, Formosa, China, India an[d] Mexico. Hair damaged by permanent waving and tinting o[r] straightening is not used

(2) The most expensive natural colors of hair are in this order white, red, and blond.

(3) Gray hairs in a hairpiece are actually a mixture of black an[d] white or brown and white. Gray head hairpieces are made i[n] this same natural way.

(4) A toupee is a hairpiece that covers part or all of the top of th[e] head, whereas a wig covers the whole scalp area.

(5) A chignon is a roll of hair, worn at the top or back of the hea[d] by women.

(6) Wooden wig blocks are contoured to fit the exact curves of each head according to the individual measurements, and are stored on shelves to be used for new hairpieces or wigs as needed and ordered.

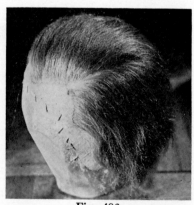
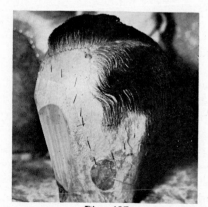

Fig. 486   Fig. 487

Hairpieces in the Making

PROCUREMENT OF HAIRPIECES

There are two general methods of procurement.

1. When a hairpiece distributor or manufacturer is located in your city, you may work out a **customer referral plan** whereby you send customers direct to him. Talk over this plan with the hairpiece concern.

2. **Mail orders:** If you are qualified to make correct fittings, you may procure hairpieces for your customers by mail. The manufacturer will provide you with instructions, equipment, ordering forms and an envelope for the hair sample. Further instructions on mail orders will be given later in this chapter.

CLASSIFICATIONS OF HAIRPIECES

There are two general classifications of hairpieces. These are:

1. **Laced hairpieces:** These are individually laced and each hair has a double-knotted anchorage to the lace base. Manufacturers of laced hairpieces contend that they are more natural looking and have good durability. They They also contend that laced hairpieces have definite individualization and are successfully styled to suit the individual. Such hairpieces take longer to make because of the merits just mentioned, and also because they are **tailored** by hand. Laced hairpieces cost more than non-laced. Many movie and TV actors wear laced hairpieces.

2. **Non-laced hairpieces:** In non-laced hairpieces, hairs are sewed and knotted into the base three to six at a time. Even though the sewing and knotting are done by hand they are completed more quickly than laced hairpieces and sell for less. Non-laced hairpieces may be worn by men of all ages and professions, but they are especially practical for the premature bald who have a substantial amount of hair and by those in heavy and out-of-door occupations. They are sold at economy prices. The front portion of non-laced hairpieces are usually laced.

RECONDITIONING HAIRPIECES

Hairpieces damaged by exposure to the sun and wind, prolonged use and improper care can be reconditioned. If the color is faded, the hairpiece can be tinted or recolored. Faded effects can also be concealed by adding hairs of the original color. Depending on proper care, hairpieces will need **resetting** and **restyling,** due to normal usage, about every two to three months. Return or have them returned to the manufacturer for this service and any needed reconditioning.

BAKING OF HAIRPIECES

After the hair has been attached to the base of the hairpiece and tentatively styled, it is placed in a thermostatically controlled oven or incubator for two reasons:

1. To completely remove all moisture.

2. To stabilize the general shape and style. This stabilizing is semi-permanent and with proper care lasts from two to three months.

SELLING HAIRPIECES

Display different available styles, showing **before** and **after.** Encourage your hairpiece customers to tell interested friends. If you yourself need a hairpiece, wear one. Extend your service to include complete care and cleaning. (Refer to the section in this chapter on "care and cleaning of hairpieces." Read the chapter in this book on salesmanship.) Impress upon your customer this slogan: "If you look good, you'll feel good." Emphasize that present-day hairpieces are casual and natural looking. Hairpieces today are not unnatural and artificial looking like they used to be. Show him a photograph of a before and after of a person approximately his age. Have at least two or three hairpieces in stock to try on and to prove to the prospective customer how his personal appearance would be enhanced.

Be sure to know your product. Show the customer how practical it is. Know the answers to such questions as "Can I sleep in it?" "Can I swim in it?" "Can I shower in it?" "How long will it last?" "How much does it cost?" "How

soon can I get it?" "Will the hairline look natural?" "Will I be embarrassed?"

A man who is partially or completely bald need not display this fact to the world. New techniques and materials successfully conceal all degrees of baldness. Completely natural-looking hairpieces are available and they even prove that baldness can be kept a secret. So natural in appearance are they that a man may wear one without his closest associates knowing it. Men in all walks of life—all over the world — wear hairpieces with complete satisfaction. The price of a hairpiece is determined by the color, quality and area to be covered. Manufacturers will give you a price list.

Measuring and sizing of bald areas: Instructions are provided by hairpiece manufacturers for measuring and sizing bald areas as well as measuring equipment. An equipment kit consists mainly of a special large, soft black pencil, a measuring tape, Saran Wrap, and flexible lead wire. Use the instructional literature and equipment of the manufacturer whose hairpieces you are featuring.

After a hairpiece is manufactured, fitting it to the head may require terminal shaping and blending. This is accomplished mainly with the thinning shears and the razor. Be extremely careful when doing this and proceed very slowly and gradually. The length of the ends must blend uniformly into the patron's hair. All hairpieces come with extra length to allow for any necessary cutting, shaping, blending, and styling. Manufacturers provide fitting instructions.

SYSTEMS OF SIZING BALD AREA FOR HAIRPIECES

There are two widely used methods of sizing the bald area for a hairpiece.

1. Measurement system.
2. Pattern system.

Only the pattern method of sizing bald areas will be explained and illustrated on the following pages. Before determining the pattern, free the bald area of all isolated and frizzy hair with a fine tooth clipper blade and a safety razor. By this same process establish the outline of the bald area.

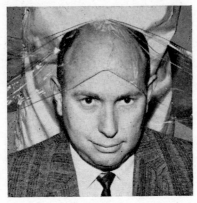

Fig. 487-A

Step 1

Covering bald area with clear plastic (Saran) wrap, with about two-foot strip and then detach it from the wrap roll.

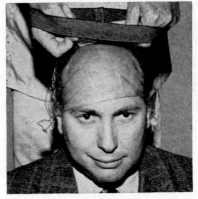

Fig. 487-B

Step 2

Fit wrap to head and hold in place by twisting sides. Secure twisted wrap with rubber bands. An elastic band may be placed around the head to assure a snug fit.

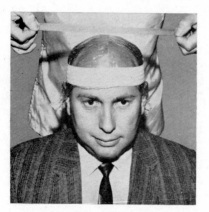

Fig. 487-C

Step 3

Criss-cross scotch tape from front to back and side to side, covering bald area. Extend tape well beyond bald area.

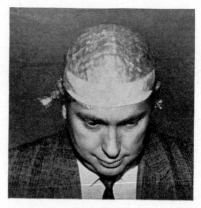

Fig. 487-D

Step 4

Scotch tape covering completed.

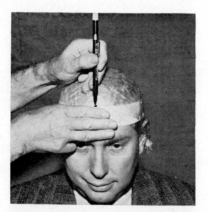

Fig. 487-E

Step 5

Place three middle fingers slightly above bridge of nose in a straight line with eyebrows. Indicate **hairline** with horizontal marking. Form a letter "T" with perpendicular line which should be in line with center of nose. Perpendicular line indicates **center of forehead.**

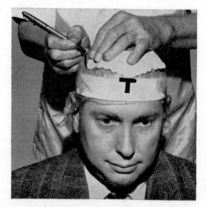

Fig. 487-F

Step 6

With felt tip pen outline front hairline and bald area. The outline may be designed with heavy paper. Before using, reinforce paper with dull scotch tape. Hold it at desired position with tape.

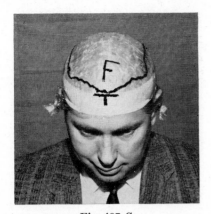

Fig. 487-G

Step 7

Designate front with "F" and back with "B"

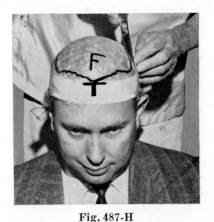

Fig. 487-H

Step 8

With shears gently and carefully cut away the excess wrap and tape beyond the marked outline while the taped-wrap is still on the head. The cut-away can also be done off the head, but the tapedwrap is difficult to hold.

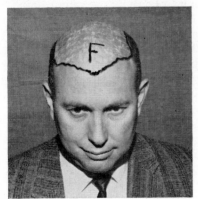

Fig. 487-I

Step 9

Check carefully pattern and measurement for fit.

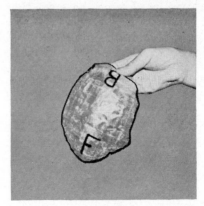

Fig. 487-J

Completed

Patern outline of hairpiece.

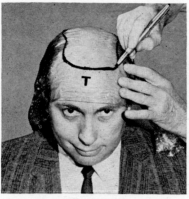

Fig. 487-K

The bald area may be outlined without securing the plastic wrap with an elastic band and before applying scotch tape. This is more difficult to do. The outline of the bald area is more easily visible through the plastic wrap than the scotch tape.

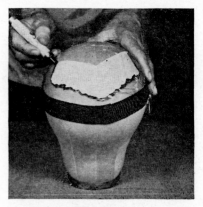

Fig. 487-L

Practice on a canvass blockhead or manikin covered with Plastic Wrap is recommended.

FITTING AND STYLING A HAIRPIECE

A new hairpiece usually needs fitting even though the measurement and description of the bald area are accurate. If the hairpiece is a **non-laced** type, be sure that the bald area is free from any new growth of hair since the original sizing of that area. Full clearance is not necessary for a **laced** hairpiece. Hairpieces come with sufficient length to allow for the final touches of fitting and styling. When shortening and blending these ends proceed very gradually. In fact, two fittings are recommended, because at first the hairpiece may look too heavy or bulky to the patron since he is changing from baldness to hair. Remember that removing hair from a hairpiece is a one way street—it will not grow back. Refrain from blunt cutting. While plain shears may be used for sizing and feathering, terminal thinning and blending are best accomplished with the thinning shears and razor. If a razor is used, be sure to dampen the hair. Reduce the unwanted bulk on top and in back by removing hair from the under side, thus preserving the length on the top side. Dampen the strand, lift it with a comb and diminish with a razor. In this way some uneven ends will be created but they will blend into the person's own hair. Bulky hair at the temples may be removed by either a razor or the thinning shears. After the unwanted hair is removed, comb the hair into its final direction or into the desired style and then remove the overlapping ends with a razor, directing the razor on the surface or top side to achieve the finished blend. The hairpiece may now be styled with an electric comb, a blow waver or finger wave. Guard against damaging the hair with excessive heat.

FOUNDATION OF HAIRPIECES

The foundation of hairpieces is made from Swiss gauze or imported English materials, such as gauze and silk. Some manufacturers use a very thin but strong laced net for the front portion of the hairpiece; others use the same material over all the bald area.

HOW HAIRS ARE ANCHORED TO FOUNDATION

Hairs are anchored to the foundation with a needle directed to make a crochet stitch or ventilated spider stitch. In the front portion of the bald area hairs are anchored individually and in the remaining area two to three hairs may be anchored in the same stitch.

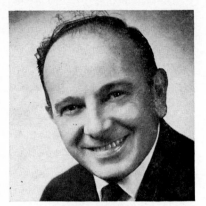

Fig. 487-M
Before

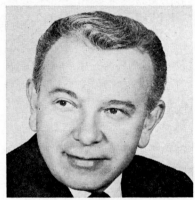

Fig. 487-N
After

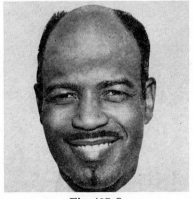

Fig. 487-O

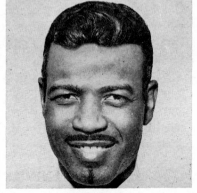

Fig. 487-P

THE CARE OF HAIRPIECES

Manufacturers of hairpieces furnish instructions on the care of their hairpieces. Follow their instructions carefully.

A new hairpiece may go through a series of adjustments to the scalp, over a few weeks. When needed remove any new growth of hair with a safety razor.

SOME IMPORTANT POINTERS ON CARE OF HAIRPIECES

All pointers are given subject to manufacturer's instruction.

1. Use manufacturer's tape, antiseptic, cleaner and softener.

2. When the hairpiece is taken off at night or any longer period of time it should be placed on a hair block. For hairpieces a semi-moon-shaped block suffices. These are available on the market and are inexpensive. They are compact enough to take on trips. It is not too damaging to a hairpiece to lay it down without placing it on a block for an hour or so, even for a few nights. While manufacturers of hairpieces instructions vary, the best practice is to remove the hairpiece when taking a shower or swimming.

3. Daily comb with a large comb with widely spaced teeth. Proceed slowly from the ends to the base.

4. As needed, apply a light base hair-dressing creme sparingly and distribute with a gentle pinching technique with the first and second fingers and the thumb. A suitable hair conditioner may also be used. A light hair spray may be used.

5. Clean after the first week and then as needed. (Refer to cleaning instructions.) Daily combing and brushing suffice between cleanings. Clean regularly about every three or four weeks, depending on your occupation.

6. When having a hair cut always tell or remind the barber that you wear a hairpiece. The barber should not remove any of the hairpiece hair.

7. Several important "Do nots":
DO NOT ever fold as it will injure the shape and damage the base to which it is anchored.
DO NOT remove in any other manner except according to instructions.
DO NOT wash with soap, shampoo or detergent.
DO NOT use a sharp tooth comb or use a stiff brush in cleaning.
DO NOT use vaseline or other heavy base hairdressing.

CLEANING OF HAIRPIECES

Like any part of the body, hairpieces must be kept cleaned.

1. **Acetone** is recommended for cleaning; however, any good cleaning solvent may be used, such as liquid dry shampoo. Manufacturers often sell cleaning agents. Follow the manufacturer's instructions.

2. Pour solvent, about one inch in depth, into receptacle. Then place front of hairpiece, with material side facing up, into the solvent and allow to

soak for about three to five minutes. Then, with a sable brush agitate or sort of tap the edge of the hairpiece until the adhesive has been removed. WARNING: Do not rub or scrub the lace or other anchorage base.

3. Place a twice folded hand towel on a flat surface, and then place the hairpiece, with material side facing up, on the towel. Again use the brush, saturated with solvent, and gently tap on the front. This will remove any adhesive that may have coagulated.

4. At times, after cleaning, the adhesive may form a powdered appearance on the lace. If this occurs, put a little water on your finger tips and in a sliding motion allow the lace to absorb the water.

5. Clean the entire hairpiece every three to four weeks. This you will do by putting sufficient solvent in a vessel to submerge the entire hairpiece. Leave it soak for about five or ten minutes, then lift the hairpiece and allow all liquid to drain. Then place the hairpiece between the bath towel, press it gently to absorb all the moisture.

6. When it is completely dry put on a plastic block, pinning it down securely, and then gently comb it. Be careful when combing so as not to pull it too hard. Start from the very edge and keep combing back until you have eliminated any snarl that may have occurred in the cleaning. After it is combed, apply wave fluid sparingly and with the fingers reset the wave by pressing the hair between the fingers in the areas where they were formerly located.

HOW LONG HAIRPIECES LAST

With proper care a hairpiece will last for years. It is advisable that the user of a hairpiece have two hairpieces, for this assures him of always having one in good condition and one to wear while the second one is being reconditioned. When two hairpieces are worn alternately, and reconditioned as needed, the wear of both will be greatly prolonged.

Shaving

Shaving is the process of removing projecting hair from the face and neck with a razor. Shaving by some means has been practiced since recorded history began. For razors, men used just about any hard, sharp material available, including bits of flint, shell fragments, and sharks' teeth. And before there were any means of shaving at all, some men plucked out their whiskers one by one with a clam shell.

For the sake of sanitation, comfort, a clean feeling, custom, becomingness, and safety, shaving is a firmly established practice. The invention of the safety and electric razors has greatly lessened shaving in a barber shop. This consequence is only natural. But the professionally-given shave with a straight razor is unequalled. It behooves the student, therefore, to master the fundamentals of shaving. The shave might be considered a "gate-way" to facials. When the customer is enjoying the soothing effect of a warm steam towel or scientifically-executed facial movement following a shave, he is likely to yield to the suggestion for a facial.

History reveals many references to shaving. Moses commanded certain people to be shaved. Joseph had his face shaved by a barber to prevent his bearded face from offending the Pharoah before whom he was to appear. Alexander the Great commanded his soldiers to be clean-shaven, after losing several battles with the Persians who caught his soldiers by the beard and threw them to the ground and slaughtered them.

It is comparatively easy to learn to shave. It requires patience, confidence, willingness, practice, proper handling of the razor, a knowledge of the preparation of the face and of the techniques of shaving. The student should not endeavor to shave a customer until he has learned a miscellaneous number of things about shaving and practiced some exercises, such as shaving a bottle or rubber utility ball with a dummy razor, and he should also memorize the fourteen sections of the face.

Three major phases of a shave: A shave consists of many individual steps, but they may be classified under three headings:

1. Preparation
2. Actual shaving
3. Finish

To gain a good perspective of the whole process of a shave, the routine steps of a shave should be learned.

Routine Steps of preparation:

1. Seat customer in locked chair.
2. Spread haircloth.
3. Adjust headrest and partially release a four-inch strip of lather paper.
4. Recline chair and adjust it to proper height—the head should be a little higher than the feet.
5. Re-lock chair.
6. Sanitize hands.
7. Tuck towel across sides and front of neck.
8. Apply creamy lather to bearded portions of face (return lather brush to mug).
9. Brace head with wide open left hand and rub lather into the beard with cushion tips of right hand.
10. Apply moderately heated steam-towel, well wrung out, over bearded portions of face and neck, and over eyes and forehead.
11. Prepare razor and insert it into disinfectant solution.
12. Provide fresh batch of lather.
13. Remove original lather with the steamer on the face, fold steamer and lay it on edge of lavatory.
14. Re-lather face generously.
15. Check to make hands free from wetness or lather.
16. Take razor from disinfectant.
17. With left hand, tear off lather paper already partially released and tuck it under towel on patron's chest.
18. Relax. You are now ready to start shaving.

Routine of actual shaving:

1. **First time over:**
    (1) Turn patron's head to left, and shave right side of face and of neck.
    (2) Re-strop razor.
    (3) Immerse razor in disinfectant.
    (4) Turn patron's head to right.
    (5) Re-lather left side of face and neck, holding lather brush and razor in same hand.
    (6) Shave left side of face and of neck.
    (7) Turn patron's head to original position and complete first time over by shaving over chin, small strip of neck under chin, and lower lip region.

(8) Fold lather paper.

(9) Apply mildly warm steamer, wiping off any excess lather.

(10) Re-strop and disinfect razor.

(11) Shave second time over, keeping face moist with warm water.

2. **Second time over:** The second time over means that the razor is passed again over the face and sides of neck.

(1) With steamer, remove all traces of lather.

(2) Turn steamer over, and place it on face.

(3) Strop razor and insert in disinfectant.

(4) Remove steamer.

(5) Dampen the face with warm water, and redampen as needed.

(6) Face may be relathered and shaved again before dampening for final second time over and checking.

(7) With the free hand, go over the entire face and sides of neck. Start at right.Do not follow first time over procedure.

Routine steps of finish:

1. Distribute a small amount of finishing cream on the fingertips of both hands.

2. Spread face cream with cushion tips of both hands, using smooth, rhythmical, and stroking movements, over the face, neck, cheeks, nose, and forehead.

3. Apply warm steamer. Remove it after one minute. Upon removing steamer, remove nearly all cream but leave just a little for powder base and to replenish skin with lubricant.

4. Sprinkle face lotion into the palm of the left hand, distribute it on the fingertips of both hands, and spread it over the same areas covered by face cream.

5. Dry and powder (if desired).

6. Pass face towel to left hand and raise patron to sitting position.

7. Place towel across back of neck and shave down sides, or as desired.

8. Remove the remaining traces of lather with a steam towel and dry the neck.

9. Place towel neatly around neck to protect clothing, then comb hair. Remove towel.

10. Lift haircloth off patron, hand him check, and **thank** him cheerfully.

Ways of holding razor for shaving: There are two basic ways of holding a razor for shaving, namely, free hand and back hand. However, there are four recognized ways. These are free hand, reverse free hand, back hand, and reverse back hand.

1. **Free Hand:** Hold the handle and blade almost parallel. The thumb should rest on the side of the shank near the shoulder of the blade. Avoid hooking the small finger on the tang. If the razor is held properly not enough length of the tang will project to hook a finger on it. The third and fourth fingers are placed astride the handle. The fourth finger simply helps to brace the razor by resting on the tip of the tang. Bend the hand slightly outward at the wrist. The elbow should be at a level most comfortable to the individual.

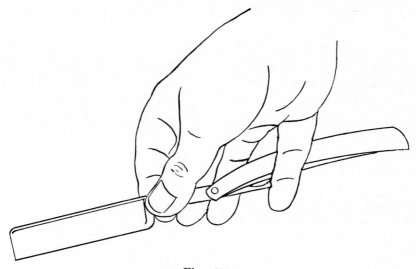

Fig. 488
Free Hand

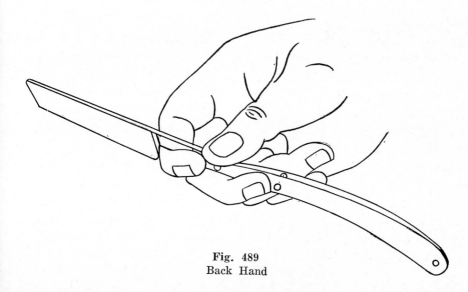

Fig. 489
Back Hand

2. **Back Hand:** The thumb rests partly on the back of the handle and on the back of the shank at the pivot. Place the first joint of the first finger in front of the shank next to the shoulder of the blade. The second finger is placed at the pivot below the thumb to assist in bracing the razor. The third and fourth fingers are placed astride the handle so that they further brace the razor.

3. **Reverse Free Hand:** This is the same as the regular Free Hand except the blade is directed upward at the base of the sides and front of the neck and at the lower lip area. In a Free Hand position, turn your hand slightly toward you so that the edge of the razor is turned upward.

4. **Reverse Back Hand:** In a Back Hand position, turn the palm of the hand upward so that the point of the razor is directed downward. Drop the elbow close to the side. This grip is used in outlining the left sideburn and in shaving down the left side of the neck.

Uses of linen in shaving: (Refer to the chapter on "Linen Uses in Common" for complete instruction. Only the general linen set-up is given here **Figs. 490 to 493.**

1. Arrange face towel across front and sides of neck.

   (1) Unfold face towel and lay it diagonally across patron's chest.

   (2) Tuck left corner section over and inside shirt collar, using a gentle sliding movement of the forefinger of the left hand to smooth it out.

   (3) Cross lower right corner section of towel over to left side of neck and arrange same as on right side, but use right forefinger to smooth out.

   (4) Do not reach over patron's face while arranging this towel. Stand at the same place. Do not move feet.

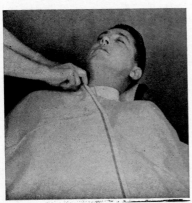

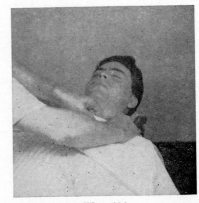

Fig. 490   Fig. 491

Making Linen Setup for Shave

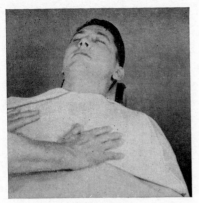

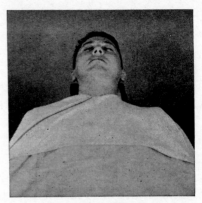

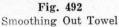

Fig. 492
Smoothing Out Towel

Fig. 493
Linen Setup for Shave

(5) With both hands, smooth out portion of towel lying across patron's chest.

(6) The lower edge of towel should be straight across chest at right angle.

Purposes of lathering for shave.

1. To cleanse the face. The physical action and the chemical reaction detach dirt and cut loose any foreign substances. This applies to the first lathering only.

2. To make the hair stand erect. This is accomplished by packing lather around the hair shafts. The theory is that an erect hair is more easily cut at the base than a slanting hair.

When to lather and relather face: Lather the face immediately prior to steaming. Upon removing the steam towel, remove this preliminary application. After shaving section five, relather the remaining sections of the face. **Keep the lather fresh and adequate** by relathering any area that becomes dry.

Number of times razor is wiped during shave: During the first-time over, the average number of wipes is seven. Guard against forming a habit of wiping unnecessarily. The usual occasions are when passing from free hand to back hand and vice versa, and after the final stroke.

Wiping lather on paper: Make the initial wipes in the center of the shave paper. It is self-evident that additional wipes can more conveniently be made from the center to the edge than from the edge to the center.

Making lather in mug:

1. Pick up the mug with the left hand, holding the brush in place with the thumb of the same hand.

2. Turn the water on with the right hand, regulating the water to a thoroughly warm temperature, remembering that too hot water wastes soap, makes lather dry quickly, and makes it sticky.

3. Rinse off the brush and the outside and inside of the mug.

4. Fill the mug almost full of water. With brush still inside of mug, drain out almost all the water. The purpose of filling the mug with water is to warm the mug. As the mug is being filled, direct the water onto the bristles of the brush to avoid wasting soap.

5. Set the mug on the work-stand. Then churm and rotate the brush to work up a creamy constituency.

6. To avoid noise when making lather, place the free end of the handle of the brush into the palm of the hand and the first two fingers and thumb about equi-distant around the lower part of the handle.

7. The right constituency of lather is important. It should not be so thin that it runs freely off the face nor so thick that it is sticky and hard to spread.

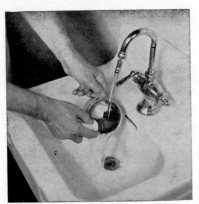
Fig. 494
Filling Mug with Warm Water

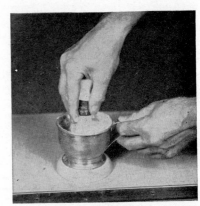
Fig. 495
Place Mug on Stand

Applying lather to face: (Figs. 496-497). When lather is made by a lather-making machine, the lather is received into the palm of the left hand and it is removed from there by the right hand and applied in the routine to be outlined for applying it with a brush.

1. Lift a generous brush full of lather from the mug.

2. Hold the lather brush in the palm of the right hand, inserting the first two fingers into the bristles to control them when lathering around the mouth.

3. Apply lather first to the right side of the neck and then proceed across the neck, up over the left side of the face, over the chin, around the mouth, and finally over the right side of the face.

4. Should you happen to get some lather on the nose or lips, or on the ears, remove it with the corner of the towel.

5. The movements for lathering are largely rotary or **circular.** This type is especially applicable to the sides of the face. Over the sides of the neck, the chin and around the mouth, the linear movements are more suitable. Around the mouth spread the bristles into a fan-like shape to facilitate lathering. The **finishing movements** may be long, sweeping, and straight; that is when leveling the lather just before shaving.

6. After the lather is applied, transfer the brush to the left hand, milk some more lather from the bristles with and into the right hand, and return the brush to the mug. Spread the left hand over the crown to brace and turn the head as needed.

7. And then work the lather well into the beard with the cushion tips of the fingers of the right hand, using rotary or circular movements on the sides of the face, and straight movements on the neck, over the chin, and around the mouth. The pressure of the fingers should be very light, say one-half the weight of the hand. One-half minute spent in so rubbing in the lather should suffice.

8. Cover the face with a steam-towel.

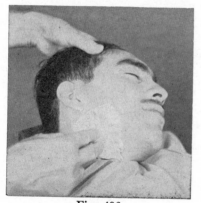

Fig. 496
Start of Lathering

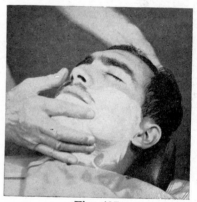

Fig. 497
Rubbing in Lather

Purposes of steaming face before shaving:
1. To soften the cuticle or outside layer of the hair.
2. To provide additional lubricant for the razor to slide over, by stimulating the oil glands to bring more oil to the surface.
3. To give a soothing feeling.

A shaving stroke: What constitutes a shaving stroke should be understood before giving the first shave. The razor's edge has formations which resembles the teeth of a saw, and so each and every stroke should be a sawing strike. A shaving stroke is explained as follows:
1. A sawing stroke.
2. A sliding stroke.
3. A leading point.
4. Laying blade almost flat.

5. Proper rate of motion—undefinable. A fast stroke can burn face; a slow stroke does not cut properly.

6. Allow just the weight of the razor to rest on the face. Figuratively speaking—CARRY THE RAZOR OVER THE SURFACE OF THE FACE; DO NOT DRAG IT.

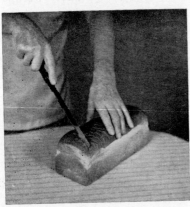
Fig. 498

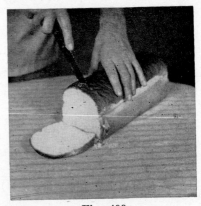
Fig. 499

Slicing Loaf of Bread Comparison With Shaving Stroke

A shaving stroke may be compared with slicing a loaf of bread. A loaf of bread is not sliced by pushing a knife straight through it; a sawing, sliding stroke is used, with practically no pressure applied. This illustrates the fundamental principle of shaving. Think of the razor's edge as resembling the teeth on a saw. **Shaving is really a process of sawing.**

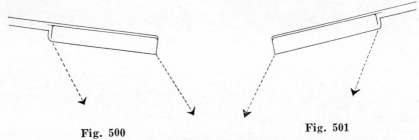

Fig. 500   Fig. 501
Point of Razor Should Lead

Importance of relaxation in shaving: Hold the razor firmly but not tightly. Holding the razor tightly tends to stiffen the whole arm. The elbow and arm should be relaxed in order that the movements may be made gracefully. Especially in the summer, a razor is more liable to drop out of a tight than a firm grasp. Hold the razor just firm enough to give a secure grasp.

Shaving sunken places: Use mainly the **heel** of the blade. The second choice is the **middle** of the blade.

Emphasize use of heel of razor: Whenever it is convenient, use the heel. Use both the middle and heel of the razor as much as convenient. There is a tendency to over use the point. Much of the trouble of keeping a razor sharp is due to an over-use of the point. Save the point for places inconvenient to shave with the middle and heel.

Wrist or arm motion in shaving: The modern tendency is to emphasize arm motion and minimize wrist motion. There is inevitably a combination of both in a shave. In wrist motion, there is more of a tendency to short, jerky strokes and of the fly-swatting variety, whereas in arm motion the strokes tend to be longer and more graceful. The fact still remains that there are many good barbers who emphasize the wrist motion. The subject is controversial—there are pros and cons for each method.

Skin should be firm: Loose skin will tend to crawl or ruffle up in front of the blade; and it is easily nicked or cut. Tight skin is easily irritated by being stretched too much. The skin, for proper shaving, therefore, should be neither loose nor tight, but firm.

How to hold or stretch skin: The left hand stretches the skin in the opposite direction that the razor is traveling. The contact is largely with the cushion tips. The **thumb and second finger** are the principal stretching team.

Ascertain degree of closeness: The barber should know whether the patron desires a close, fairly close, or very close shave. Ascertaining this is almost as important as finding out what kind of haircut the patron wishes. Remember, the first step in a scientific piece of work is to find out what is to be done. The barber will soon find out, of course, what kind of shave his regular customers prefer.

Determining the grain: There is a sort of **communication system** between the cushion tips of the fingers and both the razor and skin. The determining is made in the following ways:

1. By the sensation gained from the razor:
   (1) Shaving with the grain gives a smooth, sleek, free, or agreeable sensation.
   (2) Shaving against the grain gives a slight dragging, digging, gritty, or "traveling-up-the-hill" sensation. The degree of this kind of sensation depends upon the texture of the beard and the extent of the slant. Never should the degree equal that given by a dull razor, although, the sensation from a dull razor and those from shaving against the grain are next door neighbors. However, with the proper glide in the stroke, in the ordinary case the sensation explained is minimized and exists in a very mild degree. The above explanation of the sensation grows out of the contrast of it with the sensation rising from shaving

with the grain, and seems, therefore, to be slightly exaggerated as to terminology.

(3) Shaving crosswise the grain gives a sensation half way between the two just discussed—the grating sensation just barely registers, in fact, it may be so mild as to be entirely unnoticed.

2. By feeling with the cushion tips of the fingers.

Proper length of strokes: Smoothness, tenderness, and eruptions partly determine the length of the strokes. Tender or erupted skin cannot be stretched far without irritating. The length of the strokes also vary according to the area being shaved.

1. For the most part, the strokes should be long—from **one to three inches.** Two inches make a good average length stroke. Too long strokes are apt to pull or irritate the skin, because the cutting point is too far from the stretching point, unless the skin happens to be very firm.

2. Around the mouth, especially in the corners of the mouth, on the sides of the neck, and over the ears, the strokes will run shorter.

3. Avoid making short, jerky, choppy strokes.

4. For the second time over, the strokes will run just a little shorter than for the first time over.

Proper stroke rate of speed: The rate of speed depends somewhat upon the section of the face being shaved, because of the difference in convenience in making the strokes. Any variation in tenderness also alters the rate of speed; that is, over firm, smooth and normal skin the strokes may be faster, as is often the case on the sides of the face, but over tender, irritated, and rough skin the strokes should be slower, as is often the case at the lower lip section and on the sides of the neck.

1. A very **slow** movement or stroke will **not** cut properly.

2. A very fast movement or stroke will tend to skip beard and to irritate the skin.

3. Somewhat between these two extremes is the proper rate of speed, a rate that might be conveniently called "medium." A little study and concentration should enable the barber to determine the proper rate of speed.

Rhythm in strokes: A perfect rhythm throughout the shave would not be practical. The opposite of rhythmical strokes are jerky, irregular, and choppy. In general, the strokes can be rhythmical.

Continuing strokes: A stroke once started should **carry through to its proper destination,** whether it be a long or short stroke. A continuing smoothly executed stroke is a fundamental of shaving. A **stop and start** stroke is **amateurish.**

Original point of contact with skin: Until one has accomplished the art of shaving, make the first contact with the skin by a **short backing-up**

ovement, and then go forward. This is especially an applicable rule when assing from a sequential section of the face to another.

Light touch in shaving: A light touch really means proper touch. This means lightness of pressure, careful, gentle stroking, correct stretching f the skin, and the use of cushion tips. The term **light touch** applies to he following:

1. Mainly to the left hand, in carrying out its duty.
2. To the right hand which should carry instead of dragging the razor over the face.
3. To both hands in applying cream and lotion, in massaging, and in applying the steam towel.
4. To almost every movement that brings the hands in direct or indirect contact with the face.

Shaving with the grain: The general rule is to shave with the grain. Sections of the beard run or slant in the same direction. The fourteen sections of the face as outlined in this chapter represent the grain of the average beard. The first time over strokes are almost entirely with the grain. For close shaving, it is often necessary to shave against the grain, but mainly during the second time over. The beard may be approached from various directions:

1. With the grain
2. Against the grain
3. Crosswise of the grain
4. From any direction

Shave clean as you go: This expression does not refer to the closeness of cutting the beard, but rather to making the strokes so that no traces of lather are left behind. If there are traces of lather, the left hand cannot properly stretch the skin. In case any lather by accident remains behind the stroke where it will interfere with stretching the skin, remove it at once either with the left hand (and then dry the hand) or with the corner of the face towel across the neck. Another reason for shaving clean is that it gives a better appearance to the working process: If the fingers of the left hand get into the lather you are not going over the face in the correct sequence of sections.

Strokes lead into lather: Execute the strokes so that they lead into the lather—from the clean surface into the lathered surface. This principle also means that the lead is point-wise, that is, proceed in the direction of the point of the blade of the razor. This is opposite to having the heel of the razor lead.

Checking face for missed patches: Whether it is a once-over or a twice-over shave, the face should be checked closely to find out if there are rough places or patches of remaining beard. The particular places to check are:

1. Just below the nostrils.
2. The edge of the upper lip.

3. The corners of the mouth.
4. The edge of the lower lip.
5. The whole lower lip.
6. The crease in the center of the chin.
7. Just in front of the lower tip of the ear, including the corner of the lower jaw bone.
8. All the way across the base of the neck.

Removing lather or excessive cream from face: Grasp each end of the steamer and, using both hands simultaneously, with gentle, stroking movements remove the lather or any excess preparation from the various sections of the face in the following order:
1. The forehead.
2. The eyes.
3. The temples and sides of the face.
4. Around the nostrils and mouth.
5. The chin.
6. The front and sides of the neck.
7. The extreme back sides of the neck and regions around the ears, for good measure.

Temperature of steam towels: Some customers like to have a barber shave them for the soothing and relaxing effect of the steam-towel. This towel should be comfortably hot but not hot enough to be uncomfortable. If two preliminary steamers are used, the first one should not be as hot as the second one. Steaming should be emphasized for the following conditions:
1. Coarse texture beard.
2. Excessive density of beard.
3. Neglected or long beard.
4. Excessively dirty face.

A sensitive tender face should be steamed only moderately and a chaffed or irritated or blistered skin should not be steamed at all.

Removing steamer from face: Gather the ends into the hands as you work down over the face, and then lift the steamer off the face and place the middle portion over the forehead, bring the two ends up and overlap in such a way that the ends just come together. Place both hands on top the steamer and remove it by sliding it firmly backward onto the frontal area of the hair.

Proper height of chair: The proper height places the face about three-fourths the arm's length downward. Such position is advised for these reasons:
1. It makes for gracefulness of movements.
2. It exposes the face to easy visibility.
3. It allows the barber to avoid the awkwardness of positions in trying to shave a face elevated too high.

Distance of barber from patron: The barber should stand at an average of three-fourths of his arm's length. This will give freedom and gracefulness in executing the various strokes. Watch that the stomach does not touch the head of the patron when executing strokes that require a standing position behind the patron. The amateur hovers over his work; the master stands back away from it.

Applying powdered or liquid alum or styptic: Such items are used to check the bleeding from a nick.

1. When to apply. If it is a slight nick, let it go until after the cream and lotion are applied, or apply it just before the powder. In such a case, however, the bleeding may stop entirely, making styptic powder unnecessary. On the other hand, if the nick is pretty deep and it is bleeding freely, apply styptic immediately.

2. How to apply: Sift it into the palm of the left hand, remove it from the palm with the corner of a dampened small towel and apply it to the nick. If it is a very slight nick, apply the agent with the cushion tips.

Once-over: A patron who requests just a once-over shave desires to have a smooth face without having a very close shave. He may just want the "five o'clock shadow" removed. In such a shave, the barber may feel free to check to see whether any hairs or patches of beard were missed. Survey the whole bearded portion of the face in this checking. If the patron acts as though he thinks you are going to shave the second time over, assure him that you are merely checking over the shave to make sure that no hairs were missed. In giving this "once over" type of shave, aim to shave just a little closer than when giving a once over to be followed by a second time over in the ordinary shave.

Second-time over: The purpose of the second time over is to check for missed patches and to achieve the desired closeness. Proceed over the face systematically, from left to right, using only the free hand. Work out your own system.

Dampening face for second-time over:
1. Water may be obtained direct from the faucet.
2. Water may be dispensed from a water bottle.

Undesirable things noticeable to patron: Because of the delicacy and personal contact with the patron in a shave, there is a number of things that irritate the patron. The barber should try to avoid these:

1. Failure to wash your hands.
2. Uncomfortable position in chair.
3. Heavy touch of hand.
4. Cold or too hot water.
5. Improperly heated steamers.
6. Insufficiently wrung-out steamers.
7. Non-disinfected razor.
8. Skipping over areas.
9. Too much conversation.

10. Bad breath.
11. Cold fingers.
12. Offensive body odor.
13. Unshaved patches.
14. Glaring lights.

15. Loud music.
16. Scraping the skin.
17. Shaving too close.
18. Dull or rough razor.

Inserting razor in disinfectant: Open the razor "back to back." Insert the blade so that the pivot rests on the edge of the container. It is left in this position until used, but do not leave it thusly between customers.

Upon removing razor from disinfectant: Do not take the razor straight from the disinfectant to the skin of the patron. Do one of the following:

1. Run hot water over the blade and shake excess water off at the bowl.
2. Wipe it on the corner of the face towel across patron's neck.
3. If the disinfectant is non-poisonous, it is sufficient just to shake of the excess solution at the bowl.

Folding and discarding shave paper:

1. Upon completion of the final stroke of the first-time over, fold shave paper in the middle. Leave it on chest.

2. Upon completion of the final stroke of the second-time over, remove the shave paper and deposit it in the receptacle.

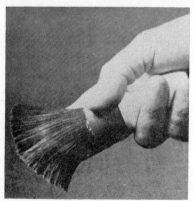

Fig. 502
Proper Way to Hold Brush

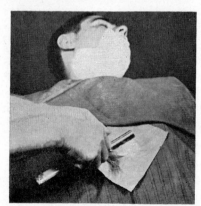

Fig. 503
Use Center of Paper First

Sectionization of the face: Shave strokes should be given systematically over the face. Therefore a blueprint of the areas has been drawn, setting forth the sequence in which the various sections should be shaved. The blueprint is intended to allow for flexibility, because the grain on faces vary. Whether the stroke is downward or upward depends largely on how the particular grain grows. The face is divided into fourteen sections. Section No. 1 is shaved first, and Section No. 2 is shaved next, etc. These regular sections are applicable only to the regular first-time over. It is recommended that the student memorize the fourteen sections before he does his first shave.

Resume of the fourteen sections

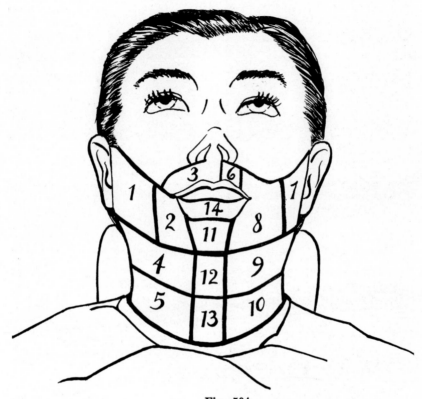

Fig. 504
Fourteen Sections
For Right Handed Barbers

Names of strokes:

1. Free Hand.
2. Back Hand.
3. Free Hand.
4. Free Hand.
5. Reverse Free Hand.
6. Back Hand.
7. Back Hand.

8. Free Hand.
9. Back Hand.
10. Reverse Free Hand.
11. Free Hand.
12. Free Hand.
13. Reverse Free Hand.
14. Reverse Free Hand.

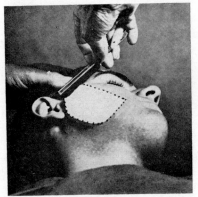

Fig. 505
Section No. 1, R.H.

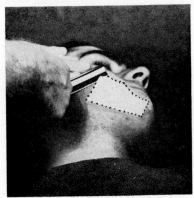

Fig. 506
Section No. 2, R.H.

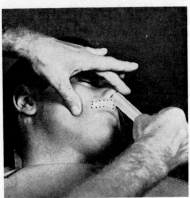

Fig. 507
Section No. 3, R.H.

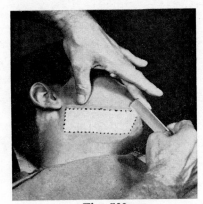

Fig. 508
Section No. 4, R.H.

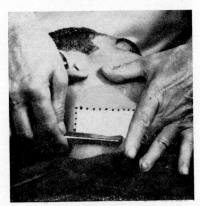

Fig. 509
Section No. 5, R.H.

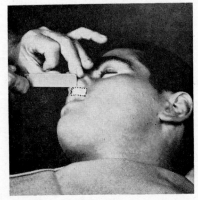

Fig. 510
Section No. 6, R.H.

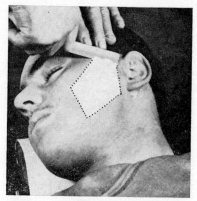

Fig. 511
Section No. 7, R.H.

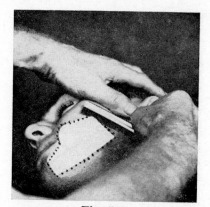

Fig. 512
Section No. 8, R.H.

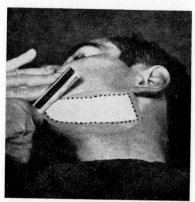

Fig. 513
Section No. 9, R.H.

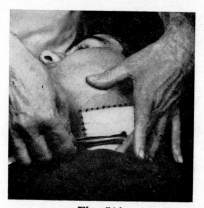

Fig. 514
Section No. 10, R.H.

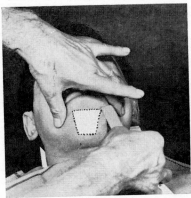

Fig. 515
Section No. 11, R.H.

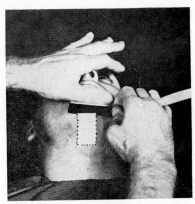

Fig. 516
Section No. 12, **R.H.**

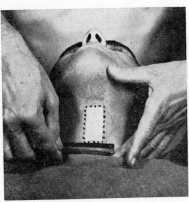

Fig. 517
Section No. 13, R.H.

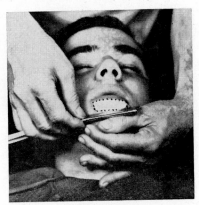

Fig. 518
Section No. 14, R.H.

Shaving Instruction for the Left Handed

The following drawings and pictures are designed for the left handed barber. The left handed person should learn to shave left handed. A person's dexterity has no relation to left-handedness or right-handedness. The letters "L.H." are used to designate left hand.

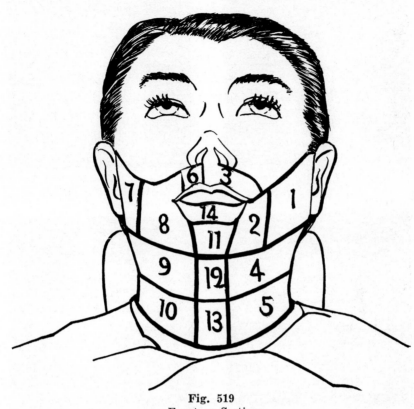

Fig. 519
Fourteen Sections
For Left Handed Barbers

Names of strokes:

1. Free Hand.
2. Back Hand
3. Free Hand.
4. Free Hand.
5. Reverse Free Hand.
6. Back Hand.
7. Back Hand.
8. Free Hand.
9. Back Hand
10. Reverse Free Hand.
11. Free Hand.
12. Free Hand.
13. Reverse Free Hand.
14. Reverse Free Hand.

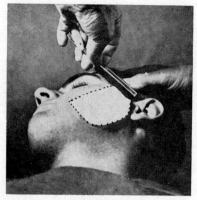

Fig. 520
Section No. 1, L.H.

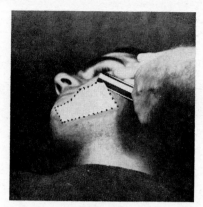

Fig. 521
Section No. 2, L.H.

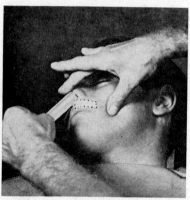

Fig. 522
Section No. 3, L.H.

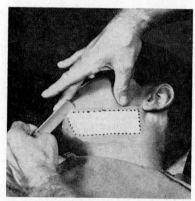

Fig. 523
Section No. 4, L.H.

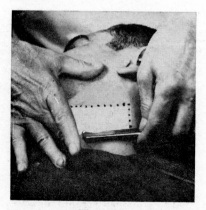

Fig. 524
Section No. 5, L.H.

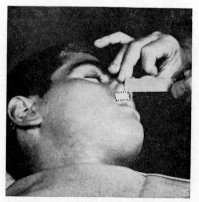

Fig. 525
Section No. 6, L.H.

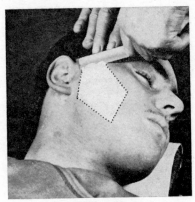

Fig. 526
Section No. 7, L.H.

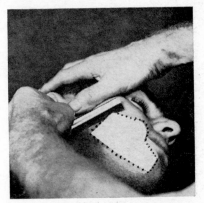

Fig. 527
Section No. 8, L.H.

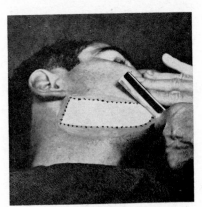

Fig. 528
Section No. 9, L.H.

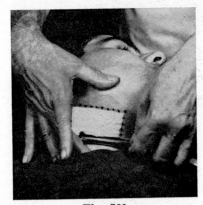

Fig. 529
Section No. 10, L.H.

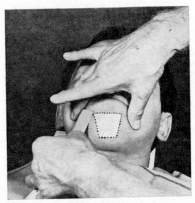

Fig. 530
Section No. 11, L.H.

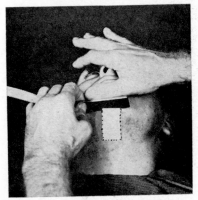

Fig. 531
Section No. 12, L.H.

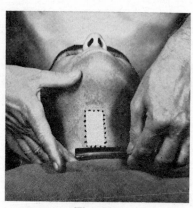

Fig. 532
Section No. 13, L.H.

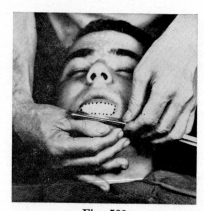

Fig. 533
Section No. 14, L.H.

Shampoos

A shampoo is a special preparation for cleansing the scalp and hair. When given correctly it can be a business builder. The barber should know what kind of shampoo to recommend for a given condition and also how to administer it scientifically. Since there are innumerable shampoos on the market, no attempt will be made in this chapter to specify them as to name or brand.

Chief purpose of shampoo: The chief purpose of any shampoo is to cleanse the scalp and hair.

Stimulation incidental: Stimulation should not be regarded as a major purpose of shampoos. The incidental stimulation from a shampoo results from the shampoo movements and steaming regularly involved in the process of shampooing.

Necessity of shampoos: The hair is vulnerable to flying particles in the air and eventually becomes heavy laden with dirt and foreign matter. Natural oil from the sebaceous glands and dead cells of the skin accumulate on the scalp. The dirt, excessive oil, and shedding cells are injurious to the scalp. Shampoos are also given for such conditions as dandruff, excessive oiliness, and itching. While shampoos are given for scalp and hair ailments, they are also necessary to keep a healthy scalp healthy.

1. When natural oils are allowed to remain on the scalp too long, they tend to coagulate into tallow, waxy-like substances which mix with natural scales that tend to clog and choke the hair follicles. Consequently, the hair is deprived of the proper oxygen and nourishment and at length baldness begins to appear.
2. Perspiration, mingled with dirt and dust, also collects and becomes sandwiched in with the oils and they together lead to the same consequences as stated above.
3. Disease producing bacteria find a happy home in the stifled conditions just described, and these agents begin their deadly work of breeding scalp diseases.

Cleansing and corrective shampoos:
1. Regular shampoos just cleanse.
2. Corrective shampoos are given not only to cleanse but also to correct some scalp or hair disorder. These shampoos have medicinal properties and are recommended for such conditions as dandruff, dryness, oiliness and itching.

Shampoo as preliminary service: Shampoos are also given as a preliminary to such services as follows:

1. Scalp treatments.
2. Hairstyling.
3. Blow waving, hot comb waving, and finger waving.

Some preliminary essentials to know about a shompoo:

1. Purpose.
2. Procedure.
3. Why certain ingredients are in shampoos.
4. Probable results.

Some types of shampoos:

1. **Liquid soap shampoos.** These are **foaming** shampoos that contain such oils as cocoanut and olive oils. Some of these may be called foaming oil shampoos that are made from the saponification of certain vegetable oils and fatty acids. (Refer to soaps in chapter on Cosmetic Chemistry). Example: Castile Soap Shampoo. Unless a liquid soap shampoo is especially for oily hair, **give one extra application for oily hair.**

2. **Medicated Shampoos.** These are usually liquid soap shampoos that contain such medicinal properties as tar, sulphur, and alcohol. Example: Tar shampoo.

3. **Egg shampoos.** While actual eggs may be used, commercially prepared egg shampoos in which dehydrated eggs are used have become the standard egg shampoos. The manufactured product is more convenient and economical. Follow the manufacturer's instructions. When the actual whole egg is used, it is called **Liquid Egg Shampoo,** because water is used to rinse it off. When only the albumen (white) is used, it is called **Dry Egg Shampoo,** because no water is used to free it from the hair—just a brush). Egg shampoos cleanse without removing the natural oils from the hair and add softness and glossiness. Recommend such shampoos for dry, brittle, dyed, over-bleached hair, and for a tender, sensitive scalp.

4. **Cream shampoos.** These shampoos are a creamy substance in liquid or semi-solid form. They are prepared in bottles, tubes and jars. Some cream shampoos are medicated and some are not.

5. **Hot oil shampoos.** This shampoo includes the application of some oil such as olive oil, special oil, or a lanolized oil, followed by a liquid soap shampoo. Actually, the oil should be just soothingly warm. The oil may be applied unheated, but in this case increase the time of steaming or dermal light.

6. **Soapless oil shampoos.** These are sulphonated oil shampoos. There

are two kinds of soapless oil shampoos, (1) soapless oil non-foamy shampoo and (2) soapless oil foamy shampoo.

7. **Dry shampoos.** Such shampoos may be given when the patron's health makes it inadvisable to give a wet shampoo. Two examples of dry shampoos are:

(1) Dry egg shampoo, already explained. It is excellent for a sensitive, tender scalp.

(2) Dry powder shampoo In this shampoo, orris root powder is used. Sprinkle it freely into the hair. Brush out with a long bristled brush. This powder readily absorbs oil. Do not apply any dry powder shampoo to a sensitive scalp since it would irritate it.

(3) Dry liquid shampoos. These are similar to dry cleaning fluids. Such shampoos are evaporative and inflammable. They are no longer used on human beings, but they are used to cleanse toupees and wigs. (Refer to chapter on Toupees and Wigs.)

Selecting a shampoo: If a shampoo has a special purpose, it is usually stated on the container. There are, however, some general guides. One can rely largely on shampoos labeled for a given purpose if manufactured by a reputable concern. A barber should become familiar with many shampoos on the market. Learn to observe closely what is written on shampoo bottles, jars, and other containers. Occasional visits to your supply dealer are recommended.

1. For excessive dryness, select an oil shampoo or one with a neutralized base. Cocoanut and olive oil base shampoos, hot oil shampoos, and most cream shampoos are examples.

2. For oiliness, select green soap or tar shampoos.

3. For a tender scalp, select a soothing cream or egg shampoo.

4. For a sensitive scalp, give an egg, oil or mild soothing shampoo.

Freqency of shampoos: One should have a shampoo whenever the scalp and hair need it. The proper shampoo correctly given will not be harmful and neither are frequently given shampoos injurious. It is not the frequency of shampoos that is harmful, but rather the wrong choice of a shampoo and the improper manner of administering it. As a general recommendation, one should have a shampoo every week or ten days. One's occupation has a lot to do with it. The most suitable time to have a shampoo, except when a definite need exists, is immediately after a hair cut. The factors that determine the recommended frequency of shampoos are:

1. The degree of exposure to dust, dirt, and flying particles.

2. The season—perspiration accumulates with dust and natural oil more in summer than in winter.

3. The locality—in smoky localities the hair needs cleaning more frequently than in a meadowy country or on a ship.
4. The physical condition of the hair—oily hair needs shampooing oftener than dry hair. Oily hair accumulates dirt readily and quickly forms waxy-like material that clogs the pores of the scalp.
5. The state of general health.

Preliminary scalp manipulations: When the scalp is very dirty, preliminary manipulations should be light The time to emphasize them is after scalp has been cleansed, since heavy, prolonged manipulations can push dirt, sand, or other foreign matter into the pores of the scalp Omit them when the scalp has ailments that would be aggravated. One school of thought is that the scalp should not be manipulated prior to a shampoo. Manipulations may be given by hands or electric means.

Purposes:
1. To loosen up the scalp to make it less sensitive to shampoo movements.
2. To loosen up dirt, scales or dandruff.

Supplement to manipulations: Supplementing the scalp manipulations by a "scratching" movement with the blunt coarse teeth of a large comb is recommended to loosen up dirt, scales or dandruff. Lay the teeth almost flat and make a scratching, scraping movement without much pressure. This method should not be used over a tender, irritated scalp. Light linear and rotary shampoo movements will also loosen up debris.

Kinds of rinse water:
1. The water should be comfortably warm. (Cold water rinses may be given with permission of patron.)
   (1) Cold water hampers maximum foaming, and it is uncomfortable.
   (2) Hot water tends to cause a flaking and drying effect.
   (3) Test the temperature of water by spraying it on the wrist.
2. **Soft water** is better. It makes a shampoo foam more and helps remove any soap curd. Hard water does not help these merits, since it contains minerals.
3. Rain water and distilled water are **examples of soft water.** Natural soft water is found in some areas.

Ways to soften water:
1. The simplest method is distillation. Such preparations as borax and Washing soda may be used as a softener; most of them, however, tend to dry out the hair; in fact, borax tends to discolor hair and

should not be used as a softener only on black hair when a reddish tinge is desired. The discoloring effect is more marked on hair of light shades of hair.

2. The best means of providing soft water in a barber shop is to have a water softening installation.

Steaming in tonics, oils and ointments: The method of steaming in these preparations is illustrated with the use of the steam towel in the chapter on Scalp Treatments.

Methods of applying oil to scalp: Refer to chapter on Scalp Treatments where these methods are illustrated.

Linen Set-ups for Shampoos

There are several good linen setups. Make sure that the clothing of the patron is protected. A special shampoo apron is recommended for economy.

1. Most economical linen set-up (Figs. 534, 535). This is called the **Hood** set-up. With a steamer fully open, grasp each end and form a sort of bonnet-effect over the head, bringing the two lower ends together in front and holding them in place while the right hand places wings of the apron around the lower ends of the steamer enveloping the neck; release the left hand to help fasten the apron in back, and turn the steamer down all around into a cuff-arrangement with the surplus portion spread out over the shoulders and back.

2. Two-towel **Diagonal** set-up. This is a unique linen set-up. **Place the small towel** around the neck in a diagonal **double fold,** then bring haircloth up so that the towel can be turned down in an overlapping cuff-like manner. Preferably use a hair-cloth clasp for security. Place an open **steam-towel** on the right shoulder and tuck a portion of it, single thickness, between the small towel and the neck. Now lift up the **diagonally** corresponding portion and tuck it between the towel and the neck of the left side. (Figs. 536-539)

3. Two-towel square set-up. This set-up is the same as the diagonal set-up except the steamer is not folded diagonally. (Fig. 590)

4. The linen set-ups may be the same for both the Inclined and Reclined methods. There is a slight preference for the Hood set-up for the Reclined method. A small towel should be placed around the neck while combing or dressing the hair.

Linen Set-ups for Shampoos

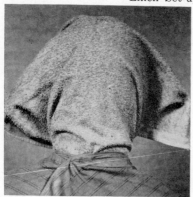

Fig. 534
Start of Hood Method

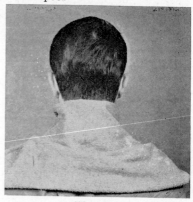

Fig. 535
Hood Method Completed

Done with One Steam Towel Only.

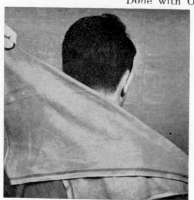

Fig. 536
Step One

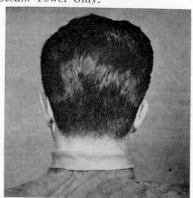

Fig. 537
Step Two (Small Towel)

Diagonal Towel Set-up

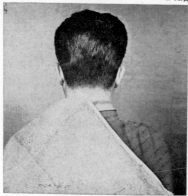

Fig. 538
Step Three (Steam Towel)

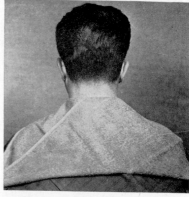

Fig. 539
Completed Set-Up (Steam Towel)

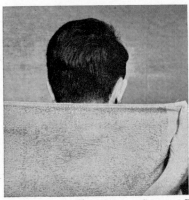 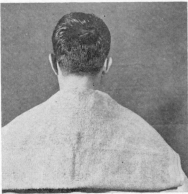

Fig. 540   Square Steamer Set-up   **Fig. 541**
Step One   Completed Set-Up
Refer to Figs. 536-37 For Use of Small Towel

How to apply shampoo. This depends somewhat upon the kind of shampoo. As concerns the kind that is applied from the bottle, the following instruc-tion is applicable:

1. Pick up the bottle with the right hand.
2. Step to the **left side** of the patron.
3. Separate the hair with **thumb** and **second** finger of left hand.
4. **Apply the shampoo first at the crown** and proceed forward along the vertex to hairline in spots about two inches apart. Then start at the crown and proceed in like manner across the back. This procedure helps to prevent shampoo from running below the hairline. Then deposit a few drops of shampoo in the hand and work it into the edges of the scalp, especially behind the ears. (Figs. 542, 543)

Applying water before shampoo: In a majority of shampoos water should be applied immediately before the shampoo. Of course this depends on

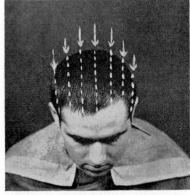 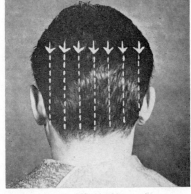

Fig. 542   **Fig. 543**
From Crown to Front Hairline   From Crown to Back Hairline
Procedure of Applying Shampoo

the shampoo and the instructions on its label. Water is not applied first in giving a hot oil shampoo or in the soapless oil and dry shampoos.

Chin and neck rest towels at bowl: Follow established shop practice.

1. In inclined method, place small towel on edge of bowl for chin rest. This is not necessary if patron holds his chin above bowl.
2. In reclined method, pull steamer over nape of neck.

How water is applied over shampoo:

1. From regular water bottle, when patron is in barber chair.
2. With the shampoo spray, when at the shampoo bowl.

Chin-Neck Rest Towels at bowl:

Applying shampoo at bowl: Apply shampoo at the crown and proceed in all directions to the hairline.

Removing lather when more water is to be added at the barber chair: Palm off the lather with the palm of the right hand, starting at the front hairline. Work in strips from right to left until the entire head is covered. Transfer the lather from the right to the left hand at the end of each strip. When sufficient lather has been removed, empty it into the bowl and rinse off both hands. Then apply more warm water.

Number of shampoo applications: The number of shampoo applications depends upon the kind of shampoo and upon the condition of the scalp and hair. **Two applications** are the standard number for most shampoos, especially for the soap and cream variety. If the head is extremely dirty, three applications are recommended. Only one applicaiton of soapless is usually given. Every previous application should be **rinsed out before making another one.**

Shampoo movements: There are **three types** of widely used shampoo movements. These are movements that are executed to distribute the shampoo. Each of these movements should be given several times and until the shampoo is thoroughly distributed on the scalp and through the hair. Shampoo movements are different from scalp manipulations. Shampoo movements merely slide over the surface of the scalp, and they are designed to distribute preparations over the scalp and through the hair. They may be vigorously given over the shampoo.

1. The Shuttle Movement.
   (1) Stand directly behind the patron. Place the finger tips of both hands at the hairline just above the ears and at the temples, proceed upward with firm pressure, gradually spreading the fingers until those of each hand interlock at the top. The movement is executed on both sides of the head at the same time. Repeat this movement several times.
   (2) Now step to the left side of the patron. Place the finger tips of

the left hand at the hairline at the forehead and the tips of the right hand at the crown. With the fingers separated proceed along the roof of the head until the fingers interlock. Repeat this movement several times.

2. Linear Movement. Remain standing at the left side of the patron. Brace the head with the open left hand placed across the frontal area. Place the finger tips of the right hand in a vertical position at the hairline on the neck just behind the right ear. Slide upward to the crown area. Continue in this manner across the back of the head. Repeat this movement several times. (This type of movement can also be used on the sides of the head).

3. Rotary Movement. Take a position behind the patron. Place the finger tips of both hands at the hairline just behind the ears. With a continuous rotary movement proceed up and along the edge of the head to the temples and then up to the center of the forehead. With large rotary movements cover the sides of the head between the edge and center, continue back over the crown, down the back, and across the neck to the original starting position. Repeat this movement several times.

Use of cushion tips in fingers: When executing the shampoo movements, use the cushion tips of the fingers.

Two methods of shampooing:

1. Inclined method (Fig. 476). When using this method, the shampoo and necessary water for the first application are applied while the patron is still in the barber chair or in other suitable chair. If a second shampoo application is to be given, it may be given while the patron is in the chair, in which case the lather is first palmed off. In most shampoos the second application is given at the bowl. In either case, the patron is invited to a stool by the bowl at the proper time. The inclined method is still the prevailing barber shop method for men, but it is unsuitable for women, since too much hair would fall over the face.

2. The reclined method is given entirely at the shampoo bowl, except when some preparation other than the shampoo itself is used in which case such shampoo is applied while patron is in the barber chair. This is the preferred method, because it affords greater comfort to the customer and gives him a feeling of luxury. This method means that the patron is laid down somewhat after the fashion of the shave position with his head lying upon the headrest of either a shampoo tray or of a shampoo bow. Draw up a part of the bowl, stand on the left side of patron.

Movement **No. 1**

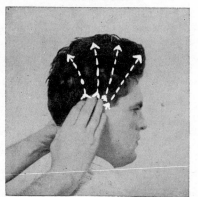

Fig. 544
Shuttle on Sides

Movement No. 2

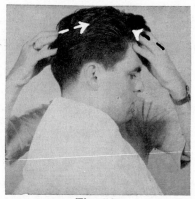

Fig. 545
Shuttle Forehead-Crown

Movement **No. 3**

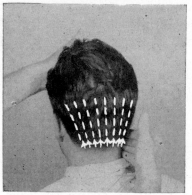

Fig. 546
Linear Movement

Movement No. 4

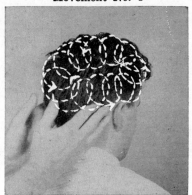

Fig. 547
Rotary Movement

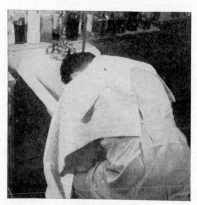

Fig. 548
Inclined Method

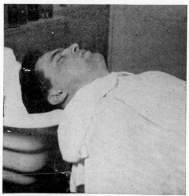

Fig. 549
Reclined Method

Evidence of clean hair: Hair that is thoroughly clean **squeaks** and tends to stick to the fingers on final rinsing.

Thorough rinsing important: Make sure that the hair is rinsed well. All traces of soap or foam or any shampoo preparation must be entirely rinsed out.

How shampoo is rinsed out: By the shampoo spray. Hold the spray **close** to the hair but not firmly enough to pull the hair. Keep the water guarded from running down on the face and neck and into the ears by the left hand.

Rinses: (See chapter on rinses). A plain water rinse regularly follows a shampoo. A special rinse is not always necessary if a good shampoo preparation is used, especially if soft water is used. A special rinse is recommended following all shampoos if hard water is used. Shampoo does not lather freely with hard water and it is more difficult to rinse out. The mineral elements in hard water produce a soap curd when brought into contact with soap.This curd can be fully removed by the application of a special rinse made for that purpose. Some manufacturers, particularly the makers of cream shampoos, contend that they require no special acid rinses such as lemon and vinegar and that such shampoos leave the hair clean and with a natural luster. There are two kinds of plain water rinses:

1. Tepid water rinse.

2. Cold water rinse. A cold water rinse helps to close the pores.

Effects of leaving soap or soap curd on scalp and hair:

1. It tends to cause scaling of the scalp.

2. It tends to bring about some form of dermatitis on the scalp.

3. It causes the hair to become dry and brittle.

4. It adds a dull color to the hair.

Before beginning to dry hair: Press out excess water in the hair with the tips and palms of both hands sliding from crown to hairline.
Drying eyes, forehead, ears: With the steam towel, first dry the eyes then the forehead, then the ears, and then the hair.

Drying hair: The steam-towel is more suitable than the face towel for drying the hair, since this kind of towel is more absorbent. This towel may be used unfolded or folded. Grasp the two corners of the towel to prevent them from dangling on the patron's face. Spread the hands over the towel and execute drumming and zigzag movements. Turning the towel over once to take advantage of the unused side. An electric hair drier is also recommended (Figs. 550-553, p. 216)

DRYING HAIR

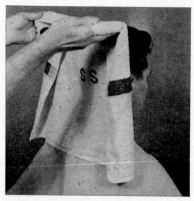

Fig. 550
Single Thickness

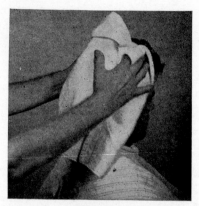

Fig. 551
Single Thickness

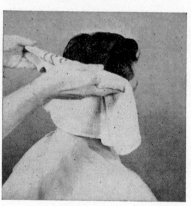

Fig. 552
Double Thickness

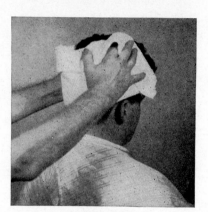

Fig. 553
Double Thickness

Combing very fine hair after shampoo:
1. Section the hair, and with the coarse part of the comb, start at the ends of small strands, and work towards the scalp.
2. As a final resort, apply a little hair oil with a fine spray or atomizer.

Why hair is sometimes badly tangled after shampoo: One or more of the following conditions may be the cause:
1. Extremely fine texture.
2. Extremely clean hair.
3. Over-steaming in a scalp treatment or in a permanent wave.
4. Too much alkali in the shampoo used.
5. Over-softening for coloring.
6. Over-bleaching.
7. Over-processing in permanent waving.

Shampooing matted hair: With a fine spray or atomizer apply a little mineral oil before applying shampoo. Separate the hair into small sections, beginning at the ends and comb through the hair with the coarse part of a large comb. Then proceed with the shampoo.

Shampooing eyebrows: When the eyebrows contain dust, dirt, or dandruff, it is a nice gesture to cleanse them. Extreme care should be used so as not to get any of the shampoo in the patron's eyes. Apply with finger tips and remove with end of dampened steam towel just used in the shampoo.

Shampoos for particular conditions: Select a shampoo according to the manufacturer's instructions, but here are a few especially recommended:

1. For **dry** scalp and hair.
   (1) Hot Oil Shampoo
   (2) Foamy soapless oil shampoo
   (3) Foaming Oil Shampoo
2. For **oily** scalp and hair.
   (1) Green Soap Shampoo
   (2) Tar Shampoo, if prepared especially for this condition. (Some so-called tar shampoos are recommended for normal conditions, but their label so indicates.)
3. For **tender, sensitive** scalps.
   (1) Egg Shampoo (manufactured).
   (2) Creme Shampoo.
   (3) Hot Oil Shampoo.

Shampoos for normal scalp and hair: Any shampoo may be used on a normal scalp and hair, except those primarily intended to be used on excessively oily conditions. Creme shampoos are very popular today. There are innumerable good shampoos on the market.

Amount of shampoo for a complete shampoo:

1. The amount of shampoo used depends on three factors, namely, the concentration of the shampoo itself, the degree of dirtiness of the head, and the quantity of hair.
2. An average amount of a liquid shampoo is one ounce.

STANDARD OUTLINE FOR LIQUID SOAP SHAMPOOS

1. Make linen set-up.
2. Systematically arrange all items to be used.
3. Manipulate scalp about one minute.
4. Dampen hair with warm water.
5. Apply shampoo.

6. Execute shampoo movements over entire scalp several times.
7. Rinse hair. (Test temperature of water.)
8. Give another application of shampoo.
9. Give shampoo movements several times. (Execute them **more** vigorously than before.)
10. Rinse hair thoroughly.
11. With hands open press down over entire head to remove **excessive** water.
12. Dry tentatively eyes, forehead and ears, with towel tucked around the neck, and pass towel over entire head to absorb excess wetness. Place shampoo towel over patron's head.
13. Direct patron back to barber chair.
14. Finish drying.
15. Dress hair.

Examples of liquid soap shampoos:
1. Cocoanut oil shampoo.
2. Olive oil base shampoo.
3. Tar shampoo.
4. Cream shampoos.
5. Any liquid foaming shampoo.

Sources of instruction for shampoo procedures:
1. Textbooks on barbering and cosmetology.
2. Manufacturers of shampoos. (Study their labels and phamplets.)

PLAIN SHAMPOO

A plain shampoo means any liquid soap shampoo such as cocoanut oil shampoo. Its name identifies it with shampoos in the low price bracket. It cleanses without any particular medicinal properties. Follow the standard outline for liquid soap shampoos.

HOT OIL SHAMPOO

Purpose: To cleanse dry scalp and hair.

Purpose of the oil:
1. To lubricate the scalp and hair so as to prevent irritating the scalp and damaging the hair shaft during the process of shampooing.
2. To alleviate a dry scalp and brittle, dry hair.
3. To aid in dislodging scales on the scalp.
4. To soothe tender, sensitive scalps.

Kinds of oil and shampoo:
1. Use either a vegetable oil, a sweet almond oil, or a specially prepared scalp oil.

2. Use any good liquid soap shampoo, such as castile or cocoanut oil shampoo.

Hot oil term a misnomer: A hot oil shampoo actually means applying oil to the scalp and hair and washing it out. Being a two-application procedure, one of oil and a liquid soap shampoo.

Procedure:

1. Arrange linen set-up.
2. Place all necessaries in readiness.
3. Manipulate scalp.
4. Apply oil direct to scalp, work it into scalp and distribute it along hair shaft with coarse comb placed flatwise with hair.
5. Encourage penetration of the oil:
    (1) By red dermal light, or
    (2) By electric steamer, or
    (3) By five steam-towel applications.
6. Shampoo with good liquid soap. (Usually, **two** applications).
7. Standard Finish—Dry and dress hair. (A few drops of oil applied with an atomizer is recommended).

NON-FOAMY SOAPLESS OIL SHAMPOO

Purpose: To cleanse the scalp and hair without soap.

Noteworthy: It is best for **oily** scalp and hair, but may also be used for normal or dry scalp. Too frequent use is drying and renders hair very absorptive. This detergent consists of olive or castor oil treated with sulphuric acid to make it water soluble.

Procedure:

1. Linen set-up.
2. Manipulate scalp.
3. Spray hair with warm water.
4. Apply about an ounce of shampoo and distribute through the hair with finger tips and coarse end of comb and massage into scalp.
5. Make two steam-towel applications.
6. Rinse hair thoroughly.

NEUTRALIZER SHAMPOO

All neutralizer shampoos are recommended following hair relaxing treatments, coloring and bleaching, and for sensitive scalp and dry hair. They are soothing, soft, suave, and unperturbing. **They are soapless.** There are many good brands on the market.

EGG SHAMPOOS

Fresh eggs were formerly used, but today manufactured egg shampoos are used. Commercially prepared egg shampoos are more economical and more convenient. Actual eggs require "kitchen work" to prepare, they are difficult to remove from the hair, and their odor is difficult to destroy.

Some conditions for which recommended:
1. Dull, lusterless hair.
2. Tender, sensitive scalp.
3. Dry, brittle hair.
4. Scalp with psoriasis or eczema.
5. Bleached or dyed hair.
6. Permanent waved hair.

Two kinds of actual egg shampoos:
1. Dry egg shampoo. Use only the white (albumen) of an egg. No water or liquid is used.
2. Liquid egg shampoo. Use whole egg. A water rinse follows.

DRY EGG SHAMPOO

Purposes:
1. To cleanse and soothe a very sensitive and allergic-to-soap scalp.
2. To add glossiness and softness to dry and dull hair.

Procedure:
1. Make linen set-up.
2. Prepare mixture. (See formula.)
3. Apply all the mixture at one time.
4. Rub the mixture into scalp as applied, using finger tips.
5. Execute shampoo movements. A comb may be used to further distribution.
6. Remove the shampoo with a dry Turkish towel or brush.
7. Dress hair dry. (A few drops of oil or creme hairdressing may be applied.)

Formula: Use only white of egg. Add one-half teaspoonful of salt and tablespoonful of witch hazel. (Use egg beater.)

Noteworthy: Especially recommended for sick persons whose hair should not be wet. Use no water or liquid. Only the albumen of an egg has cleaning ability. Salt is added to facilitate mixing and witch hazel to destroy the odor of the egg.

LIQUID EGG SHAMPOO

Purposes:
1. To cleanse and soothe a sensitive scalp that is allergic to soaps.
2. To add softness and glossiness to dry, dull hair.

Formula: Use whole egg. Add one teaspoonful of salt and tablespoonful of witch hazel. (Use egg beater).

Noteworthy: Salt is added to the egg to facilitate mixing and witch hazel as perfume to destroy the odor of the egg. A tonic or liquid hairdressing may follow the shampoo. Tepid water is used, because warm or hot water would coagulate the egg.

Procedure:
1. Make linen set-up.
2. Prepare mixture. (See formula).
3. Dampen hair with tepid water.
4. Apply about one-half of mixture.
5. Rub into scalp as applied, using finger tips.
6. Execute shampoo movements. A comb may be used to further distribution.
7. Rinse out with tepid water.
8. Apply balance of mixture.
9. Execute shampoo movements.
10. Rinse out with tepid water.
11. Dress hair.

MANUFACTURED EGG SHAMPOO

Purposes:
1. To cleanse and soothe a sensitive scalp.
2. To add glossiness and softness to hair.
3. To cleanse any kind of hair.

Noteworthy: Select creme egg shampoos. They are more convenient to give and are pleasantly scented. Besides cleasing the hair, they brighten and add manageability even with hard water rinse. The formula may contain a low percent of protein, say 5%, from actual eggs.

Procedure: Follow the manufacturer's instructions. They will closely follow the **standard outline for a liquid soap shampoo.** Typical Procedure:
1. Linen set-up
2. Massage scalp
3. Dampen hair
4. Apply shampoo and work up rich lather
5. Rinse with warm water
6. Repeat steps 4 and 5
7. Dress hair

DRY SHAMPOOS

Dry shampoos were discussed under "some types of shampoos" and one under "Egg Shampoos." They have different purposes. If a manufactured one is used, follow the manufacturer's instructions. Dry shampoos are given very rarely and for conditions that make regular wet shampoos inadviseable. In giving dry shampoos, the hair is sectioned to facilitate complete coverage of the head. When a powder preparation is used, it may be sprinkled onto the hair by a dispenser such as used for talcum powder. Use a brush for distribution of the preparation. Continue brushing until the hair is free from the preparation. Dress the hair without liquid. The standard linen set-up is used. (Refer to the chapter on Toupees and Wigs, sub-section "Care and Cleansing of Hairpieces.")

The kinds of dry shampoos:
1. Dry egg shampoo.
2. Liquid dry shampoo.
3. Powdered dry shampoo.

Conditions for which dry shampoos are especially recommended:
1. Sensitive and tender scalps.
2. Bed-fastness.
3. Physical weakness.
4. Probability of wetness causing a bad cold.

TONIC SHAMPOO

Definition: A tonic shampoo is simply a liquid soap shampoo which is immediately preceded and followed by an application of tonic.

Purposes:
1. To cleanse the scalp and hair.
2. To soothe a sensitive, tender scalp.
3. To alleviate dandruff.
4. To alleviate itching.

Noteworthy: The preliminary tonic application loosens scales and debris and provides a lubricant base for manipulations.

Procedure:
1. Linen set-up for shampoo.
2. Manipulate scalp, lightly if scalp is tender.
3. One hot steam towel application.
4. Apply tonic and massage into scalp and comb through hair. (Refer to chapter on "Tonics".)
5. Apply shampoo.
6. Rinse out.
7. Apply tonic and leave on.
8. Dress hair.

SHAMPOOS FOR SCALP WITH ECZEMA OR PSORIASIS

Kinds of shampoo: Use a mild, soothing shampoo, such as egg shampoo, cream shampoo, or mild bland shampoo. A physician's prescription shampoo is best.

Procedure:

1. Linen set-up.
2. Shampoo.
3. Soothing tonic.
4. One moderately hot steam towel application.
5. Dress hair.

SHAMPOOS SUMMARIZED

The procedures of various shampoos contain many identical steps, and many of these steps are the same. The preliminaries and finish are nearly always the same. The procedure is varied only to apply a special shampoo itself. Some preparations, such as scalp oil or soapless oil, require some means of aiding penetration, such as steam towel applications, red dermal light, electric steamer, or infra-red lamp. But these are special and different from regular shampoos.

Much about procedures may be left to the discretion of the barber. The service rendered should be commensurate with the charge. The customer is entitled to more service in a high price shampoo. Manipulate his scalp two minutes instead of one. Some **sulphonated** and some **medicated** shampoos are applied before water and massaged into the scalp with the aid of either steam or dry heat. The term "medicated" however, means little since most shampoos with the usual ingredients in shampoos may be so classified. Manufacturers are inclined to simplify procedures. The following are some of their instructions:

1. Observation number one: (a one-application shampoo)
    (1) Before using any water, apply just enough shampoo to moisten scalp and hair.
    (2) Massage until foam disappears.
    (3) Add water, a little at a time, lathering after each addition of water until all foam disappears.
    (4) Rinse with warm water.
2. Observation number two: (a two-application shampoo)
    (1) Wet hair thoroughly.
    (2) Apply a small amount of shampoo.
    (3) Work shampoo into generous lather.
    (4) Rinse with tepid water.
    (5) Repeat these steps for a thorough cleansing.
3. Observation number three: (a one-application shampoo)
    (1) Wet the hair with tepid or warm water.
    (2) Apply shampoo.
    (3) Rub with fingertips.
    (4) Rinse.

Rinses

A hair rinse is an agent that removes shampoo or soap curd, highlights the hair or imparts color. Examples of rinses are plain water, a mixture of water with an acid agent, and a temporary color rinse. Rinses follow a freshly shampooed head.

Purposes of rinse: The purposes vary according to the kind of rinse. In general, the purposes are:
1. To dissolve any soap curd after a shampoo.
2. To remove any remaining shampoo.
3. To high-light the color of the hair.
4. To tone down gray hair.
5. To cover yellowish streaks in gray hair.
6. To partially color the hair temporarily.

Soap curd: This is a residue resulting from excess alkali or hard water. But today, shampoos are comparatively free from excess alkali. Soap curd has these effects:
1. It coats and tends to make the hair lusterless.
2. It tends to clog the pores of the scalp.
3. It causes itching.

Classification of rinses:
1. Plain rinse. This is a water rinse that follows all shampoos. Use tepid water, but cold water may be used if the patron prefers.
2. Acid rinses. There are two such rinses.
   (1.) Citric rinse.
   (2.) Acetic rinse.
3. Manufactured soap curd removing rinses.
4. Creme rinses.
5. Color rinses: There are many kinds of color rinses. Manufactured color rinses are most commonly used. Three non-commercial color rinses are: (1) Peroxide, (2) bluing, (3) henna.
6. Non-stripping rinses: A non-stripping rinse is formulated to prevent stripping or streaking a tint or toner. It is also recommended for semi-permanent colored hair.

Water rinse: A water rinse follows acid, peroxide, bluing and some henna rinses. Follow the manufacturer's directions. A water rinse does not follow some color rinses.

Acid rinses: The use of lemon and vinegar in acid rinses is somewhat outmoded. They have been replaced by manufactured rinses that achieve the same purpose—to remove soap curd. Such manufactured rinses are not only superior, they are move convenient to prepare. Any such rinses have little or no purpose when good shampoo and soft water are used. There are two kinds of acid rinses:

1. Citric rinse. This is a mixture of water and strained juice of a lemon. The formula is the juice of one lemon and a quart of tepid water. Use this rinse on blonde shades of hair. Follow with a water rinse.

2. Acetic rinse. This is a mixture of water and white apple cider vinegar. The formula is a half cup of vinegar to a quart of tepid water. Use on dark shades of hair. Follow with a water rinse.

Manufactured soap curd removing rinses: These rinses have practically replaced vinegar and lemon rinses. They not only remove soap curd, they leave the hair soft and pliable and easy to comb. The use of soft water and today's improved shampoos make these rinses less valuable.

Creme rinses: These manufactured rinses contain ingredients that add "body" and luster to the hair and make it softer and easier to comb by keeping the hair from tangling. A creme rinse is especially recommended for dry, brittle, bleached or tinted hair.

Color rinses: Color rinses impart a temporary color. They are conveniently referred to as "shampoo to shampoo" rinses. They not only cover gray hair but impart natural shades. Such rinses are merely applied, distributed, and left on. Styling may follow. They do not penetrate the hair; they only **coat** the hair. There are many such rinses on the market. Their colors are labeled according to a color chart. Some examples of the colors are:

Blonde	Silver
Black	Smoky
Brown	Pearl
Medium Brown	Copper
Dark Brown	

Color rinses are usually prepared in **liquid** or **lotion** form. Do not confuse regular color rinses explained in this chapter with semi-permanent color tints that are sometimes called color rinses. Such color rinses, so-called, are tints that penetrate the hair and last through a shampoo. Do not give water rinse over a color rinse. (See chapter on Haircoloring.) A color rinse may last until the next shampoo if the interval of time is not too long.

Some purposes of color rinses are:
1. To tone down or cover yellowish streaks on gray or white hair.

2. To partially restore the original natural color.

3. To highlight the shade of hair.

4. To partially cover gray or white hair.

Manufactured color rinses: These come prepared for use and have almost **replaced** the traditional or non-commercial French bluing, peroxide, and henna rinses that require an individual mixture for each customer. However, these non-commercial rinses will be explained.

1. **Peroxide rinse:** (Manufactured peroxide rinses are available)

   (1) Purpose: To lighten the shade of hair.

   (2) Mixture: One tablespoonful of 20 volume peroxide to a quart of water. To lighten more, use two tablespoonsful.

   (3) Time: Leave on from 5 to 10 minutes, depending on the degree of lightening desired. Follow with one application of a mild shampoo to stop the action of the peroxide.

   (4) Use on blonde or light shades of hair.

2. **Bluing rinse:** (Manufactured bluing rinses are available) The French bluing rinse is seldom used today; however, French bluing rinse is explained as follows:

   (1) Purpose: To remove yellowish streaks from gray or white hair. It also achieves a silvery or slate color tone. By adding more bluing, it will achieve a slight bluish tone.

   (2) Mixture: 5 to 10 drops of bluing to a quart of water.

   (3) Follow with slight water rinse. This rinse can be removed or toned down by re-shampooing.

   (4) Use on gray, white and dark shades of hair.

3. **Henna rinses:** (Manufactured henna rinses are available). The old mixture of henna leaves is outmoded.

   (1) Purpose: To impart a slight auburn tinge to the hair.

   (2) Formula: 10 to 25 drops of henna liquid concentrate to a pint of water, depending on the degree of tinge desired.

Utensils for color rinses: Use a porcelain or plastic pan about 10 inches in diameter.

How rinses are applied: Pour onto the hair and distribute well with the fingers. Some color rinses are combed through the hair.

PROCEDURE OF APPLYING COLOR RINSES

1. Complete linen set-up. Plastic cape recommended.

2. Shampoo, rinse and towel dry the hair. Color rinses are always applied to clean hair.

3. Select color and mix rinse according to manufacturer's directions.

4. Apply as directed by manufacturer, however, it may be applied (1) by a bottle type plastic applicator, (2) formally, by a brush made for this purpose, and (3) informally by sparingly pouring it onto the hair. Distribute it through the hair with the finger tips and a medium-to-fine tooth comb. Be sure to make complete even coverage.

5. Begin application around the front hairline.

6. Continue application covering front and side areas working toward the crown.

7. Apply to nape line and work upward to the crown area.

8. Check for complete coverage.

9. Leave rinse on for the required length of time.

10. Rinse thoroughly with warm water until the excess color is removed.

11. Style hair.

NOTES

Tonics and Hairdressing Preparations

TONICS

A hair tonic is a cosmetic liquid for the scalp and hair.

Purposes:
1. To tone up the scalp and enliven the hair.
2. To help correct such conditions as dandruff and itching.
3. To antiseptisize the scalp.

A hairdressing preparation is either a liquid or solid to be used for grooming the hair. It adds glossiness and makes the hair obedient.

Some preparations are a combination scalp tonic and hair groomer. Tonics that are not intended for grooming may be called regular or straight tonics and those intended for grooming as hairdressing tonics.

Hair tonics and hairdressing preparations comprise an almost infinite variety of kinds and brands. There are several national manufacturers of such items and a large number of local manufacturers in nearly all large cities. The barber should become well acquainted with at least the most popular brands.

Only in a broad sense can all such preparations be referred to as "tonics". Tonics contain some medicinal properties, usually alcohol, whereas hairdressing preparations come in the form of oil mixtures and hair creams containing various proportions of lanolin and mineral oils, and may or may not include alcohol. These are intended only to add glossiness and hold the hair in place.

Types of tonics: Tonics are classified under four headings.
1. **Hydro-alcoholic tonic.** It is an antiseptic and contains sufficient alcohol to act as a mild irritant. ("Hydro" means the presence of water.) Its purpose is alleviation or correction of some scalp or hair condition.
2. **Non-alcoholic tonic.** It is usually antiseptic and contains medicinal ingredients. It has the same purpose as a hydro-alcoholic tonic.
3. **Oil mixture tonic.** It contains a large percentage of hydro-alcoholic solution and a small percentage of oil. (The oil in some mixtures floats to the top but reconsolidates upon shaking.) Besides an antiseptic, this tonic has **hair grooming properties.** Its purpose is to correct and groom.
4. **Cream oil tonic.** This is really a hairdressing tonic. It is an emulsion containing such grooming ingredients as lanolin and mineral oils.

General purposes of tonics:

1. To help maintain the normal health of the scalp and the hair.
2. To help correct disorders of the scalp and hair.
3. To dress the hair.

Broad purposes expressed in other terms: Tonics are applied for the following major reasons:

1. For hygienic reasons—to preserve the health of the scalp and hair.
2. For remedial reasons—to correct ill conditions.
3. For cosmetic reasons—to dress the hair.

Specific purposes of tonics:

1. To stop itching of scalp.
2. To help correct dandruff.
3. To stimulate circulation of scalp (co-incidental).
4. To give a pleasant perfume.
5. To antisepticize the scalp.
6. To control unruly hair.
7. To lubricate dry scalp and hair.
8. To give a feeling of relaxation.
9. To soothe a slightly irritated scalp.
10. To impart a tinkling effect.
11. To help check an over-perspiring scalp.
12. To add a life-like resemblance to the hair—to remove a dull and lifeless color.
13. To dress the hair.

Some **observations** of **claims made by manufacturers** of tonics and hairdressings are enlightening. These are some of the things they say:

1. Claims about tonics:
   1. For loose dandruff and dry hair.
   2. Hair tonic—for hair and scalp.
   3. A refreshing and cooling compound for head and face.
   4. Cooling for head and face—cooling—refreshing—invigorating. Apply briskly for that tingling all over good feeling.
   5. For removing dandruff scales.
   6. Removes loose dandruff, scales, and flakes.
   7. A medicine. Use freely for removal of dandruff scales, itching scalp . . .
   8. Antiseptic aid for the skin. Safe—soothing.
   9. Kills dandruff germs; removes loose dandruff; relieves itching scalp; conditions the scalp.
   10. For hair and scalp hygiene. Lubricates dry scalp. Cleansing action loosens itchy dandruff flakes.
2. Claims about hairdressing preparations:

1. To keep dry, unruly hair well groomed. Will not soil hats or pillows (Liquid cream).
2. Dampen the hair and rub on a few drops. Keeps the hair well groomed without being oily or sticky. (Oil)
3. Moisturizing hairdressing for men. Medicated ingredients to fight dandruff . . . (Liquid cream)
4. Liquid Butch Hair Wax.
5. Pomade for well groomed hair. (Solid wax)
6. Keeps hair in place all day long. Leaves no harmful stains.

How tonics preserve health of scalp and help correct scalp disorders:
Tonics are recommended to keep a scalp healthy and to correct certain disorders. By reason of their alcoholic content, their beneficial ingredients, their antiseptic power, the procedure of application, tonics are recommended.

1. Their alcohol helps to stimulate circulation which results in more nourishment for the hair.
2. Some of the beneficial ingredients used in tonics are quinine, resorcin, sulphur, borax, pilocarpine, cantharides, alcohol, as well as many vegetable substances.
3. The movements used in applying a tonic stimulate circulation, activate the metabolism of cells, relax the nerves, and loosen the scalp tissues.
4. The heat or steaming involved in the application also helps to stimulate circulation.
5. Some of its ingredients, especially sulphur and alcohol, are antagonistic to the presence and growth of disease producing germs.

Three apropo times to suggest a tonic:
1. Immediately after a shampoo; just before dressing or combing the hair.
2. While manipulating the scalp following any other order or service, just before dressing or final combing of hair.
3. Following a discussion of some particular scalp or hair ailment or need.

When not to suggest a tonic:
1. When the scalp and hair are extremely dirty.
2. When a man is obviously broke and "down and out."
3. When a man says he is in a hurry and wants only a hair cut.

Linen set-up for tonic: The linen should be set up neatly and snugly. See that the patron's clothing is protected. Fold a small towel diagonally and place around the neck, above the haircloth, and fasten it in front by a clasp. Then turn down the upper edge, forming a cuff-like effect. (Figs. 554-555).

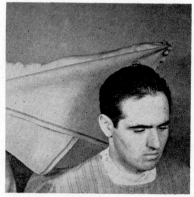

Fig. 554
First Step of Linen Set-up
for Tonic

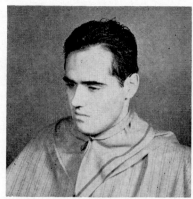

Fig. 555
Completed Linen Set-up
for Tonic

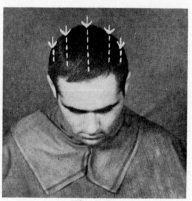

Fig. 556

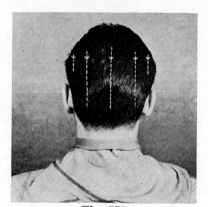

Fig. 557

Routine of Applying Tonic

PROCEDURE OF TONIC APPLICATION

1. Arrange linen set-up.
2. Manipulate the scalp, about one full minute.
3. Make one steam towel application.
4. Apply tonic and massage in.
5. Manipulate scalp for about two minutes.
6. Make one steam towel application.
7. Comb and dress hair as desired.

Reasons for prior manipulations:

1. To increase the blood supply of the scalp.

2. To make the pores more receptive to the tonic.

3. To relax the nerves and muscles of the scalp—to relax the patron.

Reasons for steaming scalp before application:

1. To open the pores for the reception of the tonic.

2. To stimulate circulation.

3. To further relax the nerves and muscles of the scalp.

4. To make the hair more controllable. Steam tends to soften brittle or stubborn hair and thus make it more pliable.

Routine of applying tonic: (Figs. 556-557).

With tonic bottle held vertically in the right hand, step to the left side of the patron. Separate the hair with thumb and second finger of left hand. Apply the tonic first at the crown and proceed forward to the front hairline. Then work across the back of the scalp in like manner. Then deposit a few drops of tonic in the hand and work it into the edges of the scalp, especially behind the ears. This principle will help prevent tonic running down over forehead. (Figs. 556-557).

Emphasize application of tonic on these areas: The edges, just behind the ears—over the mastoid regions—and the extreme front region at the center. In treating an itching scalp it is always fitting to ask which spots are itching especially, and give them particular attention.

Massaging scalp after application: After a tonic is applied, massage the scalp more than prior to the tonic. More vigorous movements are possible without irritation because the scalp now has sufficient lubrication through the tonic. But this does not mean roughly scrubbing the scalp.

Why scalp is massaged after application: For the same reasons as given for massaging it before the tonic and for two additional reasons:

1. To complete the distribution of the tonic.

2. To aid penetration of the tonic.

Apply hair oil before tonic: This is done because an oily solution clings and is absorbed more readily by a dry substance than by a wet one; and because an alcoholic or aqueous solution clings and absorbs more readily by a wet substance than by a dry one.

Tonic Steam: This simply means that steam towel applications are given both before and after the tonic is applied. (Figs.558-565).

STEAMING SCALP

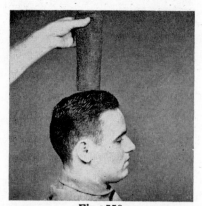

Fig. 558
Step No. 1

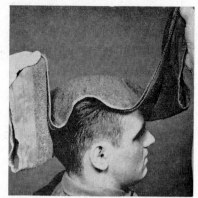

Fig. 559
Step No. 2

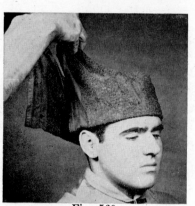

Fig. 560
Step No. 3

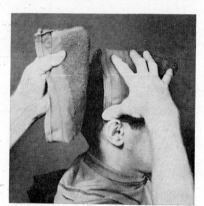

Fig. 561
Step No. 4

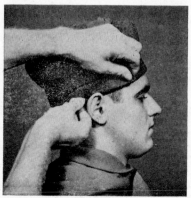

Fig. 562
Step No. 5

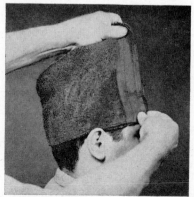

Fig. 563
Step No. 6

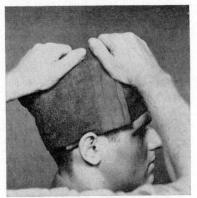 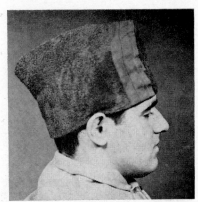

Fig. 564
Step No. 7

Fig. 565
Step No. 8

HAIRDRESSING PREPARATIONS

Types of hairdressing preparations.

1. **Oil mixtures.** Such mixtures contain a large proportion of aqueous or hydro-alcoholic solution and oil (mineral oil). In these preparations the oil may float on top and thus necessitate shaking before use.

2. **Cream oils or emulsions.** (Sometimes referred to as "creme oils.")

3. **Pomades.** These preparations are mainly petroleum jelly compounded with a scented substance and other ingredients. Pomades usually contain mineral oil.

4. **Hair wax,** frequently called "butch wax" is essentially a hairdressing in that its main purpose is grooming by causing the hair to "stay put" and add glossiness. Hair wax comes as a liquid or solid.

How to apply hair oil or hair cream: Neither oil nor cream should be applied to the scalp direct from the bottle. Douse the oil or cream into the palm of the left hand. Then distribute it over the fingers and then apply it to the hair and scalp. (Figs. 566-569, p. 234).

Distributing hair oil, hair cream or tonic to scalp and hair: Proceed according to illustrations 566-569, thus getting the preparation **underneath the hair first.** Then distribute it over the top of the hair. For massaging it into the scalp, use the finger tips.

Kind of oil best suited for hair: Use mineral oil, or an oily preparation with a mineral oil base, because it does not become rancid, it seems to add a little better gloss than the other oils, it is less absorbent, and it may be secured in the odorless form.

Hair creams: There are many good hair creams on the market. They are, of course, hairdressing preparations. Apply them as just recommended.

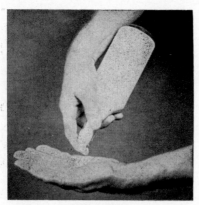

Fig. 566
Remove Oil or Cream from
Palm to Hair

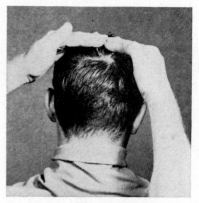

Fig. 567
From Crown to Front

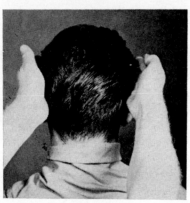

Fig. 568
From Hairline Upward
From Sides and Back

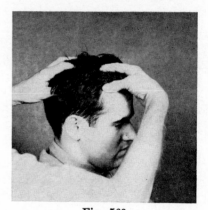

Fig. 569
Use This Movement From
Hairline to Top Around Head

Merits of hair cream:
1. It is non-greasy.
2. It is non-sticky.
3. It is easy to apply.
4. It has good grooming ability.
5. It will not soil hat, clothing, linen, etc.

Aiding the penetration of tonics and oils:
1. Use steam-towel applications to aid the penetration of hair tonics. Do not use dry heat such as produced by dermal lights, for dry heat would cause the alcoholic content to evaporate and sting the scalp.
2. Use either steam-towel or dermal lights over oils.
3. The length of time for exposure to heat is from one to three minutes. This means two or three steam-towel applications.

Massaging

Massaging is a part of every service a barber renders. Even in giving a haircut or shave a little massaging is necessary for a suitable finishing touch. In each of these services the finger tips come in contact with the scalp and face. Whenever the finger tips pass over the surface of the skin, massaging is manifest to some degree. The contact is more emphatic when giving a shampoo, tonic, facial or scalp treatment. It is therefore imperative that the barber know the principles of massaging.

Definition: Massaging is the process of stroking and manipulating bodily tissues.

Principal means of massaging:

1. By hand. (Largely by use of finger tips.)
2. By mechanical devices. (The electric vibrator is the main device.)

Major purposes of massaging:

1. To help maintain the health of the face and scalp.
2. To help correct an unhealthy condition of the face and scalp.

Specific purposes of massaging:

1. To stimulate circulation.
2. To induce relaxation.
3. To activate the oil glands.
4. To promote metabolism.
5. To tone up muscles.
6. To coax away wrinkles.

Scope of massaging in barbering: The conventional scope of massaging in barbering is the head, face, and neck.

Prerequisites to understand massaging: It is not enough to know how to execute the various methods of massaging. One must have some knowledge of the nerve points, cells, the structure of the skin, muscles and blood circulation. (Study chapters on these subjects.)

Bad effects of prolonged massaging:

1. Irritation or inflammation of the tissues.
2. Fatiguing and wasting of cells.
3. Paralyzation of cells.
4. Unpleasant sensation.

Hippocrates' theory of massaging: (Hippocrates, the father of medicine, lived around 400 B. C.)

1. "Hard rubbing binds, soft rubbing loosens, much rubbing causes parts to waste, and moderate rubbing makes them grow."
2. **Essence of the theory of Hippocrates:** Prolonged, over-vigorous massaging of the tissues injures and breaks them down, whereas moderate pressure of proper duration builds up tissues.

Types of massage movements:

1. Effleurage. (This is a stroking movement.)
2. Petrissage. (This is a kneading movement.)
3. Percussion (This is a tapping movement.)
4. Tapotement. (Alternate name for percussion.)
5. Vibratory. (This means vibrations.)
6. Rotary. (This means rotation movements.)

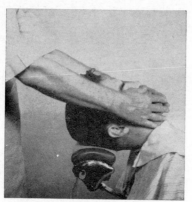

Fig. 570
Massaging Posture

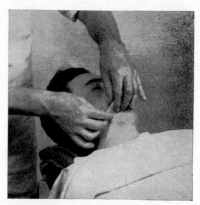

Fig. 571
Petrissage or Kneading

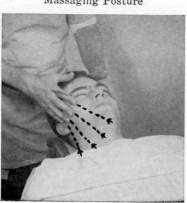

Fig. 572
Stroking Movement

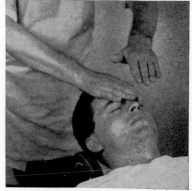

Fig. 573
Gently Stroking

Stroking (Effleurage):

1. Definition: Stroking is a linear and zigzag movement over the surface of the skin. It is executed by applying the finger tips gently and typically very lightly—with very little pressure, a feather-like kind of contact. But, when passing over the unbearded portions of the face and when massaging a lady's face, a little more pressure may be applied where the skin is fairly normal and free from any irritation. Particularly is it fitting to add more pressure when passing over such sections as the forehead, the nose, and the regions immediately behind the ears.

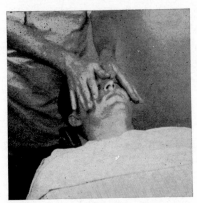

Fig. 574
Major Cushions Across Forehead

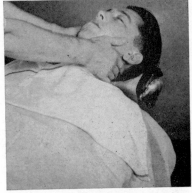

Fig. 575
Stroking

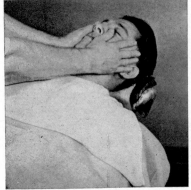

Fig. 576
Stroking

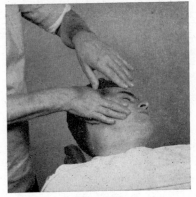

Fig. 577
Tapping

2. Methods of stroking:

    (1) Sweeping movement: These movements are made with the cushion tips almost flat against the skin and with the fingers held as closely to one another as convenient. The fingers may be

lifted and reapplied for each stroke. The movements of this method are comparatively long, graceful and sweeping. This kind of movement may be called "linear," especially when it is more fitting to use one or two finger tips as in massaging around the eyes or just back of the ears. The sweeping strokes are made:

    a. To spread or distribute creams and solutions.

    b. To give a mild, soothing effect as a finish.

    c. To relieve pain or aches, making the strokes sidewise on the forehead and lengthwise just behind the ears.

    d. To remove pink rolling cream.

(2) Rotary movement: The rotations vary from small to large, but they should be small on the scalp and on sensitive face areas.

(3) The Zigzag movement: The Zigzag movements are "to-and-fro" without breaking contact with the face.

Uses of stroking movement: Stroking is used for all general purposes of massaging, but more especially when doing the following:

1. When applying creams and lotions.
2. When passing over sections of the skin that do not permit reasonable flexibility.
3. When giving the regular shampooing movements.
4. When making the finishing strokes of a facial or of the massaging that customarily follows a shave.
5. When passing from one movement to another—forming tne transition steps between the various movements.
6. When a very slight soothing effect is desired or preferable.
7. When lathering the face.
8. When massaging to induce relaxation.

Percussion: The movements of this type are quick, short, and gently tapping, and are done entirely with the finger tips. The necessary wrist movement for this method is permissible. The patting movements are best executed by an alternating series of strokes which are made by each hand in such a way that the tips of one hand are in contact all the time during the execution. The tips of the two hands follow a single path of direction in a revolving manner as they move along. The fingers are, therefore, lifted between each stroke. The patting movements are very useful for removing pink rolling cream. It is also called **tapotement.**

Rotary Movement: Make contact with the cushion tips of two or three fingers and revolve them about four times, starting forward and then upward and continuing in a circular movement. On the fourth rotation, slide lightly over the skin into the next position and repeat the movement, etc. The number of finger tips used will depend upon the particular place being massaged; but use the number the most convenient. The first, second and third fingers are the recommended ones.

Kneading (Fig. 571): This is a process of grasping the skin with the thumb and fiingers and executing a slight pinching and rolling movement. Pass from one ridge thus formed to another without breaking contact in a manner so as to form another ridge. The successive ridges are manipulated into a sort of rolling movement. This movement is used mainly to remove rolling cream and to loosen, exercise, and stimulate the skin. It is called **petrissage.**

Vibratory movement: With the finger tips firmly against the skin, make a sort of trembling or oscillating movement without sliding over the skin. In this movement, the whole hand is shaken or vibrated. The attempt is to duplicate the vibration best represented by the electric vibrator.

1. Hand vibration: This is done with finger tips.
2. Electric vibration: This is done with an electric vibrator.
    (1) Direct: A soft or hard cup or brush-like applicator is applied directly to the skin, with the applicator vibrating under the force of electricity. This type is direct only in the sense that the applicator actually touches the skin.
    (2) Indirect: The electric vibrator is attached to the hand in such a way that only the fingers contact the skin.
3. Vibratory movements are used mainly for stimulation. Executed gently, lightly and slowly, they induce relaxation.
4. Do not use the electric vibrator on a person who has a weak heart, fever, or high blood pressure.

Movement and manipulation: These terms have a different meaning.

1. Movement means a stroking and rotary form of massaging that simply passes gently over the surface of the skin without affecting the underlying tissues. Movements are used to spread creams, lotions and shampoos and also to soothe and relax. Thus the terms "shampoo movements" and "rest facial movements" are used.
2. Manipulation means any type of massaging that moves the deep underlying tissues. Thus the term "scalp manipulation" is used.
3. Further clarification of terms: Movements are executed with light pressure whereas manipulations are executed with full moderate pressure. And so whether the execution is a movement or a manipulation is a matter of pressure. It is a manipulation when it is executed strongly enough to stimulate the deep tissues.
4. Movement an inclusive term. It is now clear that a movement becomes a manipulation when more than light pressure is applied. And so it is correct to use such a term as "massage movements."

Factors that determine effects of massaging:
1. The degree of pressure.
2. The duration of time.
3. The tempo or rate of speed.
4. The type of massaging.
5. The agent of contact.
6. The direction of pressure.

Massaging for stimulation: The general theory is:
1. Comparatively fast speed (not too fast).
2. Comparatively more pressure.
3. Comparatively long duration.
4. Comparatively more vigor.
5. Comparatively less rhythm.

Massaging for relaxation: The general theory is:
1. Comparatively less speed.
2. Comparatively less pressure.
3. Comparatively short duration.
4. Comparatively less vigor—they should be light, soft, and gentle.
5. Comparatively more rhythm.

Massaging scalp:
1. To stimulate scalp, use firmer touch than used to stimulate face.
2. To relax scalp, use slightly firmer touch than to relax face.

Finishing touches of massaging: The finishing touches are used in finishing a shave or facial and in the application of a tonic.

Proper degree of pressure over various conditions:
1. The thinner the skin the less the pressure:
   (1) Apply less pressure around the chin, especially on each side.
   (2) Apply less pressure on both sides of the neck.
2. The thicker the skin the firmer the pressure:
   (1) Apply more pressure around the cheeks and over the forehead.
   (2) Apply more pressure on the scalp than anywhere on the face and neck.
3. Over slight irritations, apply the minimum of pressure, if any.
4. The beginning strokes of massaging are with a little more pressure.
5. The finishing strokes of massaging are with a little less pressure.
6. The pressure is comparatively less right after a shave, on the bearded portions of the face.
7. The pressure is less when making sidewise than when making lengthwise strokes, because in the former case the movements are apt to be somewhat crosswise the tissues.
8. The pressure should be less over a face that is kept saturated with cosmetics.

9. Apply firm pressure when massaging the back of the neck.
10. Short, fast, light strokes are best for massing—in tonics and shampoos.
11. Movements involved in shampooing are vigorous.

How to determine degree of pressure:
1. Very light pressure means about one-fifth the weight of the fingers.
2. Light pressure means about one-third the weight of the fingers.
3. Moderate pressure means about the full weight of the fingers.
4. Heavy pressure means about the weight of the whole hand.
5. Very heavy pressure means more than the weight of the hands.
6. The amount of pressure suitable with an electric vibrator can be estimated in light of these pointers for the hand pressure.

Fundamental rule on pressure: The fundamental rule is to apply the pressure in the upward direction when massaging any part of the head, face and neck. This is true whether the purpose is relaxation or stimulation. The direction of a rotary movement is not important; the important thing is to apply pressure on the upward swing.

Massaging not recommended over some conditions: Manipulations more especially should not be given over the following conditions:
1. When there is an inflammation, because it would intensify it.
2. When there are pimples containing pus, because the massaging is liable to spread the infection.
3. When the patron is suffering from high blood pressure, because it would merely aggravate this trouble.

Base on face for massaging: The skin of the face should be lubricated with cream, oil, or other suitable emollients as base for massaging (1) to prevent irritation and (2) to facilitate the executions of the movements.

Essential contact with cushion tips:
1. Because these tips are soft, pliable, and cushion-like, and are, therefore, soothing and non-irritating.
2. Because the finger tips are better suited to the delicacy.
3. Massaging over the forehead, the chin, and the sides of the neck, the palm of the hand may be used frequently with preference, as well as the major cushion of the hand.

Continuous and broken contact:
1. When massaging for relaxation, contact should be continuous and unbroken. Sometimes this means keeping one hand on a given area until the other hand has made contact.
2. When massaging for stimulation, contact may be broken without violating any principle of massaging. In fact, breaking contact is inevitable when executing tapotement. But contact should not be broken in the execution of a single line of movements as in stroking,

kneading, rotation, and push-ups. At the end of a completed row or line of movements the hands may be lifted and placed for continuation.

Massage according to physical structure:
1. Massage over arteries in the upward direction.
2. Massage muscles from their insertions to their origins as a general rule.
3. Massage gently over nerve points.
4. Massage gently over thin skin.

Massaging to alleviate a headache:
1. Use light, slow, rhythmical movement.
2. Massage between the eyes, behind the ears, and on sides of neck.
3. Behind the ears and on the back sides of the neck, the pressure should be very firm.

Lips not massaged: Lips are self massaged through normal function.

Masseur and masseuse:
1. Masseur is a male practicioner of massaging.
2. Masseuse is a female practitioner of massaging.

Reasons for systematized massaging: Massaging should be systematically performed. It should not be a hit-and-miss performance. A systematic procedure has the following advantages:
1. To assure the proper apportionment of the movements—not to give some portions more than are advisable and to others fewer.
2. To assure the practice of the right type of movements over the different sections being massaged.
3. To save time—know where to begin and where to end the movements and know when the whole area is covered.
4. To impress the patron with your knowledge.
5. To be able to determine the proper duration of the massaging.
6. To assure that all sections receive equal or proper attention.

Balanced movements: This term means the pressure and duration of the movements on corresponding areas of the face and scalp are identical. This is an important principle when massaging both sides of the face simultaneously and likewise when massaging both sides of the scalp at the same time.

Routine series of movement recommended: A given set of movements should be given in series. That is execute the complete set once as outlined and then again begin and proceed in the same manner. Likewise, do not massage the same spot too long. The reason for this procedure is to prevent irritation.

Movements to improve facial expressions:

1. A drooping mouth effect can be somewhat corrected by massaging the zygomatic muscles upward and outward to strengthen these muscles to hold up the corners of the mouth.

2. The contours of the cheek can be improved by massaging the masseter muscle upward, backward, and sidewise toward the ear.

3. An extreme double chin can be lessened by massaging from the mouth and the chin to and under the chin.

4. Hollows in the neck under the ear can be lessened by massaging the sterno-cleido mastoid muscle backward, downward, and upward.

5. Youthfulness of expression can be kept or gained by building up the general health of the muscles of the face through proper massaging of those muscles.

6. Wrinkles can be postponed or lessened by massaging muscles.

Scalp Manipulations

Scalp manipulations play an important role in the rendering of various services of barbering. They are used in conjunction with every service in which it is proper to manipulate the scalp. They are especially a component of scalp treatments. They fittingly follow such services as the application of tonics, oils, hairdressing, and shampoos. The barber should master the fundamental principles of manipulations and be able to administer them scientifically. There are various systems of manipulations. Some of them are equally good. Regardless of the system of manipulations, they should be given systematically and scientifically. Any prescribed set of manipulations may be varied or modified at the discretion of the barber or to suit the policy of a particular barber shop or the needs of a particular customer.

Purposes of scalp manipulations:
1. Chief purpose: To stimulate blood circulation in the scalp.
2. Some other purposes:
   (1) To activate or normalize the function of the oil glands of the scalp.
   (2) To increase metabolism of the scalp.
   (3) To relax the nerves of the scalp.
   (4) To exercise and strengthen the muscles of the scalp.
   (5) To bring nutrition to the scalp and hair.
   (6) To help eliminate slight headaches.

Means of executing manipulations:
1. The scalp may be manipulated with the hands.
2. The scalp may be manipulated with an electric vibrator applied direct to the scalp or indirectly depending on the type of vibrator. The indirect method is preferable.

Pointers on executing manipulations:
1. **Except when one hand is used to brace the head, each hand manipulates corresponding scalp areas simultaneously.**
2. All scalp manipulations should be given slowly.
3. Over a tender scalp or over a thin scalp, the manipulations should be gentle and the series given only once.
4. Over a scalp with excessive oiliness, execute the manipulations gently and only once.
5. Over a dry scalp, the pressure should be firmer and the series given two or three times.

6. The pressure should be progressive; that is, begin lightly and gradually increase the pressure with each operation.

7. Apply pressure in the upward direction.

Scalp manipulations with vibrators: A single vibrator or twin vibrators may be used to manipulate the scalp. The general procedure is from the hairline upward to the vertex, emphasizing the areas of the arteries. The vibrations should be mild and never harsh. Vibratory manipulations increase metabolism and glandular activity as well as circulation. Such manipulations are also psychologically good.

Contact of hands during manipulations: The general rule is to keep contact with at least one hand throughout a series of manipulations. When returning to the starting position of a manipulation or when passing from the position of one manipulation to that of another manipulation, at least one hand should keep light contact with the head as the hand or hands are moved downward, sidewise, or otherwise.

Series of manipulations: A series of manipulations means the execution of the whole set of manipulations as illustrated. Executing them again constitutes a second series. The number of series given depends upon the purpose for which they are given. Following a tonic, one series is sufficient. The standard number in a scalp treatment is two series, given at intervals. In a dry scalp treatment, three to five series are recommended. Emphasize manipulations according to the need of the scalp.

Number of times to execute each manipulation: In a single series, execute Nos. 1, 2, 3 and 7 **four** times, and the rotary manipulations Nos. 4, 5, and 6 only **once**, but four rotations are made at each point. **FOUR is the key number.**

Manipulation No. 1: Stand directly behind the customer. This is a **linear** manipulation. Place the cushion tips of the fingers of the right hand at the hairline around the right ear, and place the cushion tips of the fingers of the left hand at corresponding positions on the left side. The positions of the fingers of both are taken simultaneously. Apply sufficient pressure to move the scalp, and proceed upward slowly and continuously without breaking contact, gradually spreading the fingers until the first three **fingers interlock at the vertex, as indicated in Fig. 578. Execute this** manipulation **four** times in a single series. This manipulation stimulates circulation in the superficial temporal arteries and in both of their branches, the frontal and parietal.

Manipulation No. 2: Step to the left side of the patron. Place the left hand across the forehead to brace the head. With the fingers of the right hand close together, place them at the right side of the nape well below the hairline as indicated in Fig. 579. Apply firm pressure and move upward until the small finger reaches the curvature. At this point only the small finger will be in contact with the scalp and the other fingers will be in a vertical position. Release the pressure and slide back to the starting position. Execute this manipulation **four** times. This manipulation stimulates the flow of blood in the **right** posterior auricular and the occipital arteries.

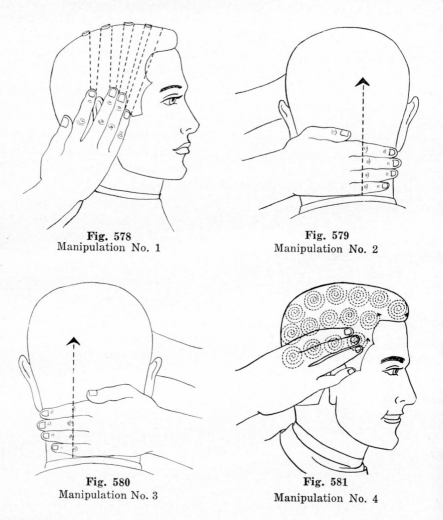

Fig. 578
Manipulation **No. 1**

Fig. 579
Manipulation **No. 2**

Fig. 580
Manipulation **No. 3**

Fig. 581
Manipulation **No. 4**

Manipulation No. 3: Step to the right side of the patron and take corresponding positions of the hands taken in Manipulation No. 2. Execute this manipulation **four** times. This manipulation stimulates the flow in the **left** posterior auricular and the occipital arteries. (Fig. 580).

Manipulation No. 4: Stand directly behind the customer. This is a **rotary** manipulation. Place the cushion tips of the first three fingers of the **right** hand at the front hairline of the right temple and at the first position of

he lowest horizontal row of rotations, as indicated in Fig. 581. Place the
:ushion tips of the first three fingers of the left hand at a corresponding
)osition at the left temple. The positions of the fingers of both hands are
aken simultaneously. Apply sufficient pressure to move the scalp, and
·otate slowly **four** times at each designated position. Start the rotations
orward and upward. Apply pressure in only the upward direction of a
·otation. Move the scalp in each individual rotation without sliding the
:ushion tips over the scalp. After the fourth rotation, move the cushion
tips backward a little more than an inch to the next position along the
;ame horizontal row. Release the pressure of the cushion tips to slide from
)ne position to another. Proceed in this manner from front to back, completing a sufficient number of rotations and rows of rotations to cover the
;ide and top portion of the scalp as indicated in Fig. 581. Complete each
·ow of rotations only **once** in a single series.

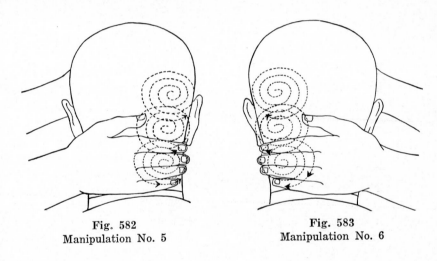

Fig. 582
Manipulation No. 5

Fig. 583
Manipulation No. 6

Manipulation No. 5: Step around to the left side of the customer. This is
a **rotary** manipulation. Place the left hand across the forehead to brace
the head. Place the cushion tips of all the fingers of the right hand well
below the hairline at the extreme right side of the nape, as indicated in
Fig. 582. Apply sufficient pressure to move the scalp, and rotate slowly
four times, moving the scalp without sliding the cushion tips over the
scalp. Start the rotations towards the ear. Apply pressure only in the upward direction of a rotation. After the fourth rotation, release the pressure and slide the hand upward about an inch to the next position
just behind the ear along the vertical row of rotations as indicated in Fig.
582. Complete this verticle row rotations only **once** in a single series.

Manipulation No. 6: Step around to the right side of the customer. This
is a **rotary** manipulation. Reverse the positions of the hands in manipula-

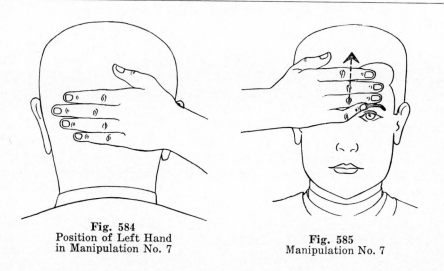

Fig. 584
Position of Left Hand
in Manipulation No. 7

Fig. 585
Manipulation No. 7

tion No. 5, placing the right hand across the forehead and the cushion
tips of the left hand well below the hairline and at the extreme left side of
the nape. Execute this manipulation in the same manner as Manipulation
No. 5. Complete this vertical row of rotation only **once** in a single series.
(Fig. 583).

Manipulation No. 7: Remain standing at the right side of the customer.
This is a **linear** manipulation. Open the left hand and place it on the back
of the patron's head near the crown to brace the head (Fig. 584). Place
the first three fingers of the right hand across the forehead so that the
third finger rests just above the eyebrows. Relax these fingers so that
they lie against and over the front portion of the forehead. Apply
sufficient pressure to move the scalp and slide the right hand slowly
upward over theforehead to about an inch past the front hairline, as
indicated in Fig. 585. As the right hand moves upward, the left hand
is kept **stationary** at the back of the patron's head to keep the head
steady. Execute this manipulation **four** times in a single series. This
manipulation stimulates the flow of blood in the supra-orbital arteries.

Scalp Treatments

The care and treatment of the scalp are well within the scope of the professional barber. The more serious and contagious conditions should be referred to a dermatologist, but there are many common and minor conditions and ailments that can be treated successfully by the barber. While the barber is limited to the treatment of certain conditions, he has almost unrestricted range in the care of the scalp. The public expects the barber to be able to give scientific scalp treatments.

The scalp is vitally related to the hair, and what is beneficial to the scalp is usually beneficial to the hair. A healthy scalp is the chief prerequisite to healthy hair. The use of the term "scalp treatment" in this book implies "hair treatment." All scalp treatments give some consideration to the hair, likewise, all hair treatments give some consideration to the scalp. The widely accepted term for a scalp treatment is "Scalpial."

Definition: A scalp treatment means cleansing, massaging, and the applying of a scalp preparation.

Major purposes of scalp treatments:
1. To maintain the health of the scalp and hair.
2. To correct unhealthy and undesired conditions of the scalp and hair.
3. To promote the growth of hair.

Requisite knowledge for treating scalp: To be able to give scalp treatments successfully and to use accurate and convincing terminology, the barber should study the following subjects which are discussed in other chapters of this book:
1. Structure and function of the scalp.
2. Structure, growth and regrowth of the hair.
3. Blood circulation of the scalp.
4. Nerve points of the scalp.
5. Metabolism.
6. Principles of massaging.
7. Shampoos.
8. Tonics, ointments and special scalp preparations.
9. Electrical appliances to be used.
10. Common scalp disorders.
11. Scalp manipulations.

Some items of which scalp treatments consist:
1. Shampoos.
2. Massaging.
3. Such electrical appliances as dermal lights, infra-red lamp, violet ray, vibrators, and electric steamers.
4. Tonics and special preparations.
5. Application of steam-towels.

Scientific basis of scalp treatment: Three types of services involved in scalp treatments are indisputably scientific. There are many more scientific services, but these are paramount and uniquely summarize the essence of the scientific aspect.
1. Cleansing the scalp.
2. Manipulation of the scalp.
3. Application of antiseptics.

Major scalp ailments:
1. Dryness
2. Oiliness
3. Dandruff
4. Falling hair
5. Itching
6. Dullness of color

Some causes of scalp ailments:
1. Personal negligence.
2. Inability of the layman completely to take care of his scalp.
3. Use of wrong kind of cosmetics.
4. Poor physical condition of the body.
5. Exposure to unfavorable climatic conditions.
6. Poor blood circulation.
7. Sluggish oil glands.
8. Over-active oil glands.
9. Invasion of germs.
10. Mechanical injury of scalp.
11. Use of improper cleansing agents.
12. Food deficiencies.

Preliminary steps to scalp treatment: These steps properly constitute a diagnosis:
1. Examine the scalp and hair carefully, trying to detect any observable difficulties such as dry, scaly dandruff, oily, waxy dandruff, the presence of some disease, dry, brittle hair, split ends of hair, apparent general neglect, tight scalp, etc.
2. By asking the patron, find out what other symptoms there are, such as itching, amount of hair that is falling out, the reaction of the hair to shampoos, etc.
3. Find out what sort of shampoo the patron has been using. And then advise the proper kind.

4. Find out how long the patron has had the condition.
5. Find out what the patron has already done.
6. Classify, if possible, the particular difficulty.
7. Assure the patron that you have scientific treatments that will greatly alleviate the condition, if such is true.
8. Make tabulations of all the significant facts of the case, along with the patron's name and address.
9. Rarely, when the case is baffling, ask the patron for his permission to work on the case by doing a little research, telling him that you are not quite sure at the moment as to all the steps to take, although you are sure of some scientific steps, and that you will be happy to do some special research on the condition.
10. Acquaint the patron with the value of proper shampooing, scalp manipulation, certain preparations, and scientific treatments.

How purposes of scalp treatments are accomplished:

1. By cleansing the scalp and hair, by means of a suitable shampoo.
2. By increasing circulation, by means of manipulation, high frequency, heat applications, and solutions.
3. By strengthening the muscles of the scalp by means of manipution, electricity, and heat.
4. By use of antiseptics.
5. By regulating glandular activity, by means of manipulation, electricity, and heat.
6. By soothing and resting the nerves, by means of manipulation, high frequency, and heat.
7. By rendering germs harmless, by means of antiseptics.
8. By nourishing the scalp and hair, by means of stimulating circulation.
9. By promoting metabolism, by means of manipulations, high frequency, and heat.
10. By stimulation, by all means of just mentioned methods.
11. By setting up natural resistance against the invasion of disease producing germs through maintaining or building up the health of the scalp and hair, and by means of all methods listed above.

Why normal scalp needs scalp treatments:

1. The scalp is the highest point from the heart and, therefore, circulation is very apt to be insufficient, especially if the physical condition generally is not up to par. Artificial stimulation, such as hand and electric manipulations bring about, is recommended.
2. Disease germs often invade the scalp and hair. Their activity should be checked.
3. Accumulations on the scalp must occasionally be cleaned off, else they will breed germs and clog pores.

4. Scalp treatments help keep the scalp loose and flexible and thus assures normal circulation.
5. A treatment serves as check-up.
6. A treatment provides an occasion for advice on care of scalp and hair.

When not to suggest scalp treatment:
1. When the patron makes known his dire poverty.
2. When serving a one-year-old child.
3. When the scalp is broken out with such ailments that should not be massaged or treated by the barber.
4. When the patron is definitely in a hurry.
5. When there is definitely no need.
6. When the patron definitely says he does not want a treatment.

Fitting moments to suggest scalp treatment:
1. When manipulating the scalp as a matter of general procedure, just before the final combing, after any service.
2. During the last half of the process of a haircut.
3. When the patron complains of an itching scalp.
4. When the patron makes a general inquiry about scalp treatments.
5. When a patron speaks of wanting to look his best.
6. During the process of conversation which you have directed to lead up to the suggestion, having observed a particular need.

Standard number of series of treatments: The average number of treatments in a series is ten. The number recommended depends on the particular condition. Even after a series of treatments has been given, an occasional treatment thereafter is advisable.

Frequency of treatments in series: Ideally, the patron should have two weekly, but he should have at least one a week as a minimum.

Purposes of manipulating scalp: The purposes are set forth in the chapter on massaging and again in the earlier part of this discussion in pointing out the purposes of massaging and the purposes of scalp treatments respectively. It might be added, however, for sake of emphasis, that the chief purpose of scalp manipulations is to stimulate circulation the value of which lies mainly in the fact that by this means the scalp and hair receive their nourishment.

1. To increase circulation of the scalp.
2. To activate the oil glands of the scalp.
3. To increase metabolism of the scalp.
4. To relax the nerves of the scalp.
5. To exercise and strengthen the muscles of the scalp.
6. To aid the scalp to absorb scalp preparations.

Number of times to manipulate scalp: The number of times a complete set of manipulations should be executed in a scalp treatment depends on the particular condition of the scalp, the treatment being given, the charge for the treatment, and the need. The following suggestions should prove helpful:

1. For the preliminary—before any preparation is applied to the scalp —execute the set of manipulations once.
2. Over the special preparation before the shampoo, execute the set once.
3. Over the final preparation, such as a special ointment, solution, or tonic, execute the set once or twice.

Difference between scalp treatment and shampoo: While there is a difference between a scalp treatment and a shampoo, some of the steps of procedure are the same. Ordinarily, a scalp treatment includes some kind of shampoo. The purpose, products and appliances used in a scalp treatment differentiate it significantly from a shampoo.

1. The essential purpose of a shampoo is to cleanse; whereas, the chief purpose of a scalp treatment, regularly, is to correct an unhealthy condition such as dandruff, dryness, oiliness, etc.
2. Scalp manipulations receive a greater emphasis in a scalp treatment than in a shampoo. In a shampoo the scalp manipulations regularly precede the shampoo only; whereas, in a scalp treatment the manipulations are regularly given at three different stages, namely, (1) as a preliminary, (2) over the preparation prior to the shampoo, and (3) over the final preparation after the shampoo.
3. Electricity enters into a scalp treatment more than into a shampoo. For instance, a scalp treatment may include the use of a high frequency current, infra-red lamp, or dermal lights.
4. Special remedial preparations are applied to and sometimes left on the scalp during a scalp treatment. The preparations used for a shampoo are typically designed for just cleansing and rinsing out.
5. A scalp treatment involves a little more careful analysis of the condition itself, its causes, and its treatment.

Words to use sparingly: Three words that should be used sparingly and advisedly are "guarantee," "cure," and "absolutely." These are the play words of quackery. Rather than guarantee the results of a treatment, it is better to assure the patron that you have faith in your recommendation and that you believe that the treatment will bring good results. You can also say that it is the best treatment for the particular condition, and that it is surely worth trying. You can also assure the patron that the scalp treatment involves the known scientific steps for treating his condition, such as those that secure thorough cleanliness, normal circulation, stimulation, relaxation, antisepsis, etc. The alleged merits of such steps are well supported by science.

Gain customer's confidence: The customer will have more confidence in the barber if he will only make truthful statements about the care and treatment of the scalp. If the area of scalp treatments is not to degenerate into quackery, the barber should practice the policy that **no guarantee** should be made to prevent loss of hair or to restore hair. Some patrons should be advised to consult a physician for certain scalp conditions, but the ills caused by the neglect of the hair and scalp, by tight scalp muscles, by over-relaxed or inactive oil glands, by tense nerves, and by retarded circulation in the scalp, can be either remedied or alleviated by proper scalp treatments, that is, by proper cleansing, scientific manipulations, and antiseptic tonics. While such treatments may only postpone baldness due to hereditary predisposition and constitutional weakness and to some other uncontrollable causes, a great deal can be accomplished to correct conditions caused by simple neglect and to other causes which can be identified and removed, such as improper cleansing, tight muscles and nerves, and poor circulation. The scalp responds to treatment in much the same way as any other part of the body—it needs to be **cleansed, ventilated, exercised** (massaged), and **antisepticized.** Keep these fundamental needs in mind when prescribing a scalp treatment. Bear in mind too that the tissues surrounding the hair papilla contain loops of tiny blood vessels, and it is from the constantly arriving blood that these tissues obtain the substances that sustain and nourish them. A proper blood supply to the scalp is indispensable, and upon this factor depend the vigor of the papilla and follicle, and the growth of the hair, its length, its life span duration, and its glossiness and health.

The scalp cannot exercise itself adequately, especially when tissues begin to shrink and harden. Mechanical means such as hand and electric manipulations must be resorted to for the indispensable stimulation.

Beneficial results of scalp treatments epitomized: Scientific scalp treatments are scientific in that they accomplish the following:
1. Thorough cleansing of the scalp.
2. Increased blood supply of the scalp.
3. Increased or normalized activity of the sebaceous (oil) glands.
4. Strengthening of the muscles of the scalp.
5. Soothing of the nerves of the scalp and the relaxing of any abnormal tension.

Ways of suggesting scalp treatments: Customer may be induced to have a scalp treatment by either direct or indirect suggestions. While the positive direct suggestion is more effective with some customers, the indirect appeals most to other customers. Use a firm but well modulated voice when suggesting a treatment.

1. Direct suggestions:
   (1) Would you like to have a scalp treatment? I notice your scalp is very dry.
   (2) Would you like to have a scalp treatment? I notice that your scalp is very oily.
   (3) Does your scalp itch? If the answer is "yes," ask him if he would like to have a scalp treatment.
   (4) Would you like to have a scalp treatment for your dandruff? We have a very good treatment.
   (5) Are you doing anything to get rid of your dandruff? Your recommendation will be determined by his answer.
   (6) I notice your hair is thinning out. Have you ever had a scalp treatment? If the answer is "no," recommend that he have a few to see what can be done.
   (7) I would like to suggest a _____treatment. I notice that your hair is _____. Would you like to have a treatment today? It would be worth trying.

2. Indirect suggestions:
   (1) Your hair is abnormally dry and brittle. A hot oil treatment would help correct this condition.
   (2) Your scalp is extremely oily. If this oil is allowed to remain on your scalp it will clog the pores and interfere with function of the sebaceous glands.
   (3) Your scalp muscles are extremely tight. A scalp treatment that includes scalp manipulations would correct this condition. These tight muscle prevent proper circulation and consequently the hair suffers from lack of sufficient nourishment.
   (4) When you can spare the time, I would like to give you a Violet Ray Scalp Treatment. Your scalp is too dry for the continuance of your fine head of hair. Eventually, this condition is going to affect the hair, and then it may be too late. This treatment will stimulate the sebaceous glands and blood circulation of the scalp.
   (5) From looking at your scalp I wonder if you have an itching scalp? If the answer is "yes," suggest scalp treatment that will alliviate the condition, but do not guarantee to stop it completely.
   (6) The best way to keep your fine head of hair is to have a scalp treatment once in a while. Such treatment preserves the

health of the scalp and hair and helps prevent scalp ailments. (If patron asks how often, recommend one a month).

(7) We have scalp treatments designed to keep the scalp and hair healthy. Sometime I would like to give you one.

(8) You know of course that your hair is falling out. We have treatments to prevent falling hair. While I cannot guarantee to stop your hair from falling out, I recommend that you take a series of these treatments. They are the result of scientific research, and they have a lot of merit. If I were you I would try them.

(9) I suppose you know you have Pityriasis. This condition usually gets worse. I recommend that you have a treatment. Pityriasis means excessive dandruff. A great deal of research has been done on this subject and as a result we have some very effective treatments.

(10) You are approaching Alopecia Prematura. This means your hair is falling out and you might become prematurely bald. As a result of scientific research, we have good preventive treatments which I believe are worth your while to try. These treatments might prevent the condition from getting worse. As yet science has done little to restore hair, but it is believed that in many instances the right treatments will postpone baldness.

Use of hair brush: The use of hair brushes is practically discontinued in barber shops, because they are very difficult to sterilize. Their use however has scientific merit, if stiff irritating bristles are not used. The brush removes flakes of dandruff, helps to cleanse the hair, and distributes sebum (natural oil) along the hair shaft. The use of individually owned hair brushes is recommended. When treating excessive dandruff, brushing the hair thoroughly is recommended prior to the application of a shampoo or other scalp preparations. Brushing also helps bring stubborn hair under control.

Use of fine tooth comb: The use of a very fine tooth comb to remove dandruff should be discouraged. The teeth are so sharp that they irritate the scalp and thus create a new crop of dead cells or dandruff. And the teeth are so close together that they might injure the hair shaft. Used gently though it will do no damage.

Applying oil to scalp: There are several good ways to apply oil to the scalp. The following are some of the methods: (Refer to p. 260).

1. By a medicine dropper—a dispenser which releases oil in drops.
2. By a spray designed to dispense oil.
3. Direct from a bottle with the proper nozzle.
4. By a cotton pledget or cotton pad. Simply immerse cotton into a pan of oil, squeeze the cotton to release the excess oil so that it will

not drip, carry it over the palm to the scalp, and rub it in.

5. Detail of application. Part the hair at center of head with a coarse comb. Keep the hair parted with the thumb and second finger of the left hand. Apply the oil as just explained, starting at the crown and working to the front hairline. Proceed in like manner, making the parts about three-quarters of an inch apart, until both sides of the head are covered. Finish one side before doing the other. At the edge where the hair is too short to part, comb it upward and hold it in place with the comb, apply the oil and immediately rub it in with the finger tips of the right hand. When the sides are completed, start at the crown area and work to the edge at the nape. Make the first part in the center of the back.

Massaging oily preparation into scalp: The regular shampoo movements may be used to further distribute the oil over the scalp, but the following recommended types of massaging are for working the oil into the pores of the scalp. The massaging should be started as soon as the oil is applied to each area or strip made by parting. This preliminary massaging keeps the oil from running and aids distribution. The general massaging is done after all the scalp has been covered and the scalp has been tentatively massaged. There are several good methods of massaging oil into the scalp.

1. With the fingers of either the left or the right hand close together, place all four finger tips firmly against the scalp at the upper end of the part near the crown, brace these fingers by pressing the thumb against the scalp, and then execute four rotary manipulations. The scalp itself should be moved and the finger tips should not slide over the scalp during the manipulations. On the fourth rotation, slide along the part and repeat the manipulations. In this way cover the whole part, and eventually the whole scalp. Alternate the hands to preserve energy, if necessary.

2. With the same placement of the finger tips as just explained, simply vibrate instead of rotating.

3. Place the thumb cushion of each hand about one inch apart right in the part near the crown and execute four semi-circular manipulations in opposite directions in such a way that the thumbs appear to be following each other. Press firmly enough to move the scalp.

Distributing scalp oil through hair: As soon as the entire scalp is saturated with scalp oil and prior to the use of some means to aid penetration, it should be distributed through the hair. Lay the comb almost flat—flatwise to the scalp—and, starting at the scalp, comb through to the end of the hair. Work from the hairline upward, from the front hairline to the crown, and diagonally across the head.

Points of similarity and differences in scalp treatments: The **beginning** and **end steps** of scalp treatments are often the same. Each treatment is in three parts—(1) Basic preliminaries, (2) body, and (3) finish. The essential variations come in the body—the middle part where there are choices of shampoos, ointments, appliances, and tonics. The purposes of the various treatments may over-lap.

1. Some **points** of **similarity** in scalp treatments are linen set-ups, manipulation, shampoos, scalp or hair preparations, electric appliances, and tonics.
2. Some **points** of **difference** in scalp treatments pertain to the degree and nature of manipulations, kind of shampoos or scalp preparations, degree and kind of electric appliances, any kind of tonics.

Types of scalp treatments: Scalp treatments may be classified according to their purpose or purposes. Not all scalp treatments have the same purpose, although the purpose or purposes sometimes over-lap and so what one scalp treatment does another one does in part. There are some common purposes, such as cleansing, stimulation or relaxation, soothing, and the checking of disease germs via antiseptics. Scalp treatments fall under four categories:

1. Preservative—to maintain the health of the scalp.
2. Corrective—to counteract or remove scalp ailments.
3. Alleviative—to relieve a scalp condition.
4. Cosmetic—to cleanse, soothe, and beautify, and includes pleasurable grooming.

Procedures of various scalp treatments: It is unnecessary to memorize the step-by-step procedure of the treatments outlined for the various scalp conditions. As just explained, the preliminary and finishing steps are either the same or approximately so. Only the body—the steps between these two divisions are different. The barber should also keep in mind the **three basic operations** of scalp treatments, namely, (1) cleansing the scalp through the medium of a shampoo, (2) stimulating the blood supply to the scalp through the medium of manipulation and massaging, and (3) the application of antiseptic preparations. In addition, corrective and alleviative lotions or ointments are sometimes applied to the scalp, and such electric appliances as the violet ray, dermal lights, and the infrared lamp are used.

With knowledge of these fundamentals, of the various products and of the electric appliances, scalp treatments can be prescribed for a particular condition. It is imperative for the competent barber to familiarize himself with the various products—tonics, oils, ointments—on the market, and to follow closely the manufacturer's directions. Give particular attention to the standard pattern procedure now to be outlined. Learning this outline will greatly simplify learning the basic steps of any scalp treatment.

1. Linen set-up.
2. Methods of applying scalp oil.
3. Steaming in oil or ointment.

Linen Set-ups for Scalp Treatment

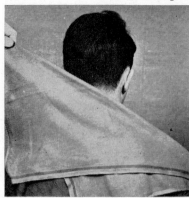

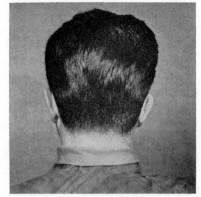

Fig. 586
Step No. 1

Fig. 587
Step No. 2

Diagonal Towel Set-up

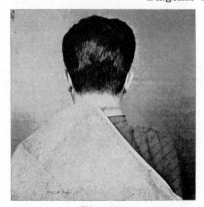

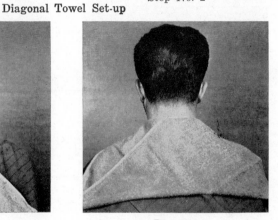

Fig. 588
Step No. 3

Fig. 589
Completed Set-up

Diagonal Towel Set-up

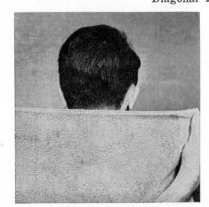

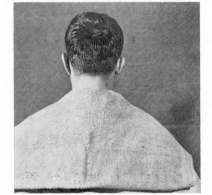

Fig. 590   **Fig. 591**
Square as Alternate to Diagonal Use of Towel in Figs. 588-89

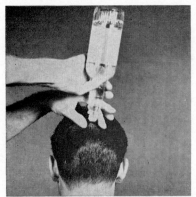
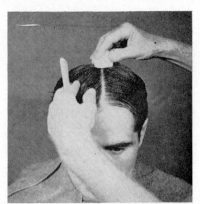

Fig. 592   Fig. 593
Methods of Applying Oil to Scalp

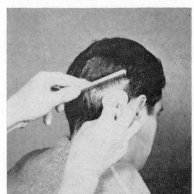
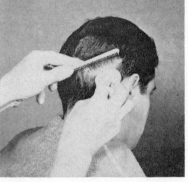

Fig. 594   Fig. 595
Applying Oil to Scalp

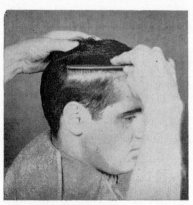
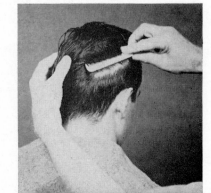

Fig. 596   Fig. 597
Combing Oil Through Hair
Comb Hair in Various Directions

Disregard Linen Set-up used in Steaming Scalp.
Pictures Taken From Chapter on "Tonics."

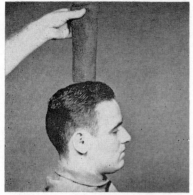

Fig. 598
Step No. 1

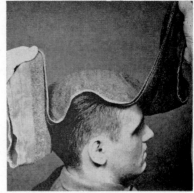

Fig. 599
Step No. 2

Steaming Scalp

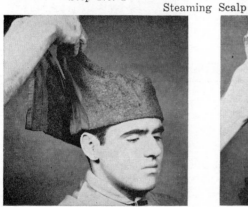

Fig. 600
Step No. 3

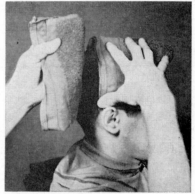

Fig. 601
Step. No. 4

Steaming Scalp

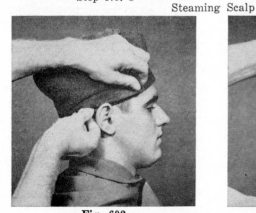

Fig. 602
Step. No. 5

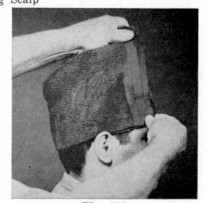

Fig. 603
Step No. 6

Steaming Scalp

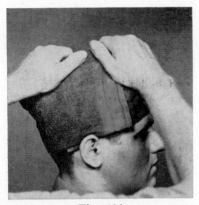

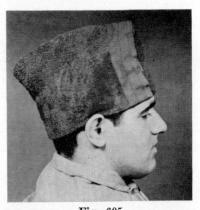

Fig. 604
Step No. 7

Fig. 605
Final Step

Steaming Scalp

STANDARD OUTLINE FOR SCALP TREATMENTS

The outline of procedure to follow sets a **pattern** or **standard** of proce
dure. It is largely a skeleton of the steps included in most scalp treat
ments. The procedure of any scalp treatment is drawn up after the manne
of this one. The different products used make the procedure for a give
scalp treatment slightly different. The kind of shampoo, the degree c
manipulation, the kind of ointment or tonic, the kind of special prepara
tion used, the use of the violet ray, will be determined by the conditio
of the particular scalp. The **purpose of this outline** is simply to set up
general pattern for scalp treatments. By selecting the shampoo, ointmen
or other special scalp preparation, and regulating the degre
and pressure of manipulations, according to the particular conditio
being treated, this treatment outline may be followed. Manufacturers c
cosmetics, such as shampoos, ointments, scalp creams, and tonics ar
glad to furnish the barber information on the purposes and the manner c
application of their products.

Purposes: (These vary according to the procedure and products but th
following are examples).

1. To preserve and build up the health of the scalp and hair in genera
2. To check falling hair.
3. To correct a dandruff condition.
4. To correct either dryness or oiliness.

How results are achieved:

1. By proper cleansing.
2. By manipulations.
3. By special preparations.
4. By use of special electrical appliances such as the high frequenc

the electric vibrator, infra-red lamp, red dermal light, and electric steamer.

Procedure:
1. Arrange linen set-up.
2. Place necessaries in readiness.
3. Execute scalp manipulations once.
4. Give proper shampoo:
   (1) If the scalp is dry, give an oil shampoo.
   (2) If the scalp is oily, give a tar or green soap shampoo.
   (3) If the scalp is tender and sensitive, give an egg shampoo, cream shampoo, or soothing foaming oil shampoo.
5. Use violet ray about three minutes.
6. Follow ONE of the following steps:
   (1) Apply a tonic of proven merit, and make two steam towel applications.
   (2) Apply an ointment, such as the sulphur ointment, and follow with the red dermal light, infra-red lamp, or steam towels.
7. Manipulate scalp from three to five minutes.
8. Dress hair as desired.

Remarks: This treatment may be called either a "General Scalp Treatment" or an "All Purpose Scalp Treatment." It is actually a treatment that leaves much to the discretion of the barber and the choice of the shampoo depends on the condition of the scalp.

PLAIN SCALP TREATMENT
(Also known as Normal Scalp Treatment)

Purpose: To keep the scalp healthy.

Procedure:
1. Linen set-up.
2. Place necessaries in readiness.
3. Shampoo.
4. Manipulate the scalp three to five minutes.
5. Apply tonic.
6. Dress hair.

Remarks: The plain scalp treatment may be given when the customer is short of time, when no particular abnormal condition exists, or when the charge has to be nominal.

HOT OIL SCALP TREATMENT

The Hot Oil Scalp Treatment consists mainly of an oil and a shampoo.

Purpose: To alleviate dryness. (It may also be recommended for a normal scalp.)

How purpose is accomplished:
1. By dislodging any scales and dirt, scientifically.
2. By unclogging the openings of the hair follicles.
3. By feeding the scalp and hair.
4. By stimulating the oil glands.
5. By providing sufficient lubrication to keep the dry hair from breaking off—replacing the deficiencies of natural oil.
6. By reducing itching.
7. By applying scientific preparations.

Procedure:
1. Arrange linen set-up.
2. Place necessaries in readiness.
3. Execute scalp manipulations once.
4. Apply oil. (Olive oil or special scalp oil) (See Figs. 592-597).
5. Execute scalp manipulations once.
6. Increase penetration of oil.
   (1) By using a red dermal light or infra-red lamp for five minutes.
   (2) By making five steam towel applications, or
   (3) By using an electric steamer from three to five minutes.
7. Give good liquid soap shampoo.
8. Complete in one of the following ways:
   (1) Apply a tonic which contains oil.
   (2) Apply a little scalp oil directly to the scalp. Use a very small cotton pledget or atomizer.
   (3) Aid penetration of preparation applied.
9. Execute scalp manipulations once or twice.
10. Dress hair as desired.

Remarks: Since excessive dryness is due to sluggishness of the oil glands this treatment is designed to activate them.

DRY DANDRUFF TREATMENT

Purpose: To remove and control dandruff.

Procedure:
1. Arrange linen set-up.
2. Place necessaries in readiness.
3. Apply direct to the scalp a vegetable oil (olive, castor, almond, or special scalp oil.)
4. Accelerate penetration by one of the following means:
   (1) Electric steamer from three to five minutes.
   (2) Red dermal light or infra-red lamp from three to five minutes.
   (3) Five to seven steam towel applications.
5. Execute scalp manipulations once.

6. Give shampoo, such as foamy soapless oil, medicated, liquid soap, creme or shampoo manufactured for dry dandruff.
7. Use the violet ray about three minutes.
8. Apply a tonic or an ointment containing sulphur, lanolin, resorcin, glycerin, ammoniated mercury, olive oil, etc. (The barber should not make up this ointment.)
9. Use red dermal light or infra-red lamp about three minutes or make five steam towel applications.
10. Execute scalp manipulations once.
11. Dress hair as desired.

Remarks: This treatment emphasizes stimulation of the Sebaceous glands. Dandruff may be oily but it is typically dry. This treatment is worth while even if it only **removes** dandruff and thus partially keeps it under control.

How Doctors' Prescriptions for Dandruff May Read

WARNING: For external use only.
POISONOUS if taken internally.
1. Wash hair with bland soap; rinse thoroughly.
2. Work 1 to 2 tsp. of medicine into scalp, using warm water to lather. Avoid contact with eyes.
3. Rinse. Repeat step 2.
4. Allow medicine to remain on scalp five minutes.
5. Rinse scalp thoroughly. Bland soap may be used to aid removal of medicine.
6. After treatment, wash your hands and under fingernails.
7. Repeat treatment as directed by physician.

ITCHING SCALP TREATMENT

In giving an itching scalp treatment, use soothing and oily substances. Itching is sometimes the result of excessive dryness. One or more of the following or their equivalents should be used: sulphur ointment, cream shampoo, special preparations to alleviate itching, tonics containing camphor or menthol or lanolin.

Purpose: To alleviate an itching scalp.

Procedure:
1. Linen set-up.
2. Comb scalp vigorously with the coarse comb.
3. Do one of the following:
   (1) Apply a preparation especially manufactured for an itching scalp, following manufacturer's directions.
   (2) Give shampoo, such as soapless oil, medicated, liquid soap, creme or shampoo manufactured for itching scalp.
4. Emphasize rinsing.

5. Apply special scalp preparation, such as:
   (1) Sulphur ointment.
   (2) An ointment or liquid labeled for this purpose.
   (3) Tonic with menthol.
6. If ointment is applied use either the red dermal light or infra-re
   lamp. If an aqueous lotion is used, such as a tonic, make three stea
   towel applications.
7. Dress hair.

Remarks: Itching may be due to excessive dryness caused by the inactivit
of the oil glands. This treatment stimulates these glands. Insufficier
rinsing and neglect can also cause itching.

DRY SCALP TREATMENT

The treatments for dry dandruff or itching scalp may be given for
dry scalp. Emphasize scalp manipulations.

Purpose: To correct or alleviate dryness.

Procedure:

1. Linen set-up.
2. Manipulate scalp.
3. Apply scalp oil and aid penetration. (This step is optional.)
4. Shampoo with foamy oil shampoo—two applications.
5. Execute scalp manipulations twice.
6. Use violet ray three or four minutes.
7. Apply suitable tonic or other preparation and aid penetration.
8. Execute scalp manipulations—twice.
9. Dress hair as desired.
10. Recommend daily use of hair creme or other suitable preparatio

OILY SCALP TREATMENT
(Also known as Oily Dandruff Treatment)

Purpose: To remove and control excessive oiliness.

Procedure:

1. Arrange linen set-up.
2. Execute the scalp manipulations once. (Execute them gently so a
   not to excite the sebaceous glands. The pressure should be sufficier
   to permit pressing and squeezing to dislodge any hardened sebu
   in the pores of the scalp.)
3. Give a tar or green soap shampoo, or a shampoo manufactured fc
   oiliness.
4. Use a mild high-frequency current for three minutes.

5. Apply a scalp astringent tonic. A quinine tonic is recommended. Massage in well. Absorb excessive moisture from hair with turkish towel. There are some ointments that may be used instead of an astringent tonic.

6. Dress hair as desired.

Remarks: Excessive oiliness is caused by accelerated action of the oil glands. The attempt here is to normalize the function of these glands. Give this treatment also for "oily dandruff".

ALOPECIA AREATA TREATMENT

The barber should not serve a patron who has a contagious kind of alopecia areata (baldness in spots). When the condition is not contagious, the following treatment is recommended, but the patron should be advised to consult a physician. The treatment should be helpful and advisedly be given in cooperation with a physician.

Purpose: To stimulate the growth of hair.

Procedure:

1. Linen set-up.

2. Cleanse scalp with a cream shampoo, egg shampoo, any good foaming oil shampoo, or soapless oil shampoo.

3. Either paint spots with iodine or a sulphur ointment, or a good ointment labeled for that purpose may be used instead of the iodine. If ointment is used, aid penetration by dermal light, infra-red lamp, or steam towels.

4. Manipulate scalp gently from three to five minutes.

5. Dress hair.

Remarks: Some cases of alopecia areata are temporary and will respond quickly to treatment. The high-frequency may be used right after the shampoo. Do not shampoo over or treat this condition unless you know it is not contagious. This treatment could advisedly be reduced to a shampoo and tonic and called "shampoo treatment".

FALLING HAIR TREATMENT

Whatever treatment helps to normalize the sebaceous glands, activate metabolism of the scalp, stimulate circulation of the scalp, and properly cleanses the scalp will help stop falling hair. That is, any treatment that makes the scalp healthy is properly a falling hair treatment. A scalp that is properly taken care of will be less likely to lose hair abnormally. Make no pre-treatment claims of assurance. Recommend the treatment on the basis of the introductory remarks and assure the customer that the treatment is based on scientific research.

Purpose: To help postpone or prevent baldness.

Procedure:

1. Linen set-up.
2. Place necessaries in readiness.
3. Execute scalp manipulations once.
4. Give a shampoo in accordance with instructions in the "Standard Procedure for Scalp Treatments", or give any shampoo or combination medicine and shampoo prepared by a physician or a manufacturer especially for falling hair.
5. Use violet ray from three to five minutes.
6. Apply a tonic suitable for the scalp and make two steam towel applications.
7. Execute the scalp manipulations three to five times. Or, complete two series, and then massage the scalp with an indirect vibrator for two or three minutes.
8. Dress hair.

Remarks: Vary the steps of procedure according to the products used. If an ointment is used instead of the tonic, use a red dermal light, infra-red lamp, or steam towels to aid penetration. The ointment should be applied after the violet ray is used.

LICE AND NITS

All lice and nit cases should be referred to a physician.

ALOPECIA TREATMENTS

Treatments for alopecia or for normal or abnormal baldness depend on the particular type of alopecia and the scalp and conditions occurring with it. In such treatments the attempt is to remove the cause or causes, if possible, and to build up the general health of the scalp. Science has not revealed absolute cures. The following recommendations should prove helpful:

1. **Alopecia Adnata.** Baldness at birth or subsequent thereafter is not treated by the barber. Refer to a physician.
2. **Alopecia Areata.** Refer to the outlined treatment in this chapter.
3. **Alopecia Prematura.** This area of baldness constitutes most of the treatments for the loss of hair. Refer to Falling Hair Treatment in this chapter.
4. **Alopecia Senilis.** Recommend either a Plain or Standard Treatment. Baldness due to senility is least likely to respond to treatment. It is advisable to confine your recommendation to a shampoo.

5. **Alopecia Universalis.** Recommend only a shampoo.

6. Alopecia may be associated with a contagious disease such as syphilis. If such is known, do not serve the patron.

Choose a treatment according to accompanying conditions, such as the following:

HAIR CONDITIONERS

Hair conditioners are usually creme preparations. They impart body to the hair, bring back natural lustre to dry, dull hair, give new elasticity to brittle, over-bleached or over relaxed hair, or damaged hair. Recommended also to insure even tints and toners. There are many brands on the market.

1. Shampoo. Squeeze out excess water.

2. Apply about ½ ounce. More for fine hair. Distribute through hair evenly with fingers and a coarse comb.

3. Leave on one to three minutes. (Follow manufacturer's instruction.)

4. Water rinse out.

Brands and Procedures: No names of products—shampoos, ointments, tonics, or any preparations—are given in this book. Instead, treatments for major scalp conditions have been outlined and procedures suggested. They are all flexible and may be varied to the degrees of the condition and according to the products used. It is better to have a knowledge of the general principles of scalp treatments than to memorize an outline of a treatment for a particular condition, or learn to apply certain brands of products. With the knowledge in this chapter, however, one should be able to follow any manufacturer's instructions for using products.

Central point of view in scalp treatments: In the final analysis the main attempt is yet to **prevent** baldness rather than to restore hair.

Rest Facial Movements

The Rest Facial Massage Movements are a set of twelve massage movements designed to cover the entire face and the neck. They are illustrated according to number and a defined area. For example, Movement No. 1 has a definite starting and terminating point and covers a specific area. The same can be said of each of the other movements. The various movements are given according to a specified sequence and each one is executed a specified number of times.

These facial movements are not confined to any one facial. They may be given in any facial in which it is proper to do massaging. When to give them and how many series to execute are largely at the discretion of the barber. In some facials only one series is given, but in the Rest Facial three series are given. The barber may elect to give part or all the movements in conjunction with some service such as a Plain Facial or a shave. Numbers 2, 4, 10, 11, and 12 may very fittingly be given as part of the finish of a shave. In fact, this set of movements is also known as the "Standard Facial Massage Movements," since they constitute a pattern of facial movements usable in so many facials. The movements are scientific in that they are designed with consideration of the nerves and muscles.

Chief Purpose of Movements: The chief purpose of the rest facial movements is to induce **relaxation.** The pointers on how to give these movements reflects knowledge of the nature of nerves and the ways of relaxing them. For example, in movements 1, 7, and 8, the cushion tips pause and vibrate over important nerve centers.

Pointers on executing movements: Execute the movements slowly, gently, rhythmically, with moderation, and continuously without breaking contact within or between movements, for the usual purpose is to relax the nerves.

Other purposes of movements: In addition to relaxing the nerves, this set of movements accomplishes the following:

1. Releases tense muscles.
2. Tones up sagging, fatigued muscles.
3. Soothes tired eyes.
4. Gives a feeling of rejuvenation.
5. Relieves the intensity of passing headaches.
6. Helps to avert wrinkles.
7. Builds up tissues.
8. Stimulates circulation. (Explanation in following paragraph).

Reverse routine of movements for stimulation: By changing the nature of executing the movements and reversing the routine, these movements may be given for stimulation. Start with No. 12 and finish with No. 1. By the reverse order the procedure is from the lower points upward in harmony with the physiology of the circulatory system. For this purpose execute the movements faster, firmly enough to move the underlying tissues, and do each movement three times instead of twice. When the movements are given in this way, they become manipulations, because they are stimulatory and affect the deeper underlying tissues.

Movements executed with hands or vibrator: These movements are designed mainly to be executed with the finger tips of the hands, but they may be given with the indirect twin electric vibrators, with one attached to the back of each hand. The use of the vibrator steps up the movements and converts their purpose to stimulation. (Refer to Amplified Facial).

Use both hands: In every movement except 3, 9, 11, and 12 both hands are used simultaneously on corresponding areas of the face and neck.

Preliminary stroking: Before doing Movement No. 1, gently stroke across the patron's forehead, from the corrugator to about two inches past the front hairline, using two alternating linear strokes with the cushion tip of the middle finger of each hand. Further the condition of relaxation by asking the patron to close his eyes.

Cream base for movements: The facial movements should never be given over a dry face. Use a good tissue or cold cream. Spread the cream over the face with light, gentle, long sweeping linear and rotary movements. Make sure the face is clean and smooth before applying this base cream.

Proper fingers to use: Use the **convenient number** of fingers. How they are used is more important than which ones are used. In Movements 3, 4, and 6 use only the second **finger.** In Movements Nos. 7, 8, 9, and 10 use fingers 1, 2, and 3. In Movements Nos. 11 and 12 use all four fingers. (In barbering the index finger is No. 1, the middle finger is No. 2, the ring finger is No. 3 and the little finger is No. 4.)

Number of times each movement executed: The number of times an individual movement is executed before passing on to the next movement varies according to the purpose. For teachability and practical purposes execute each movement **twice** except No. 5 which consists of five complete rotations.

Pause and vibrate in the following movements: In Movement No. 1 pause and vibrate each time the hands **arrive** at the right and left temples. Do not vibrate when beginning Movement No. 1. In Movements Nos. 7 and 8 pause and vibrate at the end of each movement. This means that there will be two times when vibrations are given during each of these movements.

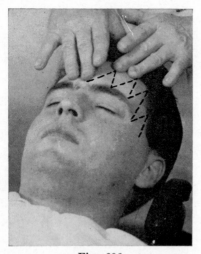

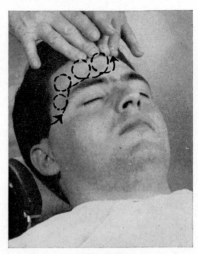

Fig. 606
Movement No. 1

Fig. 607
Movement No. 2

Passing from one movement to another: The general rule is **not to break contact.** Proceed in such a way that **at least one hand will be on the face at all times.** This is especially important if the purpose is to induce relaxation. Slide from the end of one movement to the beginning of the next whenever convenient.

Movement No. 1: Begin at the left temple with the second and third fingers of each hand and make a zigzag movement up and down completely across the forehead and return in like manner. Each time the fingers **arrive at** the temples, vibrate over the semi-lunar ganglion. Do not vibrate at the start of the movement. (The semi-lunar ganglion at each temple is vibrated over twice during this Movement.) The hands make two complete trips across the forehead. This constitutes executing this Movement twice. This movement is executed over a portion of the frontal muscle (frontalis) (Fig. 606).

Movement No. 2: Upon completing Movement No. 1 both hands are at the left temple. Leave the left hand there and slide the right hand across the forehead to the right temple. With the second and third fingers forming the contact rotate upward and over the forehead until these fingers of each hand meet. Cover the whole area between the eyebrows and the hairline. Slide back to beginning of the Movement and **repeat** this **Movement once.** This movement is executed over a portion of the frontal muscle (frontalis) (Fig. 607).

Movement No. 3: Upon completing Movement No. 2, both hands are at the center of the forehead. Retain contact with only the second finger of the left hand, and lift the right hand and place the tip of the second finger on the left side of the face against the wing of the nose. As soon as the

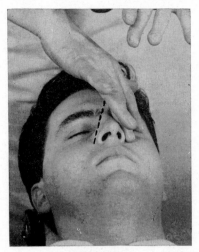

Fig. 608
Movement No. 3

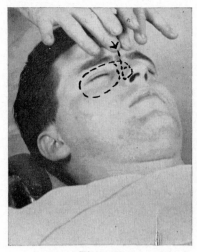

Fig. 609
Movement No. 4

second finger of the right hand makes contact against the wing of the nose, lift the left hand and proceed in slow motion to the starting point of the movement at the corresponding place on the right side of the nose. Stroke the finger diagonally upward and over the bridge of the nose to the starting point at the center of the forehead. Each hand **alternates** with the other until only two stroking movements are completed on **each** side of the nose. This constitutes doing the movement **twice.** (After the second finger of the right hand has made the second and final stroke over the bridge of the nose and returned to the original starting point at the center of the forehead, it remains there in contact until the second finger of the left hand arrives.) This movement is executed over the procerus muscle and a portion of the frontalis (Fig. 608).

Movement No. 4: Upon completing Movement No. 3, both hands are at the center of the forehead. Slide the second finger of the right hand diagonally down over the right side of the nose to the right wing of the nose, and, at the same time, slide the second finger of the left hand in like manner to the left wing of the nose. Rotate three times over the wings of the nose and then make a stroking movement over the bridge of the nose to the inner margins of the eyes. Proceed around the eyes, passing just underneath the eyebrows and returning to the inner margins of the eyes to complete the circles. From this point slide the finger of each hand to its respective wing of the nose and repeat the procedure over the wings of the nose and around the eyes. The pressure underneath the eyes should be very light. Movement No. 4 is executed **twice.** After completing two encirclements of the eyes, slide the tip of the second finger of each hand back to the original starting point at the center of the forehead. This movement is executed over the following muscles: Nasalis, procerus, corrugator, orbicularis oculi, and the dilator naris (posterior and anterior). (Fig. 609).

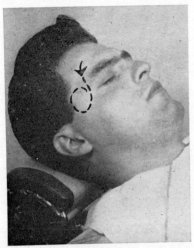

Fig. 610
Movement No. 5

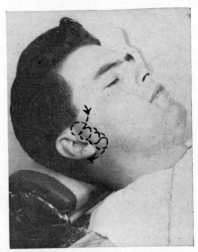

Fig. 611
Movement No. 6

Movement No. 5: Upon completing Movement No. 4, the hands are at the center of the forehead. Slide the right hand to the right temple and the left hand to the left temple. With fingers 2 and 3, rotate **five** times in circles about the size of a half silver dollar, in line with the corner of the eyes. The rotations are completed between the corners of the eyes and the hairline at the temples. **Five rotations complete** the movement. This movement is executed over a portion of the orbicularis oculi muscle and the temporal muscle (Fig. 610).

Movement No. 6: Upon completing Movement No. 5, that is, after the fifth complete rotation, slide the second finger of the right hand to the right ear as indicated in the diagram of this movement, and at the same time, slide the second finger of the left hand to a corresponding place on the left side of the face. The movement encircles the ears. Complete several rotations **immediately** in front of the ears. These rotations should be about the size of a nickel; they are executed between the beard and the ears. Behind the ears change the rotary to a linear movement until the fingers reach the starting point. **Repeat** this movement **once.** (The ear is encircled twice.) This movement is executed over the three auricular muscles (anterior, posterior, and superior), a portion of the sterno-cleido-mastoid muscle, and the masseter (Fig. 611).

Movement No. 7: Upon completing Movement No. 6 the finger tips of the right hand are at the right temple and the tips of the left hand are at the left temple. At the same time, slide the finger tips of the right hand to the right corner of the mouth and the same fingers of the left hand to the left corner of the mouth. Place the tip of the middle finger of each hand at its respective corner of the mouth. Use fingers 1, 2, and 3. Rotate from the corners of the mouth upward over the cheeks to the temples and there pause and vibrate over the semi-lunar ganglions. (Begin the rotations by starting downward.) Slide back to the beginning of the movement at the corners of the mouth and **repeat** the movement **once.** This movement is executed chiefly over the following muscles: Zygomaticus, buccinator, caninus and risorius. All of these muscles are inserted into the orbicularis oris. (Fig. 612).

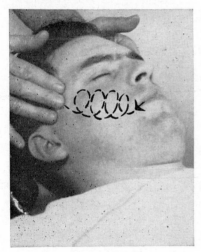
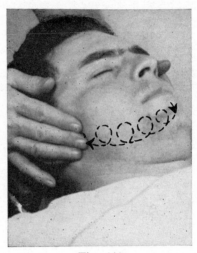

Fig. 612   Fig. 613
Movement No. 7   Movement No. 8

Movement No. 8: Upon completing Movement No. 7 the finger tips of the right hand are at the right temple and those of the left hand are at the left temple. At the same time, slide the cushion tips of each hand over the sides of the face to a place just above the middle of the chin where the tips of the second fingers meet. Use fingers 1, 2, and 3. Rotate along the lower jawbones to the ears. Just in front of the ears pause and vibrate. The vibrations will be near the **otic ganglions.** (Begin the rotations by starting downward.) Slide back to the starting point at the chin and **repeat** the Movement **once.** This movement is executed over the following muscles: mentalis, triangularis, and a portion of the masseter and platysma. (Fig. 613).

Movement No. 9: Upon completing Movement No. 8, the finger tips of the right hand are on the lower jawbone just in front of the right ear, and the tips of the left hand are at a corresponding place on the left side of the face. With the left hand retaining contact at this point, lift the right hand and place it over the chin in a cupping manner. Make a stroking movement **from the chin to the ear,** with the second finger sliding along the lower jawbone, the first finger sliding along just above the lower jawbone and the third finger sliding along just below the lower jawbone. Repeat this same procedure with the left hand. As soon as one hand contacts the chin, lift the other hand and in slow motion arrive at the cupping position just as the other hand reaches the ear. This is an alternating movement, first with the right and then with the left hand. Each hand makes **two linear strokes alternately.** This complete movement is executed **twice.** Upon completion, each hand is at its respective starting position near the ear. This movement is executed over the same muscles as Movement No. 8. (Fig. 614).

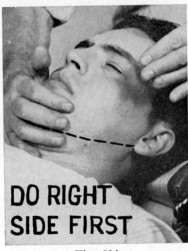

Fig. 614
Movement No. 9

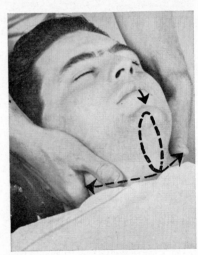

Fig. 615
Movement No. 10

Movement No. 10: Upon completing Movement No. 9, the finger tips of the right hand are on the lower jawbone just in front of the right ear and the tips of the left hand are at a corresponding place on the left side of the face. At the same time, slide the finger tips of each hand along the lower jawbone until the tips of the second fingers meet at the middle of the chin. Use fingers 1, 2, and 3. In this position make a stroking movement downward, in a semi-circular direction so as to miss the Adam's Apple and bring the tips of each hand together at the base of the neck. Then proceed along the neck until the finger tips of each hand meet at the back of the neck. In proceeding from the front to the back of the neck, the wrists and elbows should be lifted and adjusted in position so that the fingers will be pointing downward by the time the finger tips of both hands meet at the back. Make this transition gracefully and comfortably. At this point rotate, proceeding upward to back of the ear. When passing behind the ears change to a linear stroke to complete the movement at the temples. The rotations at the back of the neck are started downward. Slide back to the beginning of the movement, and **repeat** this movement **once**. The names of the muscles that this movement is executed over are: platysma, omohyoid, sterno-cleido-mastoideus, trapezius, and occipitalis. (Figs. 615-617).

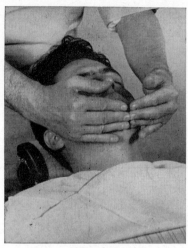

Fig. 616
Start of Movement No. 10

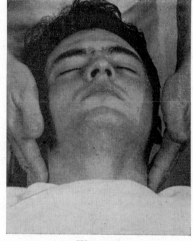

Fig. 617
Midway of Movement No. 10

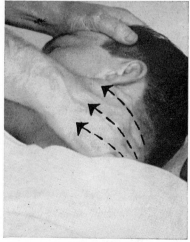

Fig. 618
Movement No. 11

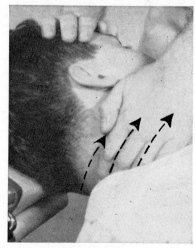

Fig. 619
Movement No. 12

Movement No. 11: Upon completing Movement No. 10 turn the head to the right. Lift the right hand off the face and step to the right side of the patron, sliding the left hand across the forehead to a bracing position just above the left eyebrow but well upon the forehead. While bracing the head with the left hand, place all four fingers of the right hand at the base of the neck on the right side, execute a stroking movement upward and across the neck almost to the Adam's Apple. Apply very firm pressure and relax the hand so that it will take the shape of the area it slides over. Slide back to the beginning of the movement and **repeat** this Movement **once.** This movement is executed over a portion of the platysma and sterno-cleido-mastoid muscles. (Fig. 618).

Movement No. 12: Step to the left side of the patron, keeping the right hand in contact with the face. Turn the head to the left. On the right side of the face, place both hands in positions corresponding with those in the last movement. Brace the head with the right hand and execute the movement with the left hand in the same manner as in Movement No. 11. **Repeat** this movement **once.** This movement is executed over a portion of the platysma and sterno-cleido muscles. (Fig. 619).

Final Touch: Manipulate the hands so that they meet and slide on the forehead into the hair line. Both hands should not be suddenly lifted straight off the face—**slide them off.**

Definition of Series: Executing the movements from No. 1 through No. 12 constitutes one series.

Number of Series to give: The number of series to give depends upon the purpose to be achieved. To induce maximum relaxation or promote maximum stimulation, execute THREE series.

Learning Movements: Learn these movements thoroughly. You should be able to do them with your eyes closed. Practice them until you have mastered them. Besides practicing them on others, you may practice them on yourself. Tracing the movements over thin paper is also recommened.

Facials

The term **facial** means a face massage. It also means face treatment. A face massage is given to cleanse and soothe, relax or stimulate, whereas a face treatment, besides accomplishing these same purposes, characteristically includes an attempt to correct some undesirable condition. Facials, however, fall under the same catagories as scalp treatments, since in a broad sense all facials are facial treatments. These categories are:

1. Preservative—to maintain the health of the face, by cleansing, relaxing the nerves, stimulating circulation, and activating metabolism.
2. Corrective—to counteract or correct some undesirable face condition, such as blackheads and Acne Vulgaris.
3. Alleviative—to relieve a face condition, such as a slightly irritated skin or Acne Rosacea.
4. Cosmetic—to soothe and beautify by such facials as the "mud pack" and "bleach pack."

General purposes of facials: The general over-all purposes of facials fall under three headings:

1. **Hygienic.** That is, facials help to maintain the health of the skin of the face.
2. **Remedial.** That is, facials help to correct or remedy unhealthy and undesirable conditions of the skin and the face.
3. **Cosmetic.** That is, facials help to beautify the skin of the face.

Specific purposes of facials:

1. To cleanse the face.
2. To increase circulation.
3. To tone up muscles.
4. To regulate glandular activity.
5. To relax the nerves.
6. To promote metabolism.
7. To soothe slightly irritated skin.
8. To reduce large pores.
9. To reduce and help postpone wrinkles.
10. To bleach skin.
11. To alleviate certain skin disorders.
12. To preserve the complexion of the skin.

13. To rest tired eyes.
14. To give a feeling of rejuvenation.
15. To reduce fat cells.

Major conditions for which facials are given:
1. Dry skin
2. Oily skin
3. Blackheads
4. Clogged pores
5. Tension and fatigue
6. Acne Vulgaris
7. Tender, sensitive skin
8. Premature wrinkles

Equipment and supplies used in facials:
1. Comfortable barber chair
2. Towels
3. Red dermal lights
4. High frequency
5. Vibrator
6. Massaging
7. Ointments
8. Creams
9. Lotions
10. Powders
11. Packs
12. Water
13. Cosmetic
   Preparations

Types of facial massage movements:
1. Effleurage. (This is a stroking movement.)
2. Petrissage. (This is a kneading movement.)
3. Percussion. (This is a tapping movement and is also known as **tapotement.**)
4. Vibratory. (This means virbation.)
5. Rotary. (This means rotation movements.)

What customers like most about facials:
1. The relaxing effect of steam-towel applications.
2. The soothing effects of creams and lotions.
3. The relaxation and stimulation from massaging.

Basis of needs for facials:
1. Negligent daily care of the face.
2. Inability of an individual to care for his face.
3. Exposure to dust, wind, and torrid sunshine.
4. Poor cosmetics.
5. Approaching old age.
6. After-effects on skin from illness.
7. Unhealthy skin.
8. Wrinkles.
9. Inalibilty of the skin to eliminate waste-matter.
10. Blackheads.
11. Poor circulation.
12. General fatigue.
13. Sluggish oil and sweat glands.
14. Excessively oily skin.

15. Excessively dry skin.
16. Sensitive, tender skin.
17. Patron's desire to beautify the face for some special occasion.
18. Poor metabolism of skin.

Scientific basis of facials: The things that are accomplished in facials have scientific merit. The following are a few of them.

1. Cleanliness. A facial cleanses the skin by creams, lotions, and steam-towel applications.
2. Stimulation. A facial stimulates the circulation of blood and activates the sebaceous glands.
3. Relaxation. A facial relaxes the nerves and reduces nervous tension by scientifically executed facial movements, steam-towel applica-
4. Strengthening of tissues. A facial builds up tissues through massaging.
5. Metabolism. A facial promotes metabolism of the cells.

Facials recommended for dry skin:

1. Dry Skin Facial.
2. Acne Facial.
3. Egg and Milk Pack Facial.
4. Rest Facial.

Facials recommended for oily skin:

1. Oily Skin Facial.
2. Clay Pack Facial.
3. Pink Rolling Cream Facial.

Facials recommended for tender, sensitive skin:

1. Egg and Honey Pack Facial.
2. Egg and Milk Pack Facial. (Use manufacturers egg and milk.)
3. Acne Facial.

Facials recommended for stimulation:

1. Combination Facial.
2. Amplified Facial.
3. Yeast Pack Facial.
4. Stim-u-lax Facial.

Facials recommended for cleansing:

1. Rolling Cream Facial.
2. Rest Facial.
3. Plain Cleansing Cream Facial.

Chief facial for relaxation: Rest Facial.

Beautifying facials:

1. Clay Pack Facial.
2. Bleach Pack Facial.
3. Egg and Milk Facial.
4. Yeast Pack Facial.

Series of facials: Ten facials constitute a series of facials.

Frequency of facials:
1. In a planned series, one to two weekly are recommended.
2. Once a month if for general purposes.
3. Luxuriously, once weekly.

Ways of suggesting facials: Before making any suggestion observe closely the condition of the face, and listen attentively to anything the customer may say about his facial needs. If you observe a definite need for a facial, pin point your suggestion accordingly. A facial may be recommended for a given condition without singling out the name of a particular facial. Customers may be induced to have facials by either direct or indirect suggestions. While positive direct suggestions are more effective with some customers, the indirect type appeals more to other customers. When suggesting a facial use a firm but well modulated voice.

1. Direct approach: The direct approach means asking a direct question. Such a question must be asked very tactfully and at the proper time. Keep in mind the pointers on selling as explained in the chapter on salesmanship. The mood and financial ability of the customer should be considered. Direct questions should be asked in such a way as not to embarrass the customer. They should be neither too forceful nor too weak. Here are some examples:

1. Would you like to have a facial?
2. Would you like to have a Rest Facial. It is very relaxing.
3. Would you like to have a toning-up facial?
4. I recommend that you have a facial to get rid of your blackheads.
5. Would you like for me to tell you about a good facial?
6. Some of our customers like our Yeast Pack Facial. Would you like one today?

2. Indirect approach: Here are some examples of how to make the indirect approach.

1. You have several blackheads on your cheeks. We have a facial in which we extract them.
2. Your face is very dry. Our Egg and Honey Facial is very soothing.
3. You said you are very tired. Our Rest Facial is very relaxing.
4. I notice you have acne vulgaris. We have a facial especially for that condition. I recommend you have one sometime.
5. I notice your skin is oily. We have a facial especially for that condition.
6. Many of our customers like our _____ facial. I recommend you have one some time.
7. Some day when you have time, I would like to give you our special _____ Facial.
8. You know it is a good thing to have a facial once in a while. It helps preserve the complexion.

Leading into indirect approach: Customers resist being harassed to buy extras. You can keep customers relaxed by the indirect approach. There are innumerable ways of making this kind of approach. You may simply say "when you have time, I would like to recommend a facial."

Fitting points to suggest facials:

1. When removing the final warm steam-towel following a shave.
2. Near the finish of most any service not within itself a finishing type of service. (Do not suggest a facial immediately upon beginning another type of service, unless you have already been serving the patron for several minutes.)
3. When a patron inquires as to his need for a facial by pointing out some condition such as blackheads, clogged pores, a dry face, etc.
4. When a patron announces that he is very tired or weary.
5. When the patron says that he is going to some auspicious affair.
6. When the patron speaks of making a lot of money.
7. During the course of conversation which you have directed to lead up to the suggestion.

When not to suggest facial:

1. When a patron has made known his frightening poverty.
2. When the patron's face is broken out with such ailments that should not be steamed or massaged. An example is severe Psoriasis.
3. When the patron announces that he has just time enough for some other service which he calls for.
4. When serving a child under ten years old.

Classification of face creams used in facials:

1. Rolling Creams—represented by the rolling or crumbling cream.
2. Cold Creams—the grease-like preparations that do not dry easily and that stand up for massage movements. They are the emollient type of creams.
3. Vanishing Creams—just what the name implies. These creams are momentarily grease-like but they dry quickly under rubbing or on exposure to air.

Kinds of grease creams: These creams are used as a base for massaging, since they retain their grease-like quality. Tissue cream is an ideal base for massaging.

1. Cleansing grease cream.
2. Tissue cream.
3. Cold cream.
4. Cocoa butter.

Standard finish to fascials:
1. One moderately hot steam towel application.
2. Finishing cream.
3. Face lotion
4. One moderately hot steam towel application.
5. Dry face and powder if desired.

Finishing creams: A tissue or cold cream may be used as a finishing especially if a little massaging is to be done. However, vanishing cream is widely used, since it forms a better base for powder.

Why vanishing cream as finishing cream is often preferred.
1. It dries and partly vanishes rapidly.
2. It makes a suitable powder base.
3. It makes a smooth pleasant finish.
4. It serves to replace the natural oil removed in shaving.

Application of creams: Preferably creams should be removed from the jar by a spatula. Place a small amount in the palm of the left hand.
1. Spot place a little cream on each cheek, on the chin, and at the middle of the forehead.
2. Use the cushion tips of both hands simultaneously on corresponding areas of both sides of the face.
3. With long stroking movements distribute the cream generally over the sides of the face.
4. Next, stroke from the base of the nose to the ear.
5. Now, work from the side of the nose, up over the bridge, between the eyebrows, across the forehead, and then to the temples.
6. Then, in long gentle strokes downward with both hands spread cream over the neck.
7. Finally, with long, gentle, rhythmical sweeping movements, work systematically over the entire face and neck, giving each corresponding area of the two sides of the face equal attention. Circle the eyes two or three times. (Refer to chapter on "Massaging.")

Select cream according to purpose: It is not always recommended that the various steps of applying cream to the face be followed. It should be more painstakingly applied when facial movements are to follow, or when finishing movements are to be given. When applied as a preliminary cleansing or after-shave application, the procedure may be abbreviated.

When to use strong and mild face lotions:
1. For a dry-like or tender face, use mild lotion.
2. For an oily-like and solid face, use the astringent lotion.

Objectionable things to avoid in giving facials:
1. Unevenly heated steam-towels.
2. Rough, heavy cold hands.
3. Cream in the nostrils and eyes.
4. Reclining or inclining patron too fast.
5. Failure to remove all traces of cream, lotion, or ointment.
6. Failure to dry facial area well.
7. Bad breath.
8. Offensive body odor.
9. Breathing into patron's face.
10. Too hot towels.

Favorable shop requirements for facials:
1. Comfortable chair.
2. Pleasant atmosphere.
3. Subdued lighting.
4. Quietness.
5. Adequate supplies.
6. Soft background music.

Combination materials for facial packs:
1. Fullers earth and almond meal.
   (1) To bleach, add one tablespoonful of peroxide or one-half ounce of lemon juice.
   (2) To soothe a sensitive skin, add one-half ounce of milk or buttermilk or the same amount of honey.
2. Barley flour and rose water.
3. White of egg and honey.
4. White of egg and milk.
5. Bran and honey.
6. Almond meal and lemon juice.
7. Any prepared pack by a reputable manufacturer.

Noteworthy points about pack mixtures: All combinations of pack materials are mixed about half and half. The above combination should be so mixed as to make a consistency that will spread quickly and evenly. Lemon juice, egg white, milk, or honey may be added to any combination not including these ingredients for the purposes stipulated above. It is to be remembered that honey is healing and soothing, lemon juice is bleaching (though slightly drying,) the white of egg is cleansing and nourishing, and milk is healing and soothing.

Five commonly known packs:
1. Clay Pack (also known as mud pack).
2. The Bleach Pack.
3. Egg and Milk Pack.
4. Egg and Honey Pack.
5. Yeast Pack.

Source of clay used in clay packs: It comes mainly from volcanic areas in the United States, Italy, Germany and Hungary.

How face packs are dried:
1. Allowed to dry naturally.
2. By red dermal light. (Be sure to cover eyes well.)
3. By fanning with small towel.

Protect eyes when dermal lights are used on face (Fig. 627): Cotton pads or neck strips soaked in witch hazel, rose water or boric acid may be placed over the eyes.

Applying pack on face: Put a bit of the pack four places on the face— one on each cheek, one on the chin, and one at middle of forehead. Now, with the cushion tips, distribute the pack evenly over the face and neck, omitting the ears and lips. Omit it from the eye lids if a dermal light is to be used. Keep it out of the nostrils.

Purposes of preliminary steaming of face:
1. To cleanse the face from foreign substances.
2. To prepare the skin for the reception of the preparations.
   (1) By relaxing the tissues.
   (2) By opening the pores.

Purpose of cool towel finish: It is given mainly to close the pores.

Methods of extracting blackheads:
1. By a special implement: the round hole at the end of such an imple-

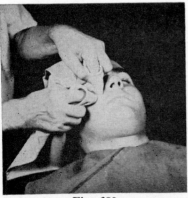

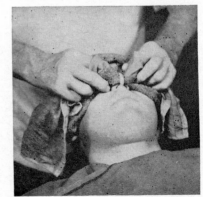

Fig. 620   Fig. 621

Removing Blackheads

Using Dry Face Towel   Using Warm Damp Steam Towel

ment is placed directly over and around the blackhead and pressure is applied.

2. By the teasing method: cover the tips of the index fingers with sterile gauze, lift the surrounding tissues up between these finger tips, and gently rotate inwardly as you apply sufficient pressure to press out the plug. The pressure should be applied as closely to the plug as possible and a little below it so as to minimize the degree of inevitable irritation. The corner of a face towel may be used instead of the gauze, although the gauze is preferable. (To reduce the amount of irritation dampen slightly the corner of the face towel: likewise, the gauze may be slightly dampened. If this dampening is done in the winter time, keep the dampened portion warm. If a little grease cream is applied before the extracting is begun, it will, of course, be unnecessary to dampen the linen.)

Preliminary steps of extracting blackheads:
1. Steam the face thoroughly, unless the skin is excessively dry.
2. Apply cold cream and use red dermal light from three to five minutes. (Minimize the use of dermal light on excessively oily skin.)

When to check for blackheads and whiteheads: Check early in the facial. It is a general practice to remove them in any facial unless doing so would interfere with the purposes of the facial. It is preferable not to remove them in the rest facial unless they are specially offensive.

When to place necessaries in readiness:
1. Right after the linen set-up, or
2. While the preliminary final steam towel is on the face.

Elaborate linen set-up (Fig. 625). This set-up is not made unless it is the regular shop practice. It consists of five towels, two steam-towels and three small towels.
1. Place one face towel across the front and sides of the neck (Fig. 625).
2. Tuck one face towel across the back of the neck, and arrange the surplus back part of the towel over the head-rest.
3. Place one face towel around the head just sufficient to cover the hair; the lower edge of the towel should trail the hairline, plus one across front and sides of neck.

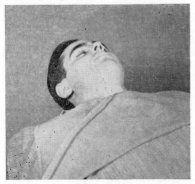

Fig. 622
One Small Towel
Across Front and Sides of Neck

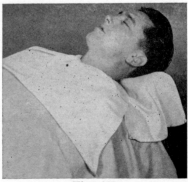

Fig. 623
Two Small Towels
One Across Front, Sides of Neck,
One Across Back of Neck

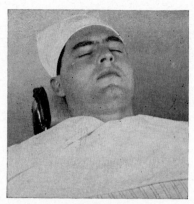

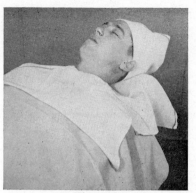

Fig. 625
Three Small Towels
One Across Front, Sides of Neck
One Across Back of Neck
One Around Scalp

Fig. 624
Two Small Towels
One Across Front, Sides of Neck
One Around Scalp

4. Use two steam towels for steaming the face.

Advantages of using two steam-towels: One steamer can be prepared while the other one is on the face.

1. To minimize the elapse of time between the application of the steamers and thus provide continuous steaming.
2. To save time, since the second steamer is prepared during the time that the barber would otherwise be idle.

Uses of steam-towels: (Refer to Chapt. on Linen Uses.)

Standard number of steam-towel applications: Three is the standard number, but when steaming is emphasized, make five.

Temperature of steamers to be progressive: The temperature should be graduated, starting with a mild steamer and ending with a slightly hotter one. Although some men patrons call for very hot steamers, an extremely hot steamer should never be applied to the face because of the resulting constriction of muscles and because of the consequent slight irritation.

Practical linen set-up: The barber should not use linen too sparingly as it is comparatively inexpensive; on the other hand he should take every opportunity to save whenever it is reasonably possible and advisable.

1. Four-towel-set-up: A small towel is tucked across the front area and sides of the neck and another one around the back of the neck. Two steam-towels are used.
2. Three-towel-set-up: There are two alternatives:
    (1) Use one small towel and two steam towels.
    (2) Use two small towels and one steam towel.
    (3) The three-towel-set-up may be used in lower price facials. There is a slight preference for the use of two small towels and one steamer.

Two ways of arranging towel across front of neck:

1. A single thickness is tucked under the collar of the shirt.
2. Make a slight diagonal fold from the lengthwise middle to the end and tuck a double thickness of the towel under the collar of the shirt. This method gives additional protection to the shirt.

Points of similarity in facials: There are many points of similarity in facials, and this makes it comparatively easy to design an original facial. With exceptions the following apply to all facials:

1. Linen set-up.
2. Preliminary cleansing of face (not after shave).
3. Three moderately hot steam towel applications.
4. The applications of special preparation, such as rolling cream, clay pack, and special face pack.
5. Aiding the penetration with a dermal light, depending on the substance used.
6. Massaging.
7. Removal of special preparations.
8. Removal of any offensive blackheads or whiteheads. Do the extracting after rolling cream is removed, but before any special pack is applied.
9. Application of grease cream.
10. Fanning and wiping face with towel.
11. Standard finish.

Facials, like scalp treatments, consist of three major divisions—the basic preliminaries, the body, and the finish. The preliminaries and finish are fairly uniform. The essential difference in facials is the body—the particular preparations used such as mud pack, yeast pack, egg and honey, etc. Whatever the procedure is it must contribute to the main purpose of the facial.

Points of difference in facials:

1. No massaging is done in some facials, such as the Acne Facial, Rosacea Facial, and Egg and Honey Facial (if skin is slightly irritated).
2. No steaming in some facials, such as the Rosacea Facial.
3. Witch hazel is usually considered an extra service.
4. The steaming is done according to the condition and purpose.
5. Some facials include more items and supplies.
6. The violet ray is used only in some facials.
7. The degree and pressure of movements vary according to the condition and purpose.

STANDARD OUTLINE OF FACIALS

The standard outline of facials is a general flexible guide or **skeletal** procedure.

It is to be changed according to the purpose of the given facial, cosmetic preparations, needs of the patron, and established shop practice.

1. Make linen set-up.
2. Cleanse face.
3. Give three steam-towel applications.
4. Apply facial preparation.
5. Remove facial preparation unless it was applied as a base for massaging.
6. Execute standard facial movements.
7. Make one to three steam-towel applications.
8. Give standard or special finish.

PLAIN FACIAL

Alternate name: Rolling cream massage.
Purpose: To cleanse the face.
Preparations: Rolling cream.

Kinds of skin for which recommended:

1. Normal skin.
2. Oily skin.
3. Thick skin.

Kinds of skin for which not recommended:

1. Excessively dry skin.
2. Skin with acne vulgaris.
3. Very tender, sensitive skin.
4. Thin skin.
5. Rough or pimpled skin.

How to apply rolling cream: Remove it from the palm in the usual manner, but distribute it in **four equal portions** over the chin, the cheeks and the forehead. Then slightly dampen with cool water the finger tips of both hands and spread it evenly over the face, using stroking movements.

Nature of massaging over rolling cream: The movements should be light, both long and short, stroking movements including the sweeping, rotary, patting and zigzag varieties. They should be executed in such a way as to cover completely both sides of the face almost simultaneously and quickly because of the drying of the cream. A suitable variation is to make some of the movements "dashy" as might be used gently to knock off drops of water from the surface of the skin. Generally, the movements should start at the base of the neck and proceed upward; but the main idea is to cover the whole face well systematically.

Procedure:

1. Linen set-up.
2. Three steam-towel applications.
3. Place all necessaries in readiness, while third steamer remains on face.
4. Apply rolling cream.
5. Execute stroking movements, rolling off cream.
   (1) With finger tips dry, and then
   (2) With finger tips dampened, and then
   (3) With mildly warm steamer.
6. Check for blackheads and extract regulation number, if any.
7. Apply mild antiseptic lotion, if any blackheads were removed.
8. Apply cold cream.
9. Execute about three minutes of massage movements, emphasizing the long sweeping and stroking rotary movements.
10. Make two steam towel applications, wiping off most of the cream with the last one.
11. Standard finish.

COMBINATION FACIAL

Alternate Name: Double Massage.
Two-fold purpose: The two-fold purpose is to **cleanse** and **stimulate**.
Definition: A combination facial is a plain facial plus the use of the electric vibrator.

Use of Vibrator (Fig. 626):

1. Employ the regular massage principles. The pressure should be in the upward direction and in only one direction.
2. Regulate the rate of vibration down to a minimum—vibrations should never be rapid. Rapid vibrations tend to tear down the tissues and to irritate the face.
3. The movements are largely stroking and rotary. Proceed slowly over the face.
4. Regardless of which type of vibrator is used, the vibrations around the eyes and the nostrils should be of the indirect nature. With the cup vibrator, this can be done by placing the cup on the back of fingers one and two of the left hand.
5. In using the cup vibrator, sort of envelop the vibrator in the right hand as holding a lather brush. Never guide it by the handle entirely.
6. The movements should be continuous without breaking contact.
7. The whole face should be gone over just twice.

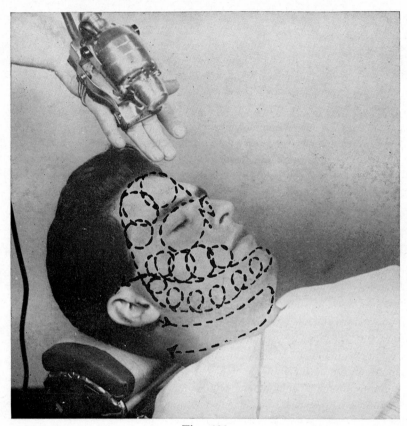

Fig. 626
Routine of Vibrator

8. Pause with the vibrations about five seconds over the temples and at the back sides of the neck; and apply more pressure when passing over the mastoid regions.

Procedure: Follow the same procedure given for the plain facial, except use the vibrator right after applying the grease cream.

Routine of vibrator: A routine is necessary for systematic procedure and so that each corresponding area of the face will receive equal attention. It is believed that twin vibrators should not be used since they might over-stimulate the face. Over-stimulation breaks down tissues. Massaging should be done with moderation.

CLAY PACK FACIAL

There are many clay packs and other face packs on the market. Unless otherwise instructed the same procedure may be followed for giving all of them.

Purposes:
1. The clay pack may be recommended for oily skin.
2. It may also be recommended as a beautifier of normal skin.

Incidental purposes:
1. To serve as a mild tonic to the tissues.
2. To promote smoothness of the skin.
3. To help prevent wrinkles.
4. To bleach or lighten slightly.

Kinds of skin for which not recommended:
1. Very dry skin.
2. Very thin skin.
3. Tender, sensitive skin.

Greek physicians praise virtues of clay or mud: Galen and Hippocrates recommended the use of mud on the face. Clean dirt, to the degree of a superstition, has been regarded as having healing properties. The clay or mud massage was very likely one of the very **first remedies** used by primitive man **to heal skin lesions.**

Manner of application: Same as the standard procedure, but use a little warm water on the hands. Do not cover the ears and be especially careful to keep the clay out of the nostrils. Applying it on the eyelids is optional. Apply none on the lips.

Procedure:
1. Arrange linen set-up.
2. Place clay in heating.
3. Make three moderately hot steam towel applications.
4. Place all necessaries in readiness, while third steamer remains on face, even putting a little of warm clay into palm of hand.
5. Apply clay. (It is fitting to cover lips slightly with grease cream just before applying clay, to keep them comfortable. Do not put any clay on lips, in nostrils, on eyebrows, on eyelashes, or on ears. You may put it on eyelids, unless pads are to be placed over eyes.)
6. Allow clay to dry naturally, or use red dermal light.
7. Remove pack with warm damp steam towel. Two applications usually suffice.
8. Apply good tissue cream.
9. Give about two minutes of exceptionally light, long stroking movements, or go through Rest Facial movements once, or some of the movements.
10. Remove excess cream with one mildly warm steamer.
11. Give standard finish.

ACNE FACIAL

Alternate name: Acne Vulgaris Facial.

Chief purpose: To alleviate Acne Vulgaris (simple pimples.)

Recommended also for:
1. Normal skin.
2. Dry skin.
3. Relaxing the tissues of the face after a hard day.
4. Soothing the face after a long ride in the wind.
5. Any minor pustular condition.
6. Acne articificialis.

Noteworthy points of Acne Facial:
1. There is no massaging.
2. Steam-towels especially should be moderately heated.
3. Stroking movements over the face to spread creams and solutions should be very light and gentle.

Procedure:
1. Arrange linen set-up.
2. Cleanse face with cleansing cream.
3. Make three moderately hot steam applications, removing all cream with last one.
4. Place all necessaries in readiness, while third steamer is on face.
5. Extract any blackheads and whiteheads; and evacuate any ripe pustules.
6. Apply mild antiseptic. (Where the face is especially tender, this lotion may be applied with piece of cotton as sponge.)
7. Apply good tissue cream and cover eyes for dermal light.

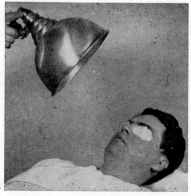

Fig. 627
Dermal Light on Face

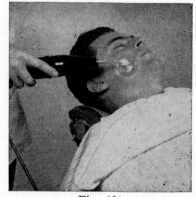

Fig. 628
High Frequency on Face

8. Irradiate face with red dermal light for about five minutes. (Fig. 627).

9. Make three to five minute application of violet ray. (Fig. 628).
10. Uncover eyes, and remove excess cream with one warm steamer.
11. Sponge face with mild antiseptic.
12. Make standard finish.

ACNE ROSACEA FACIAL

Purpose: To cleanse and soothe an acne rosacea condition.

Procedure: Use no hot towels in this facial.

1. Arrange linen set-up.
2. Cleanse face with cleansing cream.
3. Remove cream gently with warm steamer.
4. Apply soothing face lotion. A **soda** solution may be used.
5. Apply tissue or astringent cream.
6. Use blue dermal about three minutes.
7. Use violet ray about three minutes.
8. Finish:
   (1) Bathe face with witch hazel.
   (2) Dry and powder.

STIM-U-LAX FACIAL

Chief purpose: To enliven the face and refreshen the patron.

Occasions for this facial: The tired business executive or shopper feels the need of such a facial in the afternoon, about 4:00 P.M. in the hot months. The heat-weary will also like this facial.

Procedure:

1. Arrange linen set-up.
2. Make two moderately hot steam-towel applications.
3. Apply mentholated cleansing cream.
4. Execute long, rhythmical massage movements, gently and slowly. Movements 2, 4, 10, 11, and 12 may be used.
5. Remove cleansing cream with warm steam-towel.
6. Apply vanishing cream.
7. Apply mild astringent.
8. Apply a cool steam-towel.
9. Give standard finish.

EGG AND MILK FACIAL

Purposes: To cleanse and soothe sensitive skin.

Recommended especially for these kinds of skin:

1. Delicate, thin skin.
2. Tender, sensitive skin.
3. Normal skin.

Mixture:
1. Use commercially prepared egg and milk, or
2. Mix the white of an egg with one heaping tablespoonful of powdered milk and whip them into a paste.

Procedure:
1. Arrange linen set-up.
2. Cleanse face with cleansing cream.
3. Make three moderately hot steam-towel applications.
4. Place all necessaries in readiness.
5. Cover eyes for dermal light, if it is to be used.
6. Apply the mixture with finger tips.
7. Let pack dry naturally—or use dermal light or fan.
8. Remove pack with moderately hot steamer.
9. Make standard finish for facials, using muscle oil or tissue cream instead of vanishing cream.

EGG AND HONEY PACK FACIAL

Chief purpose: To cleanse and alleviate a slightly irritated face. The honey has a healing property.

Other uses: It may be recommended for emaciated skin, chafed, wind-blown or slightly sunburned face. It is also recommended as a luxury facial for a normal skin.

How this facial achieves its purpose:
1. By supplying a tonic for the cells.
2. By relaxing the tissues.
3. By cleansing thoroughly the skin.
4. By nourishing—inherent power of the ingredients.

Mixture: Mix the white of an egg already beaten with a tablespoonful of honey and just enough fine almond meal to make a good pliable paste. (Commercial powdered egg is preferred.)

Procedure:
1. Linen set-up.
2. Cleanse face with cleansing cream.
3. Make three moderately hot steam-towel applications.
4. Place all necessaries in readiness.
5. Apply mixture.
6. Prepare eyes for dermal light, if it is to be used.
7. Allow it to dry naturally, allowing from five to ten minutes. Or, dry it in about three to five minutes with red dermal light.
8. Remove pack with mildly hot steamer.
9. Bathe face thoroughly with glycerine and rose water (or some other scented lotion). The lotion may be applied with cotton pad.
10. As finish, dry face by fanning only, and apply powder if desired.

REST FACIAL

Chief purpose: To induce relaxation.

Incidental purposes:
1. To cleanse the skin.
2. To reduce or to avert wrinkles.
3. To release tense muscles.
4. To tone up sagging, fatigued muscles.
5. To nourish the skin.
6. To improve the complexion generally.
7. To soothe tired eyes.
8. To reduce the intensity of passing headaches.

Essential feature of this facial: The scientific execution of the standard or rest facial movements.

Number of series of movements: The standard times the complete series of movements are given is **three.**

Ideal atmosphere for this facial:
1. Free from disturbing noise, such as talking, jazz music.
2. Free from tobacco smoke.
3. An atmosphere characterized by quietness and pleasantness.
4. Soft music in background.
5. Mild illumination.
6. Ask patron to close his eyes.

Attitude of barber during facial: He should be especially calm, relaxed, and pleasant. When executing the movement, he may even close his own eyes.

Nature of movements:
1. Make the movements continuous, without losing contact throughout.
2. Make the movements as rhythmical as possible.
3. Employ very light pressure, because the chief purpose of the facial is to relax.
4. Execute the movements with the cushion tips.
5. Place the pressure on the upward stroke, generally.
6. Execute the movements slowly.

Procedure:
1. Make linen set-up.
2. Cleanse face tentatively with cleansing cream, and remove cream with soft, sterile paper napkin towel, or smooth, well padded dry face towel, or gently applied warmed steam-towel.
3. Make three moderately hot steam-towel applications.
4. Place all necessaries in readiness.
5. Apply an extraordinarily good grease cream.
6. With warm, thoroughly clean finger tips, softly stroke forehead,

working diagonally up and to sides from the inside ends of eyebrows, and ask patron to close his eyes. You may say, "You may close your eyes; this facial is going to be very relaxing and restful."

7. Go through whole set of pattern facial movements three times.
8. Apply moderately hot steamer.
9. Remove excess cream either with steamer just applied or some other convenient means already suggested. To complete removing of cream, a cotton sponge saturated in witch hazel may be used.
10. Ideally, make witch hazel steam finish. Although, standard finish may be given.

DRY SKIN FACIAL

Chief Purpose: For abnormally dry skin.

Recommended for other skin conditions: Tender, scaly, or very thin or delicate skin.

How the facial achieves its purpose:
1. By activating the sebaceous glands.
2. By stimulating circulation.
3. By increasing metabolism.

Procedure:
1. Arrange linen set-up.
2. Cleanse face with cleansing cream.
3. Remove cream gently.
4. Sponge face with witch hazel.
5. Make three moderately hot steam towel applications.
6. Apply tissue or nutriment cream.
7. Massage face with circular and deep stroking movements for about three minutes.
8. Use red dermal light about two minutes.
9. Use violet ray about two minutes.
10. Finish with three warm towel applications, removing cream. Apply one cold towel, and few drops skin oil or tissue cream sparingly. Blot, fan, and wipe face with face towel. Apply very little powder.

OILY SKIN AND COARSE PORE FACIAL

Alternate name: Astringent Facial.

Recommended: For excessively oily skin with large pores.

Probable causes of oily skin and large pores: Excessive eating of starchy and fatty substances and insufficient elimination.

Procedure:
1. Arrange linen set-up.
2. Cleanse face with cleansing cream or soothing soap and warm water

3. Make three warm steam towel applications.
4. Evacuate engorged pores gently.
5. Apply antiseptic and cream.
6. Massage face from three to five minutes with moderate pressure.
7. Use mild degree of violet ray two minutes.
8. Finish:
    (1) Apply astringent lotion through face towel.
    (2) Two steam towel applications.
    (3) One or two cold towel applications.
    (4) Apply lotion, dry, and powder.

BLEACH PACK FACIAL

Purpose: To whiten the outer layer of the skin.

Noteworthy:
1. This pack diminishes color of mild freckles.
2. Not recommended for excessively dark skin.
3. Peroxide is the main bleaching agent.
4. Commercially prepared packs are recommended.

Bleach pack formula: Mix one tablespoonful of starch and an equal amount of fine almond meal, 10 drops of tincture of benzoin, two tablespoonsful of citric acid, and two or three tablespoonsful of peroxide.

Procedure:
1. Arrange linen set-up.
2. Cleanse the face with cleansing cream.
3. Make three steam towel applications.
4. Protect eyes and apply cold cream on the eyebrows.
5. Apply pack.
6. Leave pack on 8 to 10 minutes.
7. Hasten drying of pack with red dermal light.
8. Remove pack gently with warm towels.
9. Apply face cream and massage face gently.
10. Apply mild lotion, dry, and powder.

YEAST PACK FACIAL

Purposes: People who do not have sufficient exercise and who have sedentary positions may find their pores clogged, face dry and rough, and their facial muscles sagging. This facial is designed to accomplish the following:
1. To cleanse the face gently and thoroughly.
2. To remove impurities.
3. To further skin nutrition.
4. To tone up face muscles.
5. To stimulate the flow of blood in the face.
6. To help to prevent wrinkles.

Procedure:

1. Arrange linen set-up.
2. Cleanse face with cleansing cream or bland soap.
3. Remove cleansing agent with warm steam-towel.
4. Apply emollient cream.
5. Execute Rest Facial movements once with double regular pressure
6. Remove all traces of cream by two warm steam-towel applications making second one hotter to open the pores for the reception o yeast.
7. Apply yeast paste. (Preferably use commercially prepared paste) Spread the yeast over the entire facial area. Work it into the ski gently with the cushion tips of the fingers.
8. Either allow the yeast to dry naturally, or aid the drying by rec dermal light or by fanning.
9. Remove dried yeast gently with one or two steam-towel applica tions.
10. Give standard finish.

STEAM FACIAL

Purpose: To tone up the face.

Noteworthy: A facial steam may follow a shave, an ordinary facial, o given as an independent service. Chiefly, the customer desires to enjoy soothing steam-towel applications, fragrant face lotion, the relaxing ap plication of a face cream, and the "velvety" finish of a gentleman's talc And the customer desires a feeling of restfulness and invigoration without the formality of a facial. It is a "quickie refresher."

Procedure:

1. Simple linen set-up.
2. Place over face a face-towel saturated with mild antiseptic or astrin gent lotion.
3. Make about five steam-towel applications, placing the final steam- towel over the last applied steam-towel, and leave one minute.
4. Remove the towels.
5. Apply finishing cream and face lotion and massage down gently.
6. Dry face and powder (if desired).

AMPLIFIED FACIAL

Chief purpose: Stimulation

Phases of stimulation:

1. Increased blood circulation.
2. Activated oil glands.
3. Promoted metabolism.
4. Toned up muscles.

Procedure:
1. Arrange linen set-up.
2. Cleanse face with cleansing cream—remove cream.
3. Make three steam towel applications.
4. Apply tissue cream or equivalent.
5. With an indirect type of vibrator attached to back of each hand, execute the movements of the Rest Facial, except the procedure may be in **reverse** order.
6. Remove the cream.
7. Give a standard finish.

Pointers on amplified facial:
1. Vibrations should be slow to moderate.
2. Pressure should be moderate.

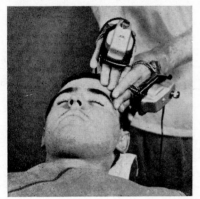

Fig. 629   Fig. 630
Amplified Facial

WITCH HAZEL STEAM

Purposes of witch hazel steam:
(1) To close the pores.
(2) To harden the tissues.
(3) To act as a mild antiseptic.
(4) To soothe the skin of the face.

Witch hazel steam defined:
1. A witch hazel steam is a service wherein a wet pad (such as a small towel) is saturated with witch hazel and is applied over the face. Make three to five steam-towel applications over this pad.

When not to give witch hazel steam: A witch hazel steam should not be given in these facials:
1. Acne Facial.
2. Acne Rosacea Facial.
3. Egg and Honey Facial.
4. Egg and Milk Facial.

Use of towels in witch hazel steam: (Figs. 631-638):

1. Place face towel across front and sides of neck.

2. **Dampen with warm water about one half of a ounce lengthwise folded face towel.** Then fold the towel lengthwise again and again until it is in a strip about three inches wide. Now roll it about one half its length. Apply witch hazel generously into the roll. Unfold the towel, and place the **dry** portion of the towel over the head and the wet portion over the face and neck. Now apply more witch hazel, patting the pad with the left hand to aid absorption. Finally make from three to five steam-towel applications.

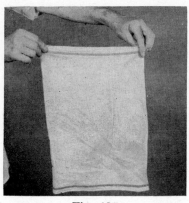

Fig. 631
Step No. 1

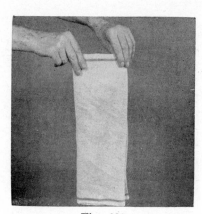

Fig. 632
Step No. 2

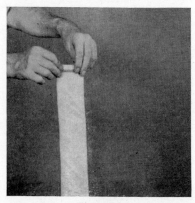

Fig. 633
Step No. 3

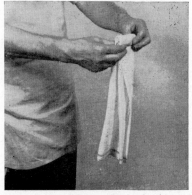

Fig. 634
Step No. 4

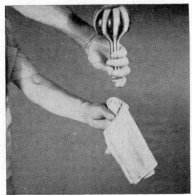

Applying Witch Hazel
Fig. 635
Step No. 5

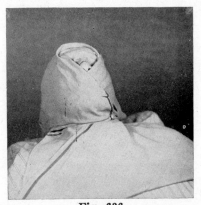

Fig. 636
Step No. 6
Towel Used as Pad

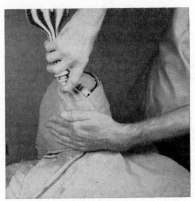

Fig. 637
Step No. 7
Applying Witch Hazel

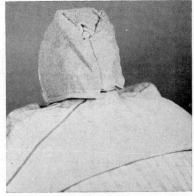

Fig. 638
Final Step
(Five Steam-towel Applications)

Complete Steaming with Two Steamers on Face

Haircoloring and Bleaching

HAIRCOLORING

The beginners course may be too short, in some states, to teach thi subject and also it may not be required. In such states schools may b obliged to teach only the HIGH POINTS of this chapter as merely a INTRODUCTION.

Haircoloring is a specialization area of barbering. There is an increas ing number of men who have their hair colored. Coloring of hair is anothe profitable source of income to the barber in the states or countries per mitting barbers to perform this service. To do haircoloring professionally one should continue to study and take special courses. Manufacturer conduct classes of instruction on the use of their products. Many har and long hours of study and practice are necessary to color or bleacl hair successfully. Like hair cuts, haircoloring has no seasons, and it is ; repeat type of business. Haircoloring patrons will return to your shop a regular intervals. The present discussion will be confined to an introduc tion and the fundamentals of haircoloring and bleaching in general, witl particular emphasis devoted to the coloring of men's hair.

Terms for coloring hair: The terms for coloring hair are Tinting or Hai Coloring. These two terms are used interchangeably. The professiona vocabulary of both the manufacturers and professional users of tint discourage the use of the word "dye."

Definition: Haircoloring is the process of changing the color of hair.

History of haircoloring: Haircoloring goes back as far as King Tut's time Egyptian women colored their hair red with Egyptian henna. The Greek used beechwood dye to color hair. During Emperor Nero's time (37 t 68 A.D.) Romans colored their hair black and auburn. Venus, the God dess of Love, bleached her hair from a dark to a golden color.

Reasons for coloring hair: The most common reason for haircoloring i to cover up gray or partially gray hair. People simply wish to make them selves look as young as possible and sometimes this is necessary for em ployment purposes, and then men who tint their hair may be prematurely gray, unmarried or married to women much younger than they. But her are some detailed reasons:

1. To change gray hair to some other color.
2. To change the natural color of hair.
3. To add a high light to the hair.
4. To bring bleached hair back to its natural color.
5. To secure a uniform color.

304

orms of coloring matter:
Coloring matter is prepared in two orms.

1. Liquid form. The aniline-derivative dyes are liquid. (Some of these are "creme" liquid and others are more aqueous-like.) The aniline derivative tints usually come in one bottle. It contains the coloring matter. The content is mixed with equal parts of 20 volume peroxide just before the mixture is applied to the hair.

2. Paste form. Egyptian and Compound hennas are examples.

Classification and Categories of Hair coloring: Hair colorings are conventionally divided into four classifications:

Classification:

1. Vegetable dyes
2. Metallic dyes
3. Compound dyes
4. Aniline-derivative tints

Vegetable dyes: Of the vegetable hair dyes, henna is the only pure vegetable dye of present-day use. Henna consists of the dried, powdered leaves of Lawsonia spinosa and produces various shades of red color obtained is relatively stable. When applied to the hair shaft. The henna is safe to use since it does not cause local or systemic toxicity. Other vegetable dyes used in the past are camomile, wood extracts and sage. Henna is a pure vegetable dye. Henna normally produces a reddish shade.

Metallic or mineral dyes: Compounds of silver, iron, copper, cobalt and nickel are often used. These dyes coat hair; make it dull and brittle; give it off-shades and metallic film. Not recommended.

Compound dyes: These are mainly a combination of vegetable and metallic materials. They coat the hair. Compound henna is an example. Not recommended.

Aniline tints: This variety may also be referred to as aniline derivatives, chemical organic derivatives, instant tints, peroxide tints, or synthetic tints. Aniline tints are the prevaling kind used and they pentrate the hair shaft. These tints are manufactured from a coal tar base and may be called "para dyes." They are classified as penetrating or oxidation tints — they penetrate through the cuticle layer of the hair into the cortex layer where they are oxidized or developed by peroxide.

Allergy: A small percent of people are allergic to aniline tints. The U.S. Federal Food, Drug and Cosmetic Act requires that a predisposition test must be given 24 hours before each application of aniline tint.

Predisposition test: This is also known as a skin or patch test. It means applying a small amount of the aniline tint to be used, mixed with an equal amount of 20 volume peroxide, on the inner fold of the elbow and allowing it to remain for 24 hours, to determine if there is any unfavorable reaction of the skin to it. Redness and swelling indicate an allergy. **Such a test should always be given prior to application of any aniline tint or toner.** A **negative** result reveals no inflammation and the tint may be applied with safety. A **positive** result reveals redness, itching, burning, and eruptions, evidencing an allergy, and the tint should not be applied. The positive effects will usually disappear of their own accord or after applying soothing skin antiseptics or ointment. If the effects do not disappear readily, a physician should be consulted. Follow the manufacturer's instruction when giving a patch test. **If a patch test is required for a coloring, it must be given not only for the original coloring** but also for subsequent applications (systemic changes may have taken place since the last application).

Penetrating tints a n d coating dyes: Aniline tints penetrate the hair; vegetable, metallic, and compound tints merely coat or color the outside of hair. If vegetable, metallic or compound dyes are present on hair they must be removed before applying an aniline tint.

Advantages of aniline tints:

1. They penetrate the hair shaft and last longer.

2. Their coloring is more natural —they can duplicate a natural color.

3. They have a larger variety of shades.

4. They can be permanent waved over successfully.

Essential ingredients of aniline tints: Paraphenylene-diamine is the essential ingredient. This chemical is an aniline derivative. When it is formulated with pigment coloring agents, various colors are achievable.

Selecting Color Shades: Color shades should be very carefully selected. Color charts are furnished by manufacturers of coloring products. Study the pointers on "Color Test" and "How to Give a Color Test" immediately following. Further in the chapter study the

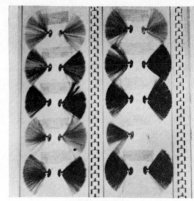

Fig. 638-A
Color Chart

pointers given under the headings "Selecting Color Shade for One step Application Tint" and "Selecting Color Shade for Two-step Application Tint." Color shades are not uniform in names. Each manufacturer uses his own color designations.

Color test: Unless the formula is known for a given patron, make a color test. This is done by applying the tint to a small strand of hair to determine the exact color effect, if the hair is damaged; and he correct length of time to retain the tint on the hair.

How to give a color test:

1. Mix ½ teaspoonful of the tint selected with the same amount of 20 volume peroxide. (**Use plastic spoon**)

2. Apply mixture to both sides of the hair strand, from scalp through ends.

3. Retain on strand until the desired color has developed.

4. Wet a piece of cotton with shampoo and remove free color.

5. Dry and examine strand.

6. If the color developed on the strand test is not desirable, select another and test again.

Ways of coloring hair: There are many ways to color hair and many products to use. The most widely used products fall under three categories — **temporary, semi-permanent** and **permanent haircoloring.**

Temporary hair coloring: Temporary coloring contains **certified colors** that are not dyes. Some merly coat the hair and so may be washed out with a shampoo, but some do not shampoo out. Temporary coloring appeals to men because it is quick to apply and easy to remove.

Temporary hair colorings are of four general kinds:

1. **The so-called 30-day color rinses:** These are especially popular with men because they achieve coverage in about ten minutes. They do not go off shade nor turn dark; will not rub off; and will endure through shampoos, require no peroxide, completely cover gray hair, look natural, and are available in a variety of colors. You may find these advertised "no patch test required." (See procedure of applying outlined elsewhere in this chapter).

2. **Color rinses:** Manufactured rinses are preferred. They are easily prepared and applied. Your local supply dealer will give you their names, literature and sell you the products. Color rinses cover yellow streaks and enhance gray hair, impart natural color to gray hair, come in a variety of shades, tone up the color of tinted or bleached hair. These rinses usually last from shampoo to shampoo. Such rinses are found to be generally satisfactory (refer to procedure of applying color rinses in chapter on RINSES).

3. **Color shampoos for highlighting:** These products are usually based upon a shampoo formulated with a synthetic detergent and the desired color added (see procedure of applying outlined elsewhere in this chapter).

4. **Crayons (powders, haircolor cremes, and mascaras):** Crayons are used mainly to retouch newly-grown gray hair between hair color applica-

tions; powders are used to cover gray streaks, mascaras to color eyelashes and eyebrows. Hair color cremes are generally used for theatrical makeup. Hair color crayons are represented as being harmless, quick and easy to apply, and easy to remove (shampoos out). S i m p l y moisten crayon and hair first. Start at the new growth and proceed along the hair shaft. Distribution may be furthered by combing. **Men find cray-**

ons handy for concealing gray hairs on moustaches, eyebrows and eyelashes. Crayons come in several basis colors: light, medium a n d dark brown; black; blonde, and auburn.

Removing temporary coloring: As just stated, some of these shampoo out and others do not. Manufacturers have products for removing temporary coloring. Free literature is available from manufacturers of all temporary coloring. Follow their directions.

CATEGORIES OF ANILINE TINTS

Aniline tints fall into two general categories according to their reaction on the hair, and they are **semi-permanent hair coloring** and **permanent hair coloring.**

SEMI-PERMANENT HAIR COLORINGS

These are neither temporary nor permanent in lasting qualities. They fill a place between these two color groups. They usually last from thirty days to six weeks. They do not shampoo out but fade gradually after application is discontinued. They are sometimes referred to as "30 day color," "six weeks color," or the "shampoo color rinse." Some semi-permanent coloring contains no peroxide and requires no peroxide developer or pre-softening. It is self-penetrating (see procedure of applying outlined elsewhere in this chapter). It penetrates the hair only into the cuticle layer. The semi-permanent hair coloring designed especially for men is mixed with 20 volume peroxide. Its application must be preceded by a patch test.

Chief characteristics of semi-permanent hair colorings are:

1. Some contain a self-penetrating coloring material.

2. The color does not rub off.

3. The color does not shampoo out.

4. The color may be removed easily.

5. The color is applied in the same way each time.

Purposes of semi-permanent colorings: Some of these are especially used for:

1. Particular colors

2. Gray hair

3. Men's hair

Whether a shampoo precedes the color application depends upon the manufacturer's instructions. The main purposes of such colorings are:

1. To cover gray hair partially or completely.

2. To highlight the natural color of hair.

3. To enhance the beauty of completely gray hair.

Semi-permanent coloring should never be applied over any other kind of tint or dye. Remove it first. **Semi-permanent coloring appeals especially to men** because when application is omitted it fades out naturally, the hair reverts to the previous shade in a few weeks, and application requires only a short service time. **A patch test** is required.

Some important hints on men's semi-permanent haircoloring:

1. If the patron has a dark skin or is partially bald — apply hair creme or vaseline to the skin around the hairline and to the bald area before color application.

2. Apply the color before giving a hair cut.

3. Apply color to temple and sideburn area first. These are resistant areas.

4. Semi-permanent haircoloring has no bleaching qualities.

5. If an undesired reddish cast appears, use hot water for both shampooing and rinsing. This will eliminate the reddish cast.

6. Use rotary motion with fingertips to work color into temple and sideburn area.

7. Use a non-stripping or mild shampoo to remove excess color. Follow manufacturer's instruction on choice of shampoo.

8. Use gloves to protect hands.

Color shade selecting for semi-permanent hair coloring:

1. Select the color closest to the patron's natural shade of hair.

2. If the hair is about 50% or more gray, select **one shade darker.**

Procedure for semi-permanent hair coloring on men:

(See also general procedure of applying outlined elsewhere in this chapter, and the one immediately following.)

1. Drape patron.

2. Examine scalp and hair.

3. Select color.

4. Pour color contents with equal amount of 20 volume peroxide into a plastic applicator bottle. Blend the mixture by gently shaking.

5. Always apply to dry hair.

6. Gently work color through hair like a shampoo until the hair is completely covered. Be sure to apply and work color through the sideburn area first.

7. Leave on the hair as prescribed. Rinse with warm water and finish with a non-stripping, mild shampoo (follow manufacturer's instruction).

SIMPLIFIED PROCEDURE OF ONE BRAND OF
SEMI-PERMANENT COLORING

Follow the standard preliminaries, such as examining the scalp, giving a patch test and a strand test. Apply on dry hair. This product contains no peroxide, penetrates the gray without coating, contains built-in shampoo, requires no pre-shampoo, requires no retouching, lasts at least 30 days, easy to apply. Apply on dry hair. If more color is desired after the process is complete, another application may follow immediately. Refer to illustrations of applying given in this chapter.

1. After shaking the bottle, pour the needed amuont into an applicator.

2. Start applying at temples and/or grayest portions and distribute throughout the hair with comb and finger tips. Use gloves. (Head may be covered with plastic cap.)

3. Leave on from 30 to 45 minutes first time and 20 to 30 on subsequent applications, depending on depth of color desired.

4. Apply sufficient warm water to work up a rich lather to cleanse the scalp and hair and then rinse thoroughly. (Patron to use a neutral shampoo, such as a creme shampoo or one recommended by manufacturer.)

5. Saturate scalp and hair with a soothing hair creme and then remove the excess creme. (There is a special "Creme After Rinse" for this purpose.)

Length of time to leave semi-permanent coloring on hair:

1. To blend gray hair leave for 7 to 10 minutes.

2. To darken hair (light coverage) leave on for 10 to 15 minutes.

3. To completely cover gray hair leave on for 30 to 45 minutes depending upon depth of color desired and texture of hair.

NOTE: On semi-permanent coloring refer to page 313-J.

PERMANENT HAIRCOLORING

The aniline tints offer the greatest success to hair coloring. They are sometimes used for men's haircoloring, but are most commonly used for women's.

TWO TYPES OF ANILINE DERIVATIVE TINTS

Aniline derivative or penetrating tints are formulated into **two distinctive types** of products. They are known as follows:

1. One-step application.

2. Two-step application.

Both of these types require a patch test (see procedure of applying outlined elsewhere in this chapter).

ONE-STEP APPLICATION TINT

The one-step application tint performs two activities. It generally **lightens** and **adds color** in one application, depending on the shade selected. One application usually suffices to make hair from one to several shades lighter. When a tint contains a bleaching agent, it is always used to lighten the shade of hair. With this type of tint, the hair is permanently colored **without** the necessity of pre-shampooing, pre-softening or pre-bleaching. These tints contain a bleaching agent, a shampoo with an oil base and the aniline derivative color.

One-step application tints have the following advantages:

1. They are time savers.
2. They color the hair lighter or darker than the natural color.

3. They do not leave a line of demarcation.

4. They can color gray or white hair to match nature's shade.

Selecting color shade for one-step application tint:

1. To cover gray hair and match the natural color of the hair, select a shade closest to the natural color. The natural shade is usually best ascertained by hair at the nape.

2. To cover gray hair and lighten the hair, select one shade lighter than the natural color.

3. To cover gray hair and darken hair, select one shade darker than the natural color.

4. Refer to the manufacturer's color chart.

TWO-STEP APPLICATION TINT

The two-step application tints require pre-softening or pre-bleaching before the tint is applied. This involves two separate steps of application. Examples:

1. Pre-softening gray hair before color application.

2. Pre-bleaching hair before a toner is applied. Toners are two-step application tints.

Two-step application tints are used:

1. To cover gray hair.

2. To produce a complete color change when applied to pre-bleached hair.

Color selection for two-step application tints: Two-step application tints come in various shades. The natural color may be matched; or by pre-bleaching the natural color may be completely changed. Use the color chart when making color selections and select the shades according to their basic tones. Examples:

1. Warm shades — contain a small amount of red or gold tones.

.2 Very warm shades — contain more red.

3. Red shades vary in intensity from light to deep and fiery reds.

4. Drab shades do not contain red or gold.

Rules to achieve these shades are:

1. Consider the percentage of gray or white in the hair.
2. Consider the natural color of the patron's hair.
3. Color added to color makes a deeper shade.
4. If the patron's hair is completely gray use the exact shade selected.
5. If the hair is about 50% gray, choose a color **one shade lighter.**
6. If the hair is about 25% gray, choose a color **two shades lighter.**

Hydrogen Peroxide: Peroxide is prepared in **several forms:** liquid, powder, cream and tablet. 20 Volume peroxide is used for the following purposes:

1. To **pre-soften** the hair. Presoftening the cuticle layer of hair makes it receptive to an aniline tine. See page 313

2. **To oxidize.** 20 volume hydrogen peroxide is mixed with all aniline hair tints. It liberates the oxygen gas which permits the coloring matter to develop.

3. **To remove hair color.** 20 volume peroxide is used in all bleaching agents.

Pre-softening: Some hair requires pre-softening to absorb a tint. Some tints do not require pre-softeners, especially semi-permanent colorings, and one-step application tints. A softener is usually required with two-step application tints. Wiry hair is usually resistant, and generally requires presoftening. The softener is left on the hair from 5 to 20 minutes depending on the resistance of the hair. 20 volume peroxide alone may be used to pre-soften the hair; or a formula of 1 ounce of 20 volume peroxide mixed with one-half ounce of neutral oil bleach. If the hair is extremely resistant use the neutral oil softener formula.

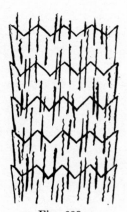

Fig. 639
Before Softening Hair

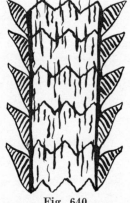

Fig. 640
After Softening Hair

Softening Opens Cells of Cuticle Layer of Hair

How to apply softener: Divide the hair into 4 quarter sections, if the hair is long enough. Follow procedure for applying softening agent and the manufacturer's instruction. Subdivide each section into small strands. Apply the softener to both sides of the strand; from the scalp to where the hair begins to show porosity, usually about 1 or 2 inches from the ends. Do not rinse out softener. Dry and apply tint. Pre-softening does not create a color change in the hair. It makes the hair more receptive to the tint. Frequent use of peroxide on the hair makes it dry and brittle.

Response of hair textures to tints: The variation in **hair porosity** will be the determining factor as to the required time for the tint to take. Successful tinting from dark to the palest shades depends on even porosity of the hair. Color Fillers used before the application of a toner or tint accomplishes this purpose.

Definition of hair porosity: The ability of hair to absorb moisture.

Definition of fillers: Fillers equalize the porosity of the hair shaft and leave the hair shaft in the same degree of porosity as is chemically possible.

Purpose of color fillers: These eliminate the problem of fadeage, control tints from darkening; and deposit a basic color to damaged or bleached hair prior to an aniline hair color application. Follow manufacturer's instruction.

How to select a color filler: The color filler must correspond to the same basic shade as the tint or toner to be used.

Timing of "take" in tinting: The time an aniline tint is left on the hair depends entirely on the product used. An aniline tint continues to take until the developer (peroxide) is completely oxidized. Aniline tints are worked out according to a time chart which may indicate from 5 to 45 minutes. When using a two-step aniline tint the hair must be kept in a moist state, with the tint product, during the timing period for good coverage. The most resistant hair is new hair near the scalp. The least resistant are the ends (especially the ends of women's hair) which as a rule are porous and very absorbent. However, the ends will sometimes reject the tint. The hair should always be put in a state of even porosity by the use of a filler. After the selected shade of tint has been applied to the re-growth for 30 minutes, add one ounce of appropriate color filler to remaining tint (instead of shampoo or water) and soap cap entire head of hair 5 to 15 minutes. Test color development at frequent intervals.

How to test for color development: With a piece of cotton moistened with bland shampoo remove tint from a small patch near the scalp or where the hair is most gray. If the gray still shows, dry the patch and re-apply the tint and leave on a few more minutes as estimated.

Removing tints: Manufactured tint removers, for aniline tints, are the best means of removing these tints. Follow this type of tint removal with a conditioning treatment for the hair. While the shade of hair can be lightened by a special aniline tint remover, the tint can hardly be entirely removed. If the original color was gray, after partial removal of the tint, the patron must be satisfied to allow the hair to grow out gray again; but any other natural color can be matched closely and applied. **Follow manufacturer's direction for any tint removal.**

Hair tint record: A written individual record of every tinting should be made. Such a record, among other items, should give the name, address and telephone number of the patron, tinting history of the patron, the dates, name and timing of the particular tint used, the texture of any preliminary correction treatments, price charged, retouch instructions and charge, and name of the barber.

Possible bad effects from tinting:

1. Excessive brittleness a n d dryness may be due to the use of too much bleaching material.

2. Vegetable henna on gray hair may cause carroty or orange tones.

3. An over reddish tinge may be caused by the use of certain hair restorers.

4. A greenish cast may be du to the use of silver restora tives.

5. A harsh black may be cause by allowing tint to stay on to long, or by compound hennas

6. A dusty gray may be cause by the use of lead prepara tions.

7. Streakiness of color may b caused by improper softenin or bleaching, improper appli cation of tint, or a weak de veloper.

8. Excessive tinting or soften ing causes hair to becom dry, brittle, and to lose it natural wave or luster.

Agents used to apply tints: Use brush, swab, or applicator bottle t apply tint to the hair.

Controlling action of tints: The ac tion of a tint may be controlled b the use of a color filler applied t the hair before the tint applicatior or the filler may be added to the tint for application.

Area tint first and last applied Tint as a rule is applied to the portion of the hair shaft closest t the scalp and to the more resistant areas, such as the sideburns. Since on men the hair ends are usually not damaged, after the scalp and sideburn areas are covered, distribute through remaining hair shaft and ends.

Items used in tinting:

1. Color chart

2. Shampoo cape

3. Towels

4. Rubber gloves

5. Dishes

6. Combs

7. Cotton

8. Shampoo

9. Tint product

10. Lightener

11. Developer

12. Tint brush, bottle applicator or swab.

A preliminary consultation: Prior to any tint application, explain the following:

1. Why a patch or predisposition test must be given.

    (1) Federal law requires it

    (2) Ascertain if patron has allergy to the tint

2. Examine the scalp for abrasions, eruptions, o r open wounds, presence of any tint, condition of hair. Do not apply tint over abrasions or eruptions since dermatitis might result.

3. Color selection.

4. Life-span of tint and upkeep.

5. Cost and time.

6. Arrange an appointment for tinting 24 hours after patch test.

Reminders on tinting:

1. Read the manufacturer's directions.

2. Examine the scalp before applying tint.

3. Protect patron's clothing by proper draping.

4. Apply color to resistant areas first.

5. Never mix tint until ready to use.

6. Do not irritate the scalp by brushing or rough shampooing prior to a tint application.

7. Use a non-strip shampoo to prevent stripping of color.

8. Use a final prepared rinse that will not strip color.

9. Color fillers are used only with aniline tints and toners.

10. Use only sterilized applicators, towels, **plastic bottles** and combs.

11. Make a customer record.

12. Sectioning of hair is done on women and on men whose hair is long enough. On men's sideburns and other short hair simply apply and gently further distribute with finger tips. Whenever the length of hair is too short to section, simply lift hair upward with a comb or tip of bottle applicator at time of applying. After sideburns are covered, proceed systematically around the head, preferably in **horizontal** strips from crown or back to front. Vertical strips are also correct, but proceed from top downward.

13. Do not leave customer while coloring is developing.

Progressive hair coloring: With some hair coloring the hair can be gradually colored to prevent a sudden change to startle friends. By following instructions the grayness can be partially colored and by repeated applications be made completely covered. One manufacturer recommends that his product be applied just like hair tonic and left and contends it will not shampoo out.

GENERAL PROCEDURE OF APPLYING HAIR COLORINGS

The steps of application as outlined are **not** equally applicable to all kinds of hair colorings. They should be varied according to the product used, the length of hair being colored, and the manufacturer's instruction. One manufacturer of semi-permanent coloring recommends that it be applied just like a hair tonic and left on and contends that color will not shampoo out.

1. Do not shampoo before coloring unless the hair is excessively soiled or instructed to do so by the manufacturer. (If a shampoo is given, use a neutral shampoo and very light movements so as not to irritate the scalp). Following the manufacturer's directions for drying the hair prior to tint application.

2. Section hair into 4 sections if hair is long enough, but this is often impractical on men (see illustrations to follow).

3. Apply softener if needed. The need is determined by the operator.

4. Apply matching shade of color filler, if needed (apply on aniline tint only).

5. Apply tint (follow manufacturer's instructions). Make about $\frac{1}{4}$ inch partings if hair is long enough. Such partings may prove impractical in men's hair coloring. In general take more care with aniline derivatives to make sure of complete coverage, especially on the early portion of the hair nearest the scalp. A thin hair coloring has to be more meticulously applied than a creamy one. In general applying coloring on men is more informally accomplished than on women, because the hair is shorter and more stubby, particularly at the edges. In all hair coloring of course strive for complete even coverage to avoid streaks and to achieve a uniform color. For men see the following illustrations.

6. Check color development at intervals as directed by manufacturer.

7. Rinse with lukewarm water as soon as color has taken.

8. Shampoo with a neutral shampoo such as creme shampoo.

9. Style hair as desired.

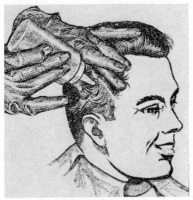
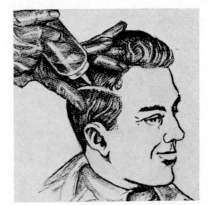

Fig. 640-A   **Fig. 640-B**

Methods of Applying Hair Coloring

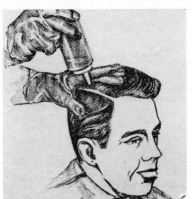
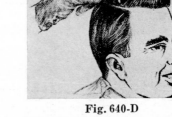

Fig. 640-C   **Fig. 640-D**

Methods of Applying Hair Coloring

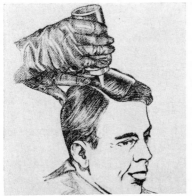
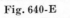
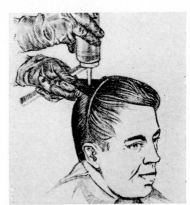

Fig. 640-E   **Fig. 640-F**

Methods of Applying Hair Coloring

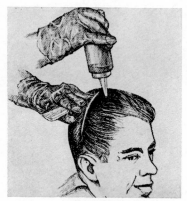

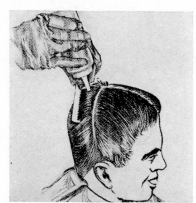

Fig. 640-G   Fig. 640-H
Methods of Applying Hair Coloring

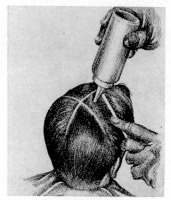

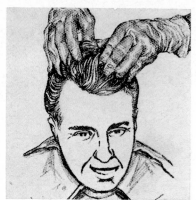

Fig. 640-I   Fig. 640-J
Methods of Applying Hair Coloring

SOURCES OF ADDITIONAL INSTRUCTION ON HAIR COLORING

Manufacturers of tints furnish, without charge, instructional material on their tints, bleaches and other coloring agents. If you cannot contact them or their retailers locally, write to them. Their products are accompanied with instructions. These manufacturers hold clinics where free instruction is given. These are found in the larger cities, but there might be one in your vicinity. Manufacturers might even send a representative to you to explain and demonstrate their products. Some local supply dealers have such demonstrations. Haircoloring manufacturers often advertise in barber and beauty magazines. Cosmetology textbooks are other good sources of instruction. Do not do hair tinting until you have adequate knowledge.

TERMS USED IN TINTING

1. **A developer** — an oxidizing agent, such as 20 volume peroxide.

2. **A retouch** — tinting only the new hair growth.

3. **Blending**—combing the color through the hair after a retouch to achieve a uniform shade throughout the hair.

4. **Virgin hair** — has neither been bleached nor tinted.

5. **Toning down** — using a particular shade of tint to drab out certain colors, such as red or gold.

6. **Oxidation** — the chemical reaction resulting from the mixture of peroxide and a tint.

7. **Pre-softening**—application of peroxide to soften resistant hair.

8. **Pre-bleaching**—removing color from the hair prior to a tint or toner application.

9. **Toner** — an aniline derivative tint, delicate in color.

10. **Porosity** — the hair's ability to absorb moisture or liquid.

11. **Patch test**—a skin test prior to tinting.

Mal-practice insurance: It is recommended that you acquire malpractice insurance before hair coloring on the public.

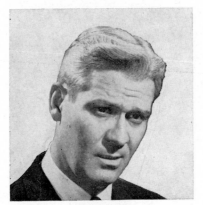 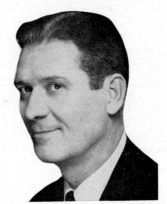

Fig. 640-K
Before

Fig. 640-L
After

Courtesy of Hoods Hair Products, Inc., Madrid, Iowa

BLEACHING OF HAIR INTRODUCTION

Bleaching means to lighten the shade of hair. It is the process of removing nearly all or part of the natural or artificial color pigment from the hair. **However,** bleaching is done mainly as a **preliminary to the application** of a tint.

Hair color pigment: The natural color of the hair is determined by the amount and kind of its pigment. Hair pigment may be brown, yellow or red or a mixture of each. During the bleaching process the pigment goes through different stages of color change. The amount of change will depend on the color of the hair, the bleaching agent used and the length of time it is left on the hair.

Forms of bleach: Bleach is prepared in two forms, liquid and paste.

Pre-bleach For Toners

Toners are delicate shades of aniline derivative tints **used only on pre-bleached hair.** They are used as a two-step application method of hair coloring. Most pre-bleaching is a preliminary step to hair coloring. **Pre-bleaching** is necessary for toner color effects. For the high fashion pastels, such as blonde, beige, platinum and silver shades the hair must be pre-bleached to gold or pale yellow.

PROCEDURE OF APPLYING TONER

1. Complete the usual preliminaries, drape, etc.

2. Section into four quarters if the hair is long enough. Otherwise lift the hair upward with the comb For men follow the illustrations in Figs. 640A to 640J. Short hair cannot be formally sectioned but systematic strips can be made by the comb or **nozzle of the bottle applicator.** On men start with sideburns and then apply to crown area.

3. Make about ¼ inch partings or strips when applying toner to the first ½ inch of hair next to the scalp. On short hair follow methods as shown in Figs. 640A to 640J.

4. Upon completing the entire scalp area, on the first ½ inch of hair, apply toner to remaining hair. Use a plastic **bottle** applicator to separate the hair on women. On men use either or both the applicator and fingers. After complete coverage, further distribute toner with finger tips. **Do not comb through hair.**

5. Leave on for about 35 minutes or as instructed by manufacturer.

6. Rinse toner out with **cool** water.

7. Shampoo lightly with a non-strip shampoo.

8. Thoroughly rinse out with cool water.

9. Style hair as desired.

Mixing a bleaching agent: Follow the manufacturer's instruction. Each manufactured bleaching agent varies in chemical contents and likewise the directions for mixture vary.

Manufactured bleaches:

1. **Oil bleaches**

   (1) **Neutral oil bleach.** Removes pigment but **does not** add color.

(2) Color oil bleach. Removes pigment and **adds some color** simultaneously.

2. **Paste or powder bleach.** It is a quick-acting agent and is recommended for use **only on strong and resistant hair.**

3. **Creme bleach.** It is the most commonly used and always used when pre-bleaching for pastel toners. This kind of bleaches have the following advantages because they contain:

(1) **Conditioning a g e n t s** which give protection to the hair.

(2) **Bluing agents** which help to drab gold and red tones.

(3) **Thickening agents** which give control when applying.

Condition of scalp: Do not bleach the hair if the scalp has abrasions or erruptions.

Coated hair: If the hair is coated with compound or metallic dyes or restorers, remove all such coating before bleaching.

Bleaching to lighten tinted hair: To achieve a lighter shade on tinted hair, the hair will have to be bleached. Tinted hair is more difficult to lighten than virgin hair. The condition of the hair itself will also be a deciding factor. As a rule, tinted hair is in a damaged condition. Re-conditioning treatments should be given prior to the bleach treatment and a creme bleach recommended for use.

Bleaching for the blonde, platinum and silver toners: These are high fashion shades and the hair will need a great deal of bleaching. The hair must be bleached to the pale yellow or almost-white stage. It must be made porous enough to accept the toner. A creme bleach is always recommended because of the previously listed advantages.

Materials and supplies for bleaching:

1. Protective cape

2. Towels

3. Peroxide (20 volume)

4. Bleaching agent

5. Mild shampoo

6. Cotton

7. Comb, clips

8. Plastic applicator bottle

9. Rubber gloves

10. Talcum powder

11. Record card

A preliminary strand test: This test should be given in order to find out the condition of the hair and to judge the length of time to leave the bleaching agent on the hair. To give a strand test follow the same procedure given for a virgin bleach, using a small amount of the bleach mixture and a small strand of hair.

PREPARATION AND PROCEDURE FOR BLEACHING VIRGIN HAIR

The general procedure given for a virgin bleach assumes the hair will receive a **toner color** treatment following the bleach, and a patch test has been given.

Prepartion:

1. Prepare patron.

2. Examine scalp and hair.

3. Do not shampoo or brush the hair.

4. Section hair into 4 quarters, if hair is long enough; otherwise lift hair with comb in systematic strips.

5. Prepare bleaching formula (follow directions).

6. Put on rubber gloves.

General procedure:

1. Begin the bleach application **one-half inch** from the scalp; on men start at sideburns; on women start at the crown. Extend the mixture down the hair shaft to where the hair begins to show porosity or damage.

2. Section each quarter into about 1/8 inch partings.

3. Apply bleach to both sides of the hair strand.

4. Continue application in same manner until the entire head is completed. Gently work the mixture into the hair with fingertips. **Do not comb the bleach through the hair.**

5. Keep the hair moist with the bleach during development.

6. Test for color by removing bleach from a small hair strand with wet cotton. Dry the strand for true color observation. If hair has not lightened sufficiently, re-apply bleach to the strand. Test frequently.

7. When the hair has lightened sufficiently, r e m o v e the bleach by thoroughly rinsing with **cool** water. Dry the hair.

8. **Scalp application:** Re-section hair into 4 quarters, if the hair is long enough. Use 1/8 inch partings. Apply the bleach over the scalp area and down the hair shaft, over the previously bleached hair, to the ends which show porosity. Cover both sides of the hair strand.

9. **Hair ends:** Apply bleach to hair ends and work through with fingers.

10. When the hair has reached the desired shade, remove the bleach by cool water rinsing and **lightly shampooing** with a mild shampoo. Towel dry or dry under a cool dryer.

Some general rules when bleaching for a toner application: The bleach is usually retained on the hair shaft from 45 minutes to one hour and 15 minutes; on the ends 30 to 45 minutes. If the scalp shows any irritation after a bleach, wait 24 hours before applying a tint or toner. Bleached hair should always be treated with the correct color filler before applying the toner.

Reminders on bleaching:

1. Always give a 24 hour patch test if a tint or toner is to follow.

2. Use only fresh bleach.

3. **Do not** irritate scalp before bleaching by brushing or manipulating.

4. Follow manufacturer's instructions.

5. Prevent dripping or over-lapping.

6. Check frequently for development.

7. **Do not** bleach hair which contains color from compound or metallic dyes.

8. Hair may be bleached if it has been colored with aniline tints.

9. Use a mild shampoo and cool water for rinsing.

10. Apply bleach to resistant areas first.

11. Use 1/8 inch strands when applying bleach.

12. Replace towel on patron's neck if it becomes moist with bleach.

13. Make and keep a customer record card.

Shampooing bleached hair:

An egg creme shampoo is recommended. Bleached hair has a tendency to mat and tangle when wet. Use luke warm water. Matting may be avoided by applying the shampoo very slowly and directing the hands under and into the hair but not from the top in the usual way. Follow with a lemon or vinegar rinse or one especially prepared for bleached hair. While the hair is still damp, apply a little lubricating dressing or other recommended preparation to aid manageability and ease in combing.

A New Semi-permanent Coloring For Men:

Made by reputable manufacturer. **Simple procedure.** Comes in 2 most popular shades for men — light to medium brown; dark brown to black. Partially or completely covers gray as it blends in with natural color. (Cut hair first.) No pre-shampoo; has built-in-shampoo. Color gradually disappears in about 6 weeks without demarcation. Partial coverage in 10 minutes; complete in 30. Gradual or partial 10-minute treatment tones down gray; repeated as prescribed, it progressively reaches full coverage, if desired. (1) Apply with applicator. Start at temples and hairline; apply against grain of hair, (2) distribute with finger tips ONLY—avoid rubbing scalp, (3) for 30-minute complete coverage use plastic cap to allow body heat to develop color, (4) with warm water work up lather; rinse well, (5) towel dry and apply Color Hold Tonic, (6) dress hair. Instruct patron not to use tonics or shampoos with alcohol or sulphur or bar soap; instead neutral or manufacturer's shampoo.

Finger Waving

(BASIC PRINCIPLES)

The purpose of this chapter is to present the basic principles of waving. These principles are a vital part of men's and boys' hairstyling. Even the youngster may be pleased with an "S" shaped wave across his toplock. The barber is chiefly interested in "S" shaped waves for styling the hair of males. This discussion, therefore, will be limited mainly to this area.

FINGER WAVING

Finger waving, formerly, was the process of forming S-shaped waves with the fingers and comb in wet hair. But its present definition is much broader and includes several kinds of **wet waving,** such as pin and sculpture curling. A pin curl is flat and over-lapping. To form a pin curl, sectionize a small strand of hair, and place the tip of the left index finger in the center of it and at right angle to the scalp. With the right hand, wind the hair flat around the index finger in the direction the curl is to be set. Hold the curl securely until it is fastened with a pin or curl clip close to the scalp. The ends of the strand are on the outside of the curl. Sculpture curls are also pin curls, but the winding begins at the ends of the strand and goes towards the scalp and the ends of the hair are on the inside of the curl. When the stem direction of a curl is toward the face, it is a **forward curl,** when away from the face it is a **reverse curl.**

Some basic points on finger waving:

1. First requisite is clean hair.
2. Naturally wavy or permanent waved hair finger waves most successfully.
3. Coarse texture hair is most difficult to wave. Medium texture waves best.
4. Hair can be made more obedient and to cling more closely to the head by slithering, thinning, or correct shaping.

5. Finger waving is preferred to marcelling, because:
   (1) It does not injure or discolor the hair, since no hot irons are used.
   (2) It is adaptable to all kinds of hair.
   (3) It produces more natural looking waves.
6. Flakiness can be caused by inferior wave fluid.
7. Matching waves means continuing the waves around and fitting them together in back. ("Horseshoe waving" means the same thing as matching the waves.)
8. A drop wave is a wave that is discontinued at the crown or part. In "S" shaped waving it is necessary to drop one wave in order that the next wave may be continued around the head after the pattern of a horseshoe, a pattern not followed on the male.
9. Deep "S" waves are made by rolling and pressing the fingers astride the ridge.
10. The average width of "S" waves is $1\frac{1}{4}$ to $1\frac{1}{2}$ inches.
11. To determine the width of waves, measure from ridge to ridge.
12 Keep the hair thoroughly wet during the waving.
13. Seat the customer in a hairdressing chair, not a barber chair. A Shampoo towel is fastened securely around the neck. Place a water repellent shampoo cape around the neck over the towel, allowing enough of the towel to protrude above the cape to absorb any draining moisture from the hair.

General procedure of finger wave:
1. Prepare customer.
2. Shampoo hair.
3. Apply wave fluid or warm water.
4. Comb hair.
5. Wave hair.
6. Place hair net over hair and dry.
7. Comb hair.

Detailed procedure of finger wave:
1. Saturate the hair with wave fluid or warm water.
2. Find the directional flow of hair by combing and moving it.
3. Comb the hair **through to the scalp in each stroke.** Do the preliminary combing with the coarse part of the comb, and follow with the fine part to form the wave, but if the thickness and volume of the hair resist, use medium tooth comb.
4. Form the waves. Refer to the explanations and illustrations on Forming Ridges and Waves.
5. Upon completion of the first ridge, form the next ridge in the same manner, but start at open end of next wave to be formed.

6. Upon completion of the whole finger wave, place a hair net over the hair. To prevent discomfort from the dryer, protect the ears and place a towel around the neck. Dry the hair thoroughly.

7. Comb hair as desired.

FORMING RIDGES AND WAVES

(1) Comb smoothly the hair of the ridge to be formed, or a portion thereof, using a semi-circular movement to position it for the direction it is to be drawn. Firmly manage the hair and keep it flowing in the desired direction and in straight lines.

(2) Place the index finger of the left hand **firmly** on the strip of hair to be moved, lengthwise with and slightly above where the ridge is to be formed.

(3) With the right hand, place the fine part of the comb firmly against the index finger ready to direct a strip of hair toward the closed end of the wave to be formed, a direction that is to the right for a right-going wave and to the left for a left-going wave. Place the teeth of the comb slightly under this finger and firmly against the scalp. Comb through the strip of hair to be moved two or three times, moulding it in the direction it is to be drawn. Comb this strip of hair **outward** about ½ inch and about one inch forward or towards the place where the first portion of the ridge is to be formed. In this way the hair is arranged in the proper **bias** direction to form the ridge.

(4) Each portion of a ridge is formed by sliding a strip of hair along the forefinger placed to hold the hair and to direct the ridge. The width of each strip should not be more than about one inch. Each strip of hair is drawn as directed from ½ to 1 inch to form each section of the ridge. If the hair is moved too far, the ridge will stand out instead of locking itself to the head. Do not slide or push the hair upward or beyond the line of the ridge; instead direct it in a tight, straight line, gradually moving the comb about one-fourth of an inch away from the guiding finger. With this strip of hair drawn to the proper place, flatten the comb against the head to hold the ridge in place and to accommodate the next position of the index finger.

(5) Next, replace the index finger with the middle finger, and place the index finger below or on the other side of the ridge. With these fingers firmly astride this portion of the ridge turn the teeth of the comb downward and comb the hair away from

the ridge in the direction the next ridge is to be formed, in a semi-circular manner, keeping in mind an "S" shaped formation. Comb through the hair in this way two or three times, arranging it correctly for forming the next ridge. The fingers are placed astride the ridge to prevent the hair slipping while combing and to assist in completing that portion of the ridge. When the hair is thin and sparse, slide it back slightly at the end of the "draw" to reduce the bare spaces and to help form an unbroken ridge.

(6) Repeat this same general process until the ridge is completed, except each additional portion of the ridge must be fitted or tied to the portion already completed so as to form a conitnuous ridge without a break. A smooth and unbroken ridge can be assured (1) by placing the index finger used to form an additional portion of the ridge so that it overlaps the portion of the ridge just completed, (2) by placing both the index and middle fingers so that they overlap the completed portion of the ridge at the end of the "draw," and (3) by overlapping the combing of these two portions of the ridge.

(7) To form a higher ridge for a deeper wave, roll and press the two fingers astride ridge while combing away from ridge.

(8) To remove a finger or fingers from a ridge do not raise them straight up, but rather gently slide them off in the direction the wave is being formed.

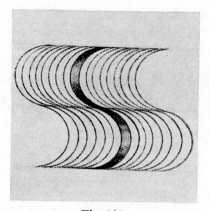

Fig. 641

Basic "S" Wave Pattern

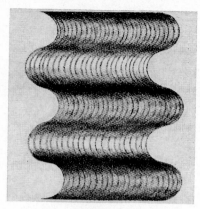

Fig. 642

S-Wave Completed

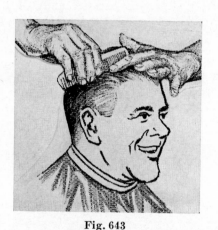

Fig. 643

Basic Step 1

Place comb under and against index finger with teeth pointed slightly forward and inserted to the scalp.

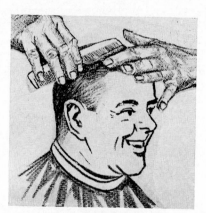

Fig. 644

Basic Step 2

At the end of the one-inch draw, flatten the comb against the head to secure the ridge until the first two fingers are place astride it.

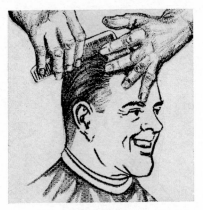

Fig. 645

Basic Step 3

Place the first two fingers astride the tentative ridge while the flattened comb is holding it secure.

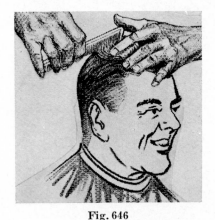

Fig. 646

Basic Step 4

Now direct the teeth of comb downward and draw the hair in the direction that the next wave is to be formed, making a semi-circular effect.

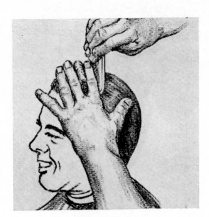

Fig. 646-A

Start the second ridge on the side of the head where the first ridge was completed. It is formed by the same procedure as the first ridge. See Fig. 129 to 133.

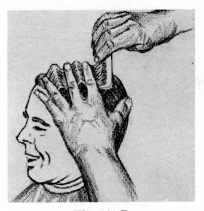

Fig. 646-B

Assuming Step 2, and 3 of forming the second ridge have been completed, complete the fourth step as already explained in forming the first ridge.

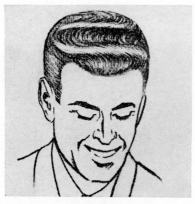

Fig. 646-C

Waves being formed. Second ridge completed. Now make third if desired. Apply net, dry and comb out.

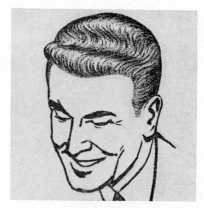

Fig. 646-D

Soft Wide Waves Completed.

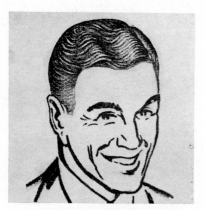

Fig. 646-E

Soft Wide Waves Completed

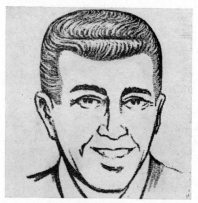

Fig. 646-F

Soft Waves Completed

NOTES

MARCELLING
(Introduction Only)

1. Definition: Marcelling is the process of making waves by heat and pressure with a marcel iron.
2. Origin of marcel: It was originated by Francois Marcel, a French man, born in 1852. It resulted from his attempt to trace and imitate the naturally wavy hair of his mother.
3. Fundamental features of marcelling:
   (1) The hair must be made to cling to the head.
   (2) The waves must be formed in curves—free from straight, hard lines.
4. Marcel iron: It consists of a groove, a rod and handles.
5. Cleaning a marcel iron:
   (1) Clean with steel wool and oil, or
   (2) Clean with a soap solution containing a few drops of ammonia, or
   (3) Clean with fine sandpaper, especially for polishing.
6. Pointers about the width of marcel waves:
   (1) The wide, soft waves are the most popular.
      a. They add naturalness.
      b. They are more artistic.
      c. They blend well with the contour of the head.
      d. They leave the hair soft and fluffy.
   (2) Strive to make every wave uniform in width.
   (3) Wide waves are most suitable for dark, coarse hair.
   (4) Narrow waves are most suitable for fine hair.
7. Coarse hair is most adaptable to a marcel; fine hair takes a marcel least successfully.
8. Wax used in marcelling:
   (1) Wax comes in solid and liquid forms. The solid kind is used by rubbing it over the face of the hot iron and also in the groove, or by rubbing the iron over it; the liquid form is applied directly to the hair with an atomizer.
   (2) Wax is used to add body to the hair, and thus assure a more lasting marcel on either fine or coarse hair. But apply only a small amount, because too much wax tends to cause the hair to break.
9. Marcelling over a permanent wave:
   (1) Shampoo the hair and dry it slowly but thoroughly.
   (2) Use an iron only slightly heated.
   (3) Spray a little brilliantine on the hair.
   (4) Wave close and flat to the head.

Conversation

Conversation can be either an asset or hindrance to success in business. It is like condiments—a little goes a long way.

Definition: Conversation is the art of conversing with people. It may also be defined as the social interchange of ideas.

Barber should know art of conversation:

1. He must make acquaintance.
2. He is continuously dealing with people.
3. The public expects it.
4. It is necessary for success.

Subjects that most interest people: For a casual conversation, you will find people most interested in talking about their own activities and achievements. Talk about the customer's interests rather than yours, at least in emphasis.

Is customer always right? It is a prevailing business principle that the customer is always right but this false assumption need not mean that a barber should accept everything the patron says. There is a sort of "professional nod of approval" that does not represent the conviction of the nodder. One either uses good business tactics or he has no business at all.

Expressing your convictions: It is sometimes inadvisable to express one's own conviction in a business relationship. A lot, of course, depends on the subject.

Desirable Subjects of Conversation: Choose subjects that are as non-controversial as possible. Arguments should be avoided at all costs. Customers usually do not wish to delve into a knotty problem of any subject. Choose a phase of a subject about which it is easy to make a few passing remarks. Most customers would rather relax and talk in the lighter vein than to become involved in a philosophical discussion. Good communication through conversation is the medium to friendly relations so necessary to success in business. It is important to choose the right time to talk about something as well as to choose the right subject. For instance, suppose that the patron in the chair is filthy and dirty, refrain from lecturing on the value of cleanliness; instead, you may even say, in case he mentions his condition, "that's O.K. It does one good to get dirty once in a while."

The following is a list of subjects that should strike a pleasant cord of conversation.

321

1. Timely information.
2. Vacations.
3. Civic developments.
4. Weather.
5. Consideration for children.
6. Honesty.
7. Punctuality.
8. Education.
9. Citizenship.
10. Travel.
11. Character.
12. Sympathy for poor.
13. Crime prevention.
14. Music.
15. Art.
16. Safety precautions.
17. Economic conditions.
18. Value of athletics.
19. Juvenile delinquency.
20. Hobbies.

Subjects on which generally a barber should not express his convictions:
1. Religion.
2. Politics—who should be elected, etc.
3. The barber trade.
4. Home troubles.
5. Love experiences.
6. Poor workmanship of other tradesmen.
7. Personal problems.
8. Ill manners of patrons.
9. Uncomplimentary rumors.
10. Financial income. (His own.)

Desirable characteristics of conversation:
1. Pleasantness.
2. Optimism. Express the bright side of life.
3. Well modulated voice—a voice with neither a very high nor a very low pitch.
4. Non-thought provoking subjects or questions. That is, do not bring up something that may cause the patron to have to think deeply. Only the rare individual cares to have his mind put to deep thinking.
5. Significance—do not talk too much about trivial things.
6. Good English. Consult a good handbook on English; read a great deal. There is no excuse for atrocious English.
7. Informality—do not be stiff in manners, voice, etc.
8. Direct the conversation away from yourself, as much as reasonably possible.
9. A smiling countenance.
10. Humor—gain the right perspective of things. Remember that all things do not have an equal value—some things are significant, and some things are insignificant.

Undesirable characteristics of conversation:
1. Unpleasantness.

2. Pessimistic attitude towards things in general.

3. High, raspy voice.

4. Argumentativeness.

5. Negative point of view.

6. Interruption of someone talking.

7. Low, extremely gutteral voice.

8. Weighty questions.

9. Triviality—excessively foolish things.

10. Bad English.

11. Formal, stiff manners.

12. Inquisitiveness.

13. Over-seriousness.

Continuous conversation not recommended: There should be restful elapses in conversation. Much depends on the customer; some customers like to chat and others prefer no conversation. There is the sin of commission and omission in conversation. It is easy to say too much or too little.

Stimulate patron to talk: Lead the patron to do most of the talking. He can be stimulated to converse by (1) asking him a good question, and (2) by listening attentively to what he says.

Be a good listener: Strangely enough, a good conversationalist is a better listener than a talker. Listening is a very important phase of conversation. A poor listener usually interrupts frequently. A good listener asks leading questions, and patiently waits for answers.

When to begin conversation: Complete the preliminaries of a service before starting a conversation. However, the time varies with the patron. The type of questions asked to put the patron at his ease are "yes and no" questions. A conversation proper is not begun until the work to be rendered is well under way.

Source of conversation material: The world is full of knowledge. Newspapers and magazines are a rich source of information. Learn to be a keen observer of life. Be interested in life itself and you can find plenty of things to talk about. Be ever eager to learn new things. Barbering affords a wonderful opportunity for a person to gain a general education through personal contact. Learn to be a good listener.

Continuity in conversation: There should be some continuity whenever possible. In asking questions you imply sufficient knowledge to talk further about the subjects brought up. Otherwise, the questions would fall flat. For instance, "Do you enjoy the movies?" implies that you have been to the theatre recently and have something very interesting to say about the picture which you saw.

General questions to ask customers:
1. How are you?
2. How is business? (If you know he is in business.)
3. Are you working hard these days?
4. Are you a native of this state? If not, ask which state.
5. How long have you lived in _____?
6. How is your family? (If you know he has one.)
7. What is your hobby?
8. Where do you like to go for vacations?

Selective questions to ask customers: The question the barber asks depends on age, sex, profession, nationality, hobbies and interests of the customer.
1. If the patron is an elderly man, ask such questions as:
    (1) Do you remember the first automobile?
    (2) Have you lived in this state a long time?
    (3) Did you take part in any war?
    (4) How many children do you have?
2. If the patron is a mother, ask such questions as:
    (1) Do you find it hard to keep your children out of the street?
    (2) Where do your children go to school?
    (3) What kind of work does your husband do?
    (4) What kind of electric refrigerator do you like best?
3. If the patron is a teenager, ask questions about school, subjects he is taking, sports and other subjects befitting his age.
4. If the patron is a sports fan, ask questions about various sports in which he is interested.

Subject of patron's family and mutual friends: If you know that a patron has a family, especially if you have met any member of his family, ask "how is the family" or about a particular member. If you know the patron is a proud father of a new baby boy, ask how the boy is. If you have mutual friends, ask about one or two of them occasionally.

Questions on occupation: Many people like to be asked about their work, others prefer to have their mind directed to other things. Learn to tell when a patron appreciates being asked about something, but do not put a difficult question. For instance, if the patron is a dentist, the barber may ask, "Do people have their teeth pulled as much today as they used to?"

Remember things said by patron: Remembrance furnishes an opening wedge for a conversation the next time he is present. In fact, this point is a great secret. Recall something told by a patron the last time he visited the shop and tie a conversational remark to it. This will greatly please the patron. A patron likes to feel that you know him, that you know something about him, provided, of course, what you know is favorable.

People's interests classified:

1. Some people like to talk about things, such as big bridges, new ships, fast trains, new cars, big towers, high buildings, large mountains, horses, farming, circuses, etc.

2. Some people like to relate narratives—to tell stories. They speak of happenings, what someone did, daring feats, races, flying exhibitions, accidents, peculiar marriages, etc.

3. Some people like to talk about people or personalities. They usually have some solid ideas about character traits. They speak of initiative, humor, brilliance, drunkenness, smoking, laziness, clever conversation, morality, success, failure, sickness, etc.

4. Some people like to talk about adventure, including such subjects as fishing, shooting, traveling, playing bridge, playing checkers, interesting books, etc.

5. Some people like to talk about ideas, such as the advantage of an education, why some people go to church, the result of the next war, careless drivers and what should be done about them, the indifference of some mothers to their children, why bachelors do not get married, the advantage of being married, better law enforcement, etc.

Study customer's reactions: If you understand what kind of a person your customer is or his present state of mind, your conversational problem is largely solved. Some customers are religious, politically minded, talkative, know-it-alls, reticent, nervous, tired, irritable, impatient, in a hurry, have time to kill, courteous, discourteous, easy-to-please, difficult-to-please, believing, skeptical, etc. Regardless of the customer's type or state of mind, the barber should be courteous, tactful, obliging, and eager to please. This will impress the customer and put him at ease, and this is of paramount importance.

Magic formula in conversation: Find out what the patron's interests are and direct the conversation around them. Make his interests first and your's secondary.

Five major faults in conversation to avoid:

1. Talkativeness. Do not be over-inclined to talk or parade your knowledge. Give plenty of opportunity for the patron to talk.

2. Impatience. Relax and give the patron your undivided attention.

3. Saying too much about yourself. Many things interesting to you about yourself are not interesting to the customer.

4. Pointlessness. While it is all right to be humorous and say a few entertaining things, do not try to be a comedian. Confine your remarks largely to significant matters.

5. Wordiness. Cultivate brevity in expression. A few words well spoken and to the point are more effective than a lot of unnecessary words.

Heedful suggestions to please customers:

1. Constantly practice friendliness.
2. Professionalize in tactful silence.
3. Never flatly contradict a customer.
4. Radiate enthusiasm.
5. Don't be didactic.
6. Don't be over-inclined to give advice.
7. Don't take yourself too seriously.
8. Manifest sincerity in listening to what people have to say.
9. Be essentially informal.
10. A well proved worthy business slogan is: "A man with a smile is a man worth while."

Thirteen brief pointers on conversation:

1. Be a good listener. Let the customer have the floor.
2. Do not interrupt a customer talking.
3. Pay attention to what is being said. Do not let your eyes drift.
4. Act interested by being interested and do not allow yourself to look bored.
5. Do not become too wrapped up in your own ideas. The opinions and ideas of others may be even more interesting than yours.
6. Be brief. Do not wrangle along merely to prolong the conversation.
7. Look pleasant and cheerful, even if it takes effort.
8. Try to end your part of a conversation on a pleasant note.
9. Put a smile in your voice. Study how to produce a pleasant sound in your voice.
10. Look into the face of the customer a reasonable amount of time when listening or talking to him.
11. Give your customer your undivided attention although you may wave at someone passing by or recognize an entering customer.
12. Do not carry on a conversation with anyone else while serving a customer.
13. Do not converse with a customer in another barber's chair, nor to the barber serving him.

Salesmanship

Anyone who serves the public is necessarily some kind of a salesman. The barber not only serves the public; he has something to sell. Services beyond the haircut and shave are services needed by the public. It is said that "Nothing happens until someone sells something."

From the cradle to the grave we are faced with the need of selling. By tears and noise, a baby induces his mother to meet his wants. A boy induces his father to buy him a new bicycle. A teenager proves his need for an automobile. An applicant for employment represents himself as qualified. When a man proposes to a woman, he assumes he has induced her to believe that he will make her a good husband. A candidate for public office campaigns on the basis of his qualifications to serve his constituency, and thus sells himself. A feeble aged man induces someone to help him across the street or off or on a bus. In the innumerable avenues of life, there is a need for salesmanship in some form. And one's success in any avenue of life depends a great deal upon his selling ability.

What the barber has to sell: A barber has many things to sell. And whatever he sells does something constructive for customers. Hair cuts add becomingness, tonics, shampoos, and treatments help preserve and restore the health of his face, scalp, and hair. Under various categories fall the items that the successful barber has to sell the public:

1. Himself—his personality.
2. His shop—its appearance and reputation.
3. His art and science of barbering.
4. Importance of good hair grooming.
5. Advisability of proper care of the scalp and hair.
6. Cosmetics and other merchandise.
7. The traditional services of barbering—hair cuts and shaves.
8. Extras. These may be called "added services," such as hairstyling, shampoos, tonics, facials, and scalp treatments.

Motivation is the basis of salesmanship: Efficient sales productivity is actuated by some motive. Basic emotions spark any planned action. Here are a few of them that prompt people to sell:

1. Desire for personal gain. This is a dominant motive.
2. Desire for recognition and praise. One likes to be recognized and praised for "doing his stuff."
3. Avoidance of monotony and boredom. All jobs sooner or later prove

somewhat monotonous and boresome. An escape from this is to develop a talent for entertaining and thrilling customers by the medium of salesmanship.

4. Pride of accomplishment. Part of the reward from selling something, especially if the customer at first did not want it, is the good feeling one has of accomplishment.

5. Desire for social prestige. One likes to be honored and respected.

6. Desire for self-confidence. Everyone has to fight the deadly gnawing of fear and worry and the inadequacies of life. Confidence built up by successful selling drives away these sapping moments.

7. Love of family or someone. The affection one has for someone else is a terrific urging impulse to be his best—this means **selling.**

A good salesman does not babble aimlessly about himself or details of no interest to the customer. A top salesman listens to everything a customer says, seeking a clue to his thinking, personality, and preference. And the salesman should know that a customer can be lost permanently if he is permitted or induced to buy something which he does not need or something that has no value or merit. It is not the "one sale" plan that makes a salesman a success, but rather the repeated business of the same customer. The style of haircut requested is in the area requiring the utmost tact and diplomacy. Some customers have a mistaken idea of how certain styles will look on them. It is up to the barber to explain this. It is easy to offend by bluntly stating "you wouldn't look good with that style". With diplomacy, however, he may be told that the style would not be becoming to him because it would make his face look too flat or his neck too long. Then, in a modulated tone of voice, suggest the appropriate style. The same tactful and sincere approach should be used in selling tonics, shampoos, facials, and scalp treatments.

Definition: Salesmanship is the art and science of selling. While salesmanship is necesarry to sell the traditional haircut and shave to maintain satisfied customers, it is indispensable for selling such extras as tonics, hairdressings, shampoos, facials, and scalp treatments. Salesmanship is the major avenue of increasing personal and shop income beyond the necessary services. In a sense, of course, these extras are necessary to the well-grooming of customers, but generally they are regarded as luxury services in contrast to the necessity of a haircut. By observing closely the condition of the customer's scalp and hair, one can point out a need for a particular service. The art, then, is to create a desire for the product or service. The elementary but important point is simply to "ask the customer" after having decided what he should have.

Sales Inducements: There are many ways of inducing customers to have extras. Only six will be mentioned in this section:

1. Serve a customer so well that he will want to benefit by more of your services. Scientifically manipulating his scalp following a haircut may suffice. Try to make him volunteer to ask about a product or service. If you see he is especially enjoying the way you service him, take the initiative of asking him. He will not be inclined to agree to any additional service if you have not already served him well and professionally.

2. By a vocabulary revealing that you know something definitely about the hair and skin, you can stimulate the customer to have extras. Such terms as "pityriasis", "sebaceous glands", "alopecia", "arterial blood", "arteries of the scalp", "acne vulgaris", and "trichoptilosis" signify that you have studied barber science and that you possess valuable information about his needs. The customer must be made to believe that you know what you are doing.

3. A well-equipped shop helps greatly to convey the idea of superior service.

4. A sanitary and comfortable shop helps to pave the way for salesmanship.

5. Inviting premises stimulate an interest in services. An attractive front, fast-moving modern barber poles, well-made signs, a cheerful shade of paint or wall finish, proper lighting, good ventilation, and thorough sanitation are associated at once with superior and satisfactory service.

6. Thought stimulating interior signs can spark the customer's interest in other services. Such signs as "try our relaxing facial", "scientific soft-water shampooing" or "stop falling hair before it stops you", should prove helpful.

Basic Factors of Salesmanship: Selling is not just babbling. Make each word count and come quickly to the point. The following are some important factors which comprise the foundation of selling:

1. Knowledge. Know what you are talking about. Know your product or service and be able to explain it in simple straight-forward language. You should be able to answer the customer's queries intelligently, fully, and interestingly. It might be safely contended that "the more you know about your services, the more you will sell". Know your customer, too, as well as possible.

2. Enthusiasm. Be enthusiastic about what you have to sell. This creates customer confidence in you.

3. Constructiveness. Never offer criticism of a condition unless you have a remedy to suggest. Make positive, constructive suggestions and point out the merits of a product or service.

4. Cheerful willingness. Be eager to serve and give the impression that you will be delighted to do it.

5. Sincerity. Earnestness of voice, tone, and attitude convinces the customer that you have faith in your services.
6. Initiative. Do not hold back or be too aggressive. Initiative means agreeable aggressiveness. In the final analysis, you must initiate the selling.
7. Determination. Resolve to make good. "Screw your courage to the sticking point". Do not be too easily discouraged. Determine to be a successful salesman. Good determination will help you to break down sales resistance. Don't be afraid to make repeat suggestions. Tactful persistence will pay off.
8. Creativeness. Study and create ways of inducing customers to buy. Be a "thinking salesman". If you are thoroughly familiar with your products and the merits of barber science services, a little concentration will enable you to create new angles and approaches by which customers can be induced to have extras.
9. Alertness. Watch for the psychological moment to make a tactful suggestion for a sale. Direct the conversation to lead up briefly and easily towards a high pitch of interest suitable for an appropriate moment to suggest a further service.
10. Workmanship. This term means "deliver the goods". Serve your customers according to the best of your ability and knowledge. Do not be a clock watcher. Instead, be a money maker, but serve the public well. The public will usually not complain about the price if they get their money's worth.

How to attract attention of patron to extras:

1. Discovering and pointing out a need.
2. Tactful suggestions.
3. Thought-stimulating interior signs. Such signs arouse curiosity and cause customer to ask questions. Examples: "Try our Scientific Dandruff Treatment," or "Let us Help You With Your Dandruff Problem".
4. Advertising.
5. Giving services so efficiently to customers that they want more and tell their friends about you.
6. Listening to the patron.
7. Rendering one service in such a manner that it calls for another.
8. Calling attention to new products or services.
9. Attractive displays of merchandise for sale. Immediately visible attractively **display cosmetic products** and other merchandise such as shaving cream, lotions, creams, tonics, and safety razor blades. These may be displayed singly or in a group. The price should be easily observable, whether the display consists of one or more items. A general sign across the top of the display, could read

"Items Every Man Needs". "Free Advice on Your Cosmetic Needs". (At the cash register have all items packaged ready to hand customer). Should the customer not already have become interested in any of the displays, merely ask him if he needs any of the items on display, but make the suggestion casual, such as "may I explain any of the items on display" or "the next time you need any of the items we have on display, I will be glad to show them to you and explain their uses". It is also effective to call his attention to a particular item or a group package deal consisting of several items. A choice place for displays is directly in front of the customer. If space permits, a middle-of-the-floor display where the items for sale are conspicuously visible to customers both while they are waiting and being served is effective. In a narrow room, the wall in front of the barber chairs is recommended for displays.

10. Cartoons, pictures, or illustrations induce customers to ask questions. Example: Have an artist or sign painter draw a picture of a man scratching his scalp in agony from itching. Have it read: "Gee! My Scalp Itches." A customer may say, "You know my scalp itches terribly." This of course is an excellent cue for the barber to sell an itching scalp treatment.

Two Types of poor salesmanship:
1. High-pressure salesmanship. This type is characterized by extravagant promises, impossible guarantees, over-enthusiasm, and unethical procedure. It is generally offensive.
2. Low-pressure salesmanship. This type is characterized by timidity, lack of confidence, lack of faith, fear, hesitance, etc.

Good salesmanship: Somewhere between the two above named extremes. Briefly, good salesmanship means selling something and keeping it sold. It is not enough to sell something just one time to a person; a desire to buy again must be created in him.

Magic Way to assure repeat sales: Sell something of genuine merit— something with self-evident value. QUALITY tells a story of success.

Fitting statements following a service: A favorable comment by the barber re-assures the customer that he will be satisfied.

Here are such statements:
1. The hair cut looks good on you.
2. The facial added color and life to your face.
3. The facial made your face look smooth and refreshed.
4. Does your scalp tingle?
5. This cream contains the best ingredients.
6. This hairdressing is very enhancing to the hair.
7. You really cannot afford to do without good face lotion.

8. This kind of hair cut compliments the contour of your head.
9. I know you will be pleased with this hair cut.
10. If you use this kind of cosmetics, your friends cannot help noticing the difference.

Use positive approach: A positive point of view in selling means emphasizing the good points and making helpful suggestions. It is a mistake to dwell on the things wrong. If possible compliment the patron; for example, you have a fine head of hair. If he has dandruff, a compliment fittingly precedes suggesting a treatment. Here are examples of usable statements:

1. You have a fine head of hair, but you have an excessive amount of dandruff. We have a good dandruff treatment.
2. Your skin is smooth and clear on the chin and forehead, but you have a lot of blackheads on the cheeks. I recommend a facial treatment.
3. We have a haircoloring rinse that would cover up your grayness, and it takes only a few minutes to give.
4. Theorize about the causes of dry hair without referring to the patron's dry hair. This stimulates him to say "my hair is very dry. What would you suggest?"
5. Have you ever had treatments for your dry hair? If the patron's response is favorable, you can tell him about your treatment.
6. If the patron states he has had an especially hard day at the office, suggest a Rest Facial.

Listen attentively after suggestions: The response of the patron is important. Link your suggestions to the interest aroused, and drive home your point. Give a patron time to become curious about your suggestions.

Do not use negative approach:

1. It is inadvisable to single out a conspicuous imperfection or defect although a sure remedy may be available. For instance:
   Barber: Your hair is very dry.
   Patron: I know it, but nothing can be done. I have tried everything.
2. It is much better for a barber to say: "You have a fine lot of hair." After such a complimentary remark, the patron may say: "But my hair is very dry." The opening wedge is then driven and the barber can "go to town," by tactfully suggesting and recommending scientific treatments for dry hair.

Suggestions for extras not made to all patrons:

1. The time, the money, the patience, and the degree of the need of the customer must be considered. When these matters are barriers, they should be minimized as far as possible. But, when a person has to board a train within a short time, do not suggest an order that

would take longer than he can spare. When the customer is positively down and out, choose fitting suggestions, perhaps they may simply lay the foundation for future sales. Additionally, certain orders may be modified somewhat to fit a particular case, both as to time and money.

2. Frequently, it is fitting and effective to point out to a customer that, in comparison with many other expenditures for securing and maintaining comfort and good appearance, the average person spends a very small amount of money on the care and treatment of his hair, his scalp, and his face, and that since these are among the most important parts of the body, especially in view of the fact that they are visible, they ought to receive a great deal or at least more consideration. The properly trained barber should be capable of meeting the patron's needs in this regard.

Winning confidence of patron:
1. Add some little touch of service that reveals your skill, such as a few movements of the Rest Facial following a shave, or a few scalp movements following a haircut.
2. Employ a few technical terms relative to the muscles, nerves, hair, or skin. Such allusions are often of inestimable force in gaining the customer's respect.
3. Make some reference to some special course of barbering that you might have had.
4. Refer to any special course on barbering you have had.
5. Be more eager to serve than to sell.

Avoid argument: Arguing with customers, except on a high plane of humor, is never recommended in business. Arguments do not lead to sales. This fact does not mean, however, that the advantages of a given product or service cannot be enumerated or tactfully laid along side of some other product or service.

Stimulating statements in selling: These statements may be either spoken or written on small signs:
1. The proper care of your hair is important.
2. Do not neglect your hair.
3. We find many people who are interested in the shampoo method of hair coloring.
4. A Rest Facial will relieve your tired feeling.
5. Your skin can be helped by an Acne Facial.
6. Your hair is so unruly I recommend a hairdressing.
7. Have you ever tried our Soapless Oil Shampoo?
8. So many of our customers like our Clay Pack Facial that we are featuring it as a special this week. Would you like to have one of these fine facials?

9. Would you like our special Holiday Facial? It is especially designed for (name any holiday).

Suggesting substitutes: A barber should attempt to sell a substitute for an article, in case he does not have the particular article the customer desires. It behooves a barber to be ready to suggest a substitute, only do not use the word "substitute." Name your article and explain the points of similarity and, if possible, make your article appear just as good or a little better than the one mentioned, although do not carry this idea to extreme and knock the one called for unless it has evident imperfections that can be clearly shown. Familiarity with your products will enable you to suggest like articles.

If patron insists on particular brand: Ask permission to secure the item, and arrange to send a card when the order is filled or to deliver it to the patron. Try to keep a customer from going elsewhere if reasonably possible.

Mailing list of customers: A mailing list is usable for announcing specials, new products, etc. And most significant of all: a mailing list is effective for reminding patrons that the date for another haircut, a facial, a scalp treatment, and-so-forth, has arrived. Such correspondence, however, should be written by an expert, for they must be tactful.

One thing at a time: Attempt to sell only one item at a time. Suggesting a whole list of items confuses the patron. Stick to one subject and allow plenty of time for response.

Display case of items for sale: Such a display is indispensable. It is often the attractive display that attracts the attention of the patron and a show-case lends the impression of a well regulated shop.

Point out patron's needs: It is the barber's duty to point out the patron's needs. It is hardly advisable to point out more than on need at one time. If the patron volunteers to state his needs, such as dandruff or dry hair, the barber has an ideal opportunity. If the patron selects the proper shampoo, tonic or service, compliment him.

Learn names of customers: Specialize in learning names. It is of supreme importance to address a person by his name. Even when explaining the benefits of additional services, occasionally, call his name.

Use Brains as well as hands: The best barbering is performed by hand-and-mind coordination. The skillful use of the hands is important but this use alone limits the barber. To be a really successful barber, he must also use his head. But more than this he should do some creative selling and this requires the use of his brains. The climax to this chapter very fittingly embraces the essence of a barber trade magazine stimulant to induce barbers to practice salesmanship. Here are the stimulating phrases used:

Barber Brains—Let's make 'em mean something!

Shape — Hair	Treat — Hair
Style — Hair	Wave — Hair
Color — Hair	Promote — Good hair grooming

Through salesmanship, make the brains pay as well as the hands. Active brains and dexterous hands spell good salesmanship.

Importance of thanking the customer: Make it an invariable rule to thank every customer as he leaves the shop. Your "thank you" should have a cheerful ring in it. It is terrifically important that the customer leave the shop feeling that the barber sincerely and keenly appreciated his patronage. Such a feeling makes him more inclined to return for future services. Never take this feeling for granted. Faithfully and invariably, regardless of the particular service, impart a feeling of thankfulness and appreciation.

Package deals: Package deals often induce customers to have something beyond a hair cut. They usually consist of a hair cut, styling of the hair, shampoo, a service to the scalp, and a hair-grooming preparation. A price is set for these combined services. In fact, barbers can make up their own package deals.

Categoriesof selling: To gain the respect of your patrons primarily confine selling to the following:

1. Services the patron requests.
2. Services the patron needs.
3. Cosmetics and other items the patron can use at home to keep himself well-groomed.

Importance of knowledge in selling: Have more than a superficial knowledge of the services you give and recommend the products you suggest. If you sell a scalp treatment mention the value of stimulating circulation and the sebaceous glands. Point out the purposes and uses of cosmetics you recommend.

Value of truth in selling: Customer must be made to believe in you. Stick to the truth, even if sometimes it is unfavorable to a sale. You may say "we don't have a sure cure for your dandruff, but we do have some treatments that may greatly alleviate the condition. I believe they are worth trying."

Three essential steps to selling:

1. Gettings the patron's ATTENTION.
2. Arousing the patron's INTEREST.
3. Creating the DESIRE to buy.

Evidence of aroused interest:
1. Interest is reflected in the patron's eyes. Do not stare at him but look into his eyes. Lifted eye lids usually indicate interest.
2. Questions by the patron. The patron whose interest has been aroused will ask questions.

Some obstacles to selling:
1. Failure to make points clear.
2. Failure to recognize mood of patron.
3. Talking too fast and too loud.
4. Lack of proper tone of voice.
5. Lack of adequate knowledge of what you are selling.
6. Bad breath.
7. Improper grooming.
8. Unshaven face.
9. Outrageous claims.
10. Cocksureness.

Good posture impresses customers:

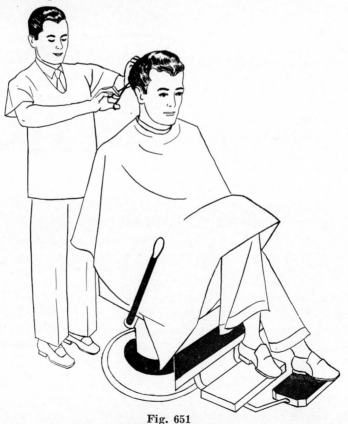

Fig. 651
Good Haircutting Posture

Shop Management

Good shop management is especially important in a trade as competitive as barbering. Good workmanship is not enough. There must also be competent management.

Definition: Shop management refers to all the principles and methods by which a business is conducted.

Some items included in shop management:

1. Services.	11. Insurances.
2. Ethics.	12. Rents and leases.
3. Shop atmosphere.	13. Utilities.
4. Bookkeeping.	14. Records of customers.
5. Advertising.	15. Wages.
6. Illumination.	16. Repairs.
7. Sanitation.	17. Hiring.
8. Ventilation.	18. Public relations.
9. Courtesy.	19. Organization.
10. Individual attention.	20 Taxes.

Good shop atmosphere characterized:

1. Wholesomeness.	6. Willingness to serve.
2. Cheerfulness.	7. Pleasantness.
3. Dignity.	8. Friendliness.
4. Humor.	9. Helpfulness
5. Courtesy.	10. Appreciation.

Bad shop atmosphere characterized:

1. Smoke from cigars and pipes is especially objectionable. No restrictions, however, can be placed upon the customer. Never smoke while serving a customer.
2. Liquor breath is very noticeable in rendering barber service. Don't mix liquor with business.
3. Profanity.
4. Loud laughing.
5. Whistling.
6. Singing or humming.
7. Questionable stories drive away more trade than they attract.
8. Gum chewing.
9. Talkativeness.
10. Indifference to customers.
11. Argumentativeness.

Greeting customers: Customers should be recognized and greeted immediately upon entrance. They should be made to feel welcome and comfortable. Speak in a pleasant tone of voice and look at the person whom you are greeting. Saying "please have a seat" is relaxing to anyone entering the shop. Newcomers are especially alert to your reception and first impressions are often lasting. If you are running an appointment shop, you can link the patron's name to the time he comes in (or glance at the appointment book). In such a shop when you are uncertain you may say "May I help you?"

Remembering names and faces: The worthwhileness of knowing the names and faces of customers is immeasureable. It will enable you to make and keep customers, and add pleasure to your profession. A very pleasant sound to a person is the sound of his own name. The recognition of a patron by name indicates to him that you appreciate his patronage and he is more likely to continue to patronize you. Learn how to remember names and faces. A few tips are:

1. Make sure you **hear** the name correctly.
2. Upon hearing a name **pronounce** it.
3. As soon as convenient **write** the name.
4. Concentrate on the name.
5. Seize every opportunity to use the name.
6. Make an effort to remember the name.
7. Learn both the first and last names.
8. Form a mental picture of the patron's face. Note all the physical characteristics of his face, such as color of eyes, size of nose, chin, ears and forehead, and the amount and color of hair.
9. If possible associate a patron's name and the shape of his face with somebody whom you already know.
10. Associate the patron's name and face with his occupation or hobby.

Answering telephone: Answer in a clear pleasant voice. Announce the name of the shop. For example: "Manhattan Barber Shop." If the cashier or secretary is answering the telephone for the shop, she need not announce her name. If she refers the call to a particular barber or person he should answer merely by announcing his name — "Mr. Cooke speaking." If a problem has been referred to him, he should add: "may I help you?" If it is necessary for you to know the caller's name, simply ask "may I ask who is calling? or "who is calling please?" Don't say "who's calling?" If the person being called is unavailable, explain to the caller by saying "he is not here right now, but he should be back shortly," or "he is away today but will be back tomorrow." Don't say "he's out," "he's busy," but you may say "he is serving a customer." Always offer some kind of assistance to the person calling, such as "may I help you?" or "may I take a message for him?" or "may he call you?" or "may I

tell him who called?" If the called party is available, either contact
him without comment, or you may say "may I tell him who is calling?"
The latter response is usually the preferred one for formal business. (If you are calling out and wish to know the name of the person
with whom you are talking, say, "may I ask your name?" or "may I
ask with whom I am talking?" **Put a smile in your voice.** Be direct.
Be brief.

Always have a paper and pencil immediately available.
If an appointment for service is requested, repeat the name of the service
desired and time, and thank the patron by name. For example: "A hair
cut, 2 p.m., Thursday, thank you Mr. Morton." Do not talk too fast or too
slowly, too loudly or too low. Your voice should be natural and express-
ive, and indicate cordiality, alertness, and interest. Make the customer
feel that his call is important and that you are giving him individual
rather than routine consideration. If you are really sincere you will not
sound artificial. If the telephone rings while you are talking with
someone,**discontinue talking or excuse yourself before lifting the re-
ceiver.** It is rude not to do so.

Importance of thanking customer: Make it an invariable rule to thank
every customer as he leave the shop. Your "thank you" should have a
cheerful ring in it. It is very important that the customer leave the shop
feeling that the barber sincerely and keenly appreciated his patronage.
Such a feeling makes him more inclined to return.

Ways to attract new customers:
1. Attractive entrance.
2. Good location.
3. Good personal appearance.
4. Window displays.
5. Meeting people socially.
6. Advertising.
7. Satisfied customers

Ways to keep customers: Customers prefer to patronize shops that are
conducted according to the principles of good management. Apply the
principles set forth in this chapter, but remember **good workmanship**
is the keynote medium. Give equal interest and consideration to all
customers.

Some illustrations of uniform service: Obviously no two barbers can perform a given service exactly the same way, but they can comply with the
same general standards. Here are ways:
1. Approximately the same length of time for certain services.
2. The same number of steam towel applications before or after a
   shave.
3. The same kind of linen set-up for certain services.
4. The same kind of face lotions, creams, etc.

5. Approximately the same type of salesmanship.
6. The same sanitation methods.
7. The same emphasis upon an attempt to please.

Ethics in management: Refer to the chapter on ethics in this book. A shop that practices ethics has met a fundamental requirement of success

By whom and when should service standards be explained:
1. By the manager.
2. The psychological times to discuss these standards are (1) upon hiring a barber, (2) early in January, when they can be set up as practices for the new and ensuing year, and (3) at business meetings of all the employees.

Blowing your lid is bad: Management entails some trying situations between the manager and employees and the public. You can best cope with these situations if you keep calm and collected. While there is no magic formula to follow, the following should prove helpful:
1. Accept the fact that you are not perfect and subject to mistakes.
2. Don't feel like you always have to get even with someone.
3. Guard against saying and doing things that you will later regret.
4. Pass over many things with a deaf ear, especially when such things might disturb your peace of mind.
5. It is often better to turn your eyes away from things that might disturb your peace of mind.
6. Do not try to convert everyone to your point of view.
7. It is better to leave everyone to his way of thinking rather than to give way to contentious discourses.
8. Rudyard Kipling, in his poem, "If," gave some advice very applicable to a shop manager:
   "If you can keep your head when all about you
      Are losing theirs and blaming it on you;
   If you can trust yourself when all men doubt you,
      But make allowance for their doubting too;
   If you can wait and not be tired of waiting,
      Or being lied to don't deal in lies,
   Or being hated don't give way to hating,
      And don't look too good, nor talk to wise!"

The person who follows this advice meets one of the important requirements of a good manager.

Some anti-social "dont's":
1. Don't try to get even or get back at people. Avoid sharp retorts.
2. Don't try to impress people with your superior learning.
3. Don't criticize one patron to another patron.
4. Don't criticize other barbers.
5. Don't urge that patrons buy extras when they don't want to.

6. Don't have a closed mind to other ways of working.
7. Don't resent suggestions from your employer.
8. Don't feel you are always right.
9. Don't be too anxious to fight to get your rights.
10. Don't manifest dullness, coldness, indifference, annoyance, apathy, or blank looks.

Term "Next": This term is still accepted in a strictly men's shop. Used as a single beckoning, it is a little too sharp, flat and abrupt. It is preferable to use it in sentence form. You may say:
1. Who is next?
2. Who would like to be next?
3. If you know the patron's name and know he is not waiting for another barber, pronounce his name and say "you are next," or simply look at him and just pronounce his name.

Managerial Duties:
1. To extend the general courtesies of the shop, especially at the door. Greetings and farewells rest mainly upon his shoulders.
2. To see that each customer's "turn" is honored.
3. To observe the character of the service received by a patron. Such observation enables him to check on the workmanship of his barbers, as well as to protect his patronage.
4. To attempt an even distribution of trade among the chairs. A manager should not employ a barber he cannot recommend. Often, a word from the manager will influence a patron in his choice of a chair. Several customers waiting for one particular barber while other barbers are idle is an unwholesome situation from a business point of view. The manager will have occasions to recommend other barbers in his shop. He may say, "you will find Mr._____ very satisfactory," or "Mr.————————— does very fine work."
5. To endeavor to secure a "shop patronage." "One man patronage" is antagonistic to general shop patronage. However, certain preferences of customers should be respected to a limited degree. The trend for preferences as to particular barbers seems to be increasing rapidly. To a great extent such preferences are justifiable.
6. To quell any momentary quarrelsomeness of a barber. Habitually quarrelsome barbers should be dismissed. Do not, however, attempt to settle disputes between barbers (1) unless you are exceedingly tactful, or (2) unless it is a matter which you can obviously clear up.
7. To provide suitable books, magazines, newspapers, etc., for both the barbers and the patrons. Recommend certain readings to the barbers. Do not have barber or beauty magazines at the convenience of patrons.
8. To have complete knowledge of supplies. Hence, he will be able to

make any necessary replacements, to buy new supplies, etc.

9. To set the atmosphere of the shop. He should see that an atmosphere of cheerfulness, decency, and wholesomeness is maintained.

10. To interview barbers seeking employment.

11. To manage the shop. Suggestions from his employees should be welcome. But he should not regularly delegate his duties to his barbers nor should he permit them to assume any of those duties. He should be in command.

12. To enforce the practice of sanitation. While each barber is individually responsible for the practice of sanitary measures, the manager should see that such measures are followed. (Refer to the chapter on Sanitation.)

13. To obtain the necessary insurance.

14. To act as a supervisor of the shop.

15. To pay or see that all operating expenses are paid.

Instructions to janitor: The manager should post a typed outline of the janitorial work and explain it to the janitor. This is particularly important when hiring a new janitor. Make sure that the janitor understands exactly what you wish him to do and when. The instructions should include a schedule of mopping, waxing and buffing of the floor, mirror cleaning, bowl cleaning, etc. Your local janitor supply store will gladly help you select the proper detergents for cleaning the floors, bowls, woodwork and other items. While a powdered detergent may be used to clean bowls, a liquid one with a mild pleasant fragrance is very popular. An immaculately clean shop reflects good management.

Storeroom: Keep an inventory of all supplies and classify them. Those that are to be used in the business are **consumption** supplies and those to be sold are **retail** supplies. Have a dispenser pad and write down every item removed from the room.

Bookkeeping: Bookkeeping books may be purchased at any stationery store. Keep an accurate record of all income and expenses. The assistance of a C.P.A. will prove valuable. Income is usually classified as Income from Services and Income from Retail Sales. Expenses have many classifications, such as salaries, rent, utilities, advertising, repairs, equipment, etc. Retain check stubs, cancelled checks, and receipts and invoices.

Sample payroll check stub: A payroll check should have a section listing necessary deductions. Such section divides itself from the other part of the check by perforations. Design your payroll checks after consulting a C.P.A., because deductions are not uniform in all the states. Your bank will make them for you. The sample to follow is usable in California.

STATEMENT FOR EMPLOYEE
Detach Before Cashing

Emp. _____

Date Paid _____

Total Compensation - $_____

Employees should keep
their pay check stubs.

S.D.I. $ _/00_

Fed. I.C.A. $_585_

Income Tax $/650_

_____ $235 235

_____ $_____

Total Deductions - - - $_____

Net Compensation - - $_____

How to pay shop expenses: Expense bills should be paid promptly and systematically. A scheduled time such as twice a month might be set. Pay wages by **check** and all major expenses. Cancelled checks are good receipts.

Leases: A lease is a written contract to use the premises for a specified purpose, time and rent. While a shop space may be occupied on a month-to-month basis, if you purchase a shop or put in a new one, a lease is advised. A lease may contain an option for an extension exercisable by the leasee. A lease usually contains the provision that it cannot be assigned to anyone else nor the premises sublet without the written consent of the lessor. It is advisable to have an attorney review a lease before you sign it.

Insurances: Some insurances are required and others are optional. State laws set the employer's required insurances. Since insurances are a technical matter, it is advisable to consult a reputable insurance broker.

1. Insurances most **states** require.
   (1) Unemployment insurance. (Refer to section on taxes.)
   (2) Disibility insurance. (S. D. I.) State Disability Insurance.)
   (3) Workman's compensation insurance (also known as **industrial** accident insurance.) This insurance provides for disability benefits due to injury on the job. Some states exempt the employer from such insurance if he has fewer than a specified number of employees, while other states exempt on the grounds that they classify barbering as non-hazardous. The penalties for failure to have this kind of insurance are often severe.

2. Optional insurances. The employer should carry most if not all these insurances.
   (1) Public Liability. This insurance protects the owner or employee against claims made by members of the public for injuries on the premises.

(2) Mal-practice. This insurance protects the employer against claims made by members of the public for injuries from the acts of barbering.

(3) Fire insurance. This insurance may be written to cover total loss or a specified percentage of the loss.

(4) Theft insurance on equipment and money. This insurance may be written for total loss or as a fifty dollar deductible policy. Under the deductible policy up to fifty dollars is not covered by insurance. This type of insurance is slightly cheaper.

(5) Money and securities insurance. This insurance protects you against the loss of money and checks from theft-burglary and robbery. Protection from such losses on the way to or from the bank is called **messenger** insurance.

(6) Health and accident insurance. The employer may carry health and accident insurance, or he may carry group insurance covering himself and his employees in case of incapacitation due to sickness or injury. A minimum number of employees is required for group insurance. There are many types of such insurance.

TAXES

Since taxes are a technical matter, it is advisable to consult your public accountant or tax consultant. Other **sources of information** are such government agencies as the Internal Revenue Service, the State Department of Employment, and the State Franchise Tax Board. Have your tax reports made out by your public accountant.

Personal income taxes: The proprietor is subject to federal and state income tax laws.

1. **Federal income tax.** This tax is based upon the proprietor's taxable income for the calendar year. To put the self-employed person on the same basis as the salaried person, the proprietor is required to file a Declaration of Estimated Tax, and pay such tax for the current year in four quarterly installments, by the fifteenth of April, June, September, and January of the following year. His income tax return is then due to be filed not later than April 15, whereon he takes credit for the aforesaid payments and pays the balance of tax due or applies for credit for any overpayment.

2. **State income tax.** This is also based upon the proprietor's taxable income for the calendar year. The rate of such tax differs in different states.

Self-employment tax: The proprietor who has self-employed income of $400.00 or more is required to pay a social security self-employment tax.

This tax is computed on the federal income tax Form 1040 (Schedule C), and paid with the filing of his income tax return.

Payroll taxes: Every employer is responsible for payroll taxes, both federal and state.

1. **Federal payroll taxes.** These taxes are paid to the Internal Revenue Service. There are four kinds of such taxes, but the employer may not have to collect or pay all of them.

   (1) Withholding income tax: This tax is based upon the employee's income and number of dependents. The rate is set by the government. Such tax must be deducted from each pay check, if due.

   (2) Social Security tax (F.I.C.A.) means Federal Insurance Contributions Act. The rate of this tax is set by the government and each payroll check must account for it. The employer must pay an alike amount as collected from an employee. That is, if the employer withholds $5.00 for this tax, he himself must also pay $5.00, making a total of $10.00. Wages above a specified sum are not so taxable. Reported quarterly on Form 941. Form 941.

   (3) When an employer withholds more than $100.00 of income and/or social security taxes for either the first or second months of a quarter, he must remit such taxes on Form 451 to the District Director of Internal Revenue in his district on or before the fifteenth of the following month. Some banks will process said tax reports for the first two months of a quarter. By the end of the month following the third month of the quarter, he must remit said taxes for the third month on Form 941, and enclose receipts for the other months of the quarter. The government sends the employers these receipts. This quarterly remittance must include employer's share of the social security tax for the quarter.

   (4) Federal unemployment tax: This tax is required of the employer only. If he employs four or more employees on at least some portion of one day in each twenty or more calendar weeks, he is liable for this tax.

2. State payroll taxes. Every employer is responsible for state payroll taxes, some of which he himself pays and some he collects from employees.

   (1) Unemployment insurance: This tax is borne entirely by the employer. His rate is determined annually by the state department according to his past unemployment experiences. There is a wage maximum above which wages are not subject to such tax.

(2) Disability insurance tax: This tax is usually deducted from the employee's wage. The rate is set by the state.

Property tax: Local governmental agencies, state, county and city, impose taxes on both real and personal property. Shop equipment and merchandise for sale and real estate are examples of property subject to such tax.

Sales tax: If you sell any merchandise of any kind to the public you are subject to sales tax if your state has a sales tax law. Be sure to obtain a sales permit from the states sales tax department. Keep all your invoices of merchandise bought for resale and carefully record all sales.

Use tax: If you elect to use in your business any merchandise purchased for resale, you will be subject to Use Tax which is reported on the same forms as the Sales Tax. The rate of such tax is usually the same as the sales tax rate.

Federal excise tax: If you sell cosmetics to the public you are subject to federal excise tax. The Director of Internal Revenue will furnish you with a quarterly report form. Number 720.

Tax on tips: Income tax must be paid on tips. If less than $100.00 yearly, report them on Form 1040; if more than $100.00 yearly, you must report them on Form ES 1040. Employer is not required to keep records of the tips of employees.

DEDUCTIBLE EXPENSES

Expenses deductible in year paid: Operational expenses are deductible in the year in which they are paid. They include license fees and organization dues, advertising, subscriptions to trade magazines, interest on business loans, business legal expense, business travel, accounting and bookkeeping, salaries to employees, rent, repairs, maintenance, barber supplies, laundry, telephone, gas, light, water, certain taxes, and miscellaneous expenses. That is, all those expenses that are both ordinary and necessary and directly connected with the business. All such deductible expenses are called **current expenses.**

License fees: The various license fees due annually include those for a state barber license, a state shop license, a city shop license, and a shop health license. In some states and cities barbers are required to have a health certificate. Some cities levy a license fee the amount of which is based upon the total of the prior year's sales of services and merchandise. Contact your city licensing department for information. Check all licenses carefully for renewal date.

Expenses pro-rated and deductible over more than one taxable year: Such expenses are called **capital expenditures.** A capital expenditure may be broadly defined as the acquisition of an asset which has a useful life of more than one year. Examples: Expenditures for new buildings, improvement on present buildings, a new roof, new furniture or fixtures, tools or instruments having a useful life of more than one year. Such Capital Expenditures are not taken as a current expense, but are Capitalized, and the cost of the same is recovered by a yearly charge to expense through depreciation. The owner is entitled to recover the cost of this Capital expenditure less the estimated salvage value, during the estimated useful life. There are several methods of depreciation. The most common one in use, and the most simple mathematically, is the Straight Line Method. By this method, a piece of equipment which costs $2,100.00, and has a salvage value of $100, with an estimated useful life in the business of 10 years, would be **depreciated** at the rate of $200 per year. At the end of ten years, the **depreciation** charge would stop, leaving an unrecovered cost of $100, which was the original salvage value. As a guide for depreciation rates for some barber equipment, the Internal Revenue Service estimates the average useful life **in years** of the following items:

Chairs: Barber	12	Massage machines	4
Bobbing	10	Mirrors	20
Waiting	8	Tables, manicure	10
Clippers, electric	4	Vibrators	4
Dryers, hair	5		

Taxpayers may determine reasonable periods for the useful life for their depreciable property on the basis of their particular operating conditions. Smaller items include razors, shears, latherizers, etc. Periods of estimated useful life are subject to review by the Department of Internal Revenue. **Leasehold improvements:** Leasehold improvements are improvements that increase the value of the property, prolong its life, or make it adaptable to a different use. Such improvements include plumbing and electrical installation, remodeling, and floor covering. The distinction between equipment and leasehold improvements depends upon the nature of the item and its final ownership. In general, leasehold improvements are items that become affixed to the property, and thus become the property of the landlord at the expiration of the lease. **Leasehold improvements are amortizable,** that is deductible, over the period of the lease. Such deductions are known as **amortizations.** For example, if a floor covering whose useful life is five or more years, is laid at the expense of the leasee and he has a five year lease, only one fifth of the cost is a deductible expense each year of the lease.

Insurance expense: Business insurances are a deductible expense. It is customary practice to write most such insurance policies to cover a period longer than one taxable year. The cost of such insurance is then prorated or deducted over the term of the policy.

Illumination for barber shops: Haircutting in particular is precision work and requires good illumination. Less light is required for facials, shampoos, and scalp treatments. Good lighting increases productivity, improves the human environment; it means stimulation, pleasantness, efficiency, and attractiveness of facilities. A light designer; the city light and power department, and manufacturers of fixtures can help you determine the proper lighting. A footcandle meter measures the number of footcandles or light units. Factors to consider are: basic room dimensions (length, width, height), color of the ceiling, walls, floors and equipment. Keep in mind the lighter colors are more reflective than dark colors. Regardless of the various colors, the proper footcandles can be obtained, although less wattage will be required when light colors are used, and more wattage when dark colors are used. The light reflected from a surface is called reflectance (formerly "reflection factor"). The **proper number of footcandles at barber chair height** is one-hundred (100). For eye comfort the difference in footcandles in the immediate room areas should not be more than (25) less. If there is too much contrast of light the eyes will suffer from strain. By having the correct footcandles, the eye strain from too much or too little light will be avoided.

The matter of color rendition is chosen according to personal preference. If a red light is turned on a green object, it will look grayish or blackish. While this is a drastic example of color effects, it illustrates a principle. A pleasing color helps to attract and keep customers. In general, choose the closest match to natural daylight.

Temperature of hot water: Set the hot water heater at normal or 140 degrees Fahrenheit.

Purchasing a shop: The buyer should require a "bill of sale." This document, purchaseable at a stationary store, should show the purchase price, the manner of payment or payments, and a detail itemization of the equipment and supplies being purchased. Certain fixtures, known as lease-hold improvements, cannot be removed from the premises unless the lease so provides. Any personal property or fixtures that are so attached to the building as to be considered permanently fixed are deemed to be a part of the building and cannot be removed by the tenant unless the lease so provides. Floor covering attached to the floor is a good example of this kind of attachment. This, along with the lease should be placed in "escrow" to make sure that the items being purchased are free from any mortgages, judgments or liens.

Consideration for new barber shop:
1. Preliminary questions:
    (1) Is my experience ample to justify an investment?
    (2) Do I have sufficient finance? You should have at least three months operating cash reserves.
    (3) Is it a good location?

(4) How many people live in the vicinity and how many people walk or ride by the location daily?

(5) What kind of potential customers are there?

(6) How many shops are in the same area?

(7) Is there a need for a new shop?

(8) Can I get a satisfactory lease?

(9) What level of prices will I be able to charge?

(10) What about parking and transportation?

2. Special recommendations:

(1) Make a list of the barber equipment to be bought.

(2) Obtain cost of the equipment from a supply house.

(3) Have an architect draw a blueprint of the complete plans. You cannot accurately determine the costs without a blueprint and specifications. A professionally drawn blueprint will save time and money.

(4) Ascertain cost of plumbing, lighting, flooring, carpentry, painting, etc. Obtain written bids.

(5) Obtain a written contract for all construction.

(6) Make a very inviting entrance.

(7) Have all signs professionally made.

3. **Location of shop:** Locate your shop where people are and at their convenience. Shopping centers, schools, factories, grocery stores and banks afford a business potential. It is better to go to the people than to depend on them to go to you. Basement locations are risky. Choose a location that matches the type of shop you will have. An inviting front, well equipped, nicely decorated and air-conditioned shop plus good service with a smile assure your success. If you locate in an office building, locate as near the elevator as possible, ideally right in front of it, and preferably on floor two or three.

Major types of business operation: There are three major types of business operations:

1. Individual ownership. In this type the owner is solely in charge of the business.

2. Partnership. In this type there are two or more owners and they must conduct the business according to the decisions of all owners. Partnership agreements should be drawn by a lawyer.

3. Corporation. This type requires a charter from the state and board of directors. To form a corporation, a lawyer should be engaged.

Points on advertising:

1. Have all signs professionally made.

2. Emphasize quality of services, variety of services, value of services, instead of prices.

3. Make only true statements.
4. Emphasize just one thing on a sign.
5. Have regular business cards giving name, location, and telephon number. Have cards made bearing the names of each individu barber in the shop.
6. Remember, it pays to advertise.

Reading material for patrons:

1. Local newspapers.
2. Magazines (no trade magazines).
3. No obscene or trashy magazines.
4. No questionable picture calendars.

Reading material for employees:

1. Magazines on barbering.
2. Textbooks on barbering.
3. Medical dictionary.

National barber magazines:

1. The Master Barber and Beautician (Published by A.M.B.B. of *
537 So. Dearborn St., Chicago, Ill.) Open subscription.
2. Barber's Journal and Men's Hairstylist. (159 N. Dearborn Stree Chicago, Ill.) Open subscription.
3. The Journeyman Barber, Hairdresser, Cosmetologist and Proprieto (1141 N. Delaware, Indianapolis, Pa.) (Subscriptions limited to men bers of J.B.I.U. of A.)

Other textbooks on barbering:

2. Standardized Textbook of Barbering. (Associated Master Barber 537 S. Dearborn, Chicago, Ill.)
3. Practice and Science of Standard Barbering, by S. C. Thorpe, Milad Publishing Corp. 3839 White Plains Ave., New York 67, New Yorl

Proper names for shops: Choose a name befitting the community or di trict in which the shop is located.

1. "Right Spot Barber Shop" would be all right for certain localitie
2. Paramount Barber Shop.
3. Jack's Barber Shop.
4. Pasadena Barber Shop.
5. Five Point Barber Shop.

Customer record card form: Put such data on a special card of the sam size as the individual record card and file both of them together or hav a separate filing index of patrons for special treatments. Such card shoul contain the name of treatment, the date given, the number probably to b taken, the apparent results or progress, the price, the name, the addres and telephone number of the patron, and name of barber, etc.

Ideal type of check pad: One which is arranged for the itemizing of particular orders with the corresponding prices. Such information enables the patron to see how the total was arrived at and it also reaches the bookkeeper in suitable form to become a part of the patron's record.

Individual patron record form:

Name and Record of Patron

Name _____

Address _____

Telephone _____

Occupation _____

Interests or hobbies _____

Patron's special desires _____

_____

_____

_____

_____

Dates of services _____

_____

Types of services _____

Kinds of cosmetics _____

Style of hair cut _____

Condition of hair _____

Condition of scalp _____

Condition of skin (face) _____

Special treatments _____

Names of equipment and supplies: Students should learn the names of some barber chairs, razors, shears, tonics, creams, and shaving soaps. These can be learned from observation, barber magazines and instructors.

Ordering supplies: Prepare your order for supplies in advance in writing. This saves time both for you and the salesman. His time is valuable too. He can write the order and give you a copy and usually deliver the supplies while you are serving a patron.

Hiring barbers: The manager should know how to interview an applicant for a job. Here are some pointers and some things to **observe** and **questions** to ask. First, put the applicant at ease. Retire to a quiet place and be seated. The employer should guard against talking too much—let the applicant do most of the talking. Give special attention to his appearance and personality. Observe whether he acts restless or relaxed, and whether he seems enthusiastic and eager to work.

Inform the applicant that you have established standard shop service procedures and all barbers are required to follow them. Inform him also that you have a set of shop regulations with which the barbers are required to comply. Later, if you decide to hire the applicant, either hand him a copy of these regulations or read them over to him; and then advise him that, upon employment, you will acquaint him with the uniform shop procedures. It is advisable to type and post the high points of shop procedures. Ask stimulating questions.

1. Questions to ask applicant:

(It is recommended that the employer have written application forms which will provide spaces for the applicant's name, address, telephone number, and which will include the questions to be asked and spaces for the answers.)

(1) From what barber college were you graduated? _____

(2) How much shop experience have you had? Give name, address, and telephone number of former employer(s) the last year.

_____

_____

(3) How is your health? _____

(4) Do you have a family? _____.

(5) How many dependents do you have?_____

(6) Where have you lived the last three years? _____

_____

(7) Do you rent or own your own home? _____

(8) How would you travel to and from work? _____

(9) What barber service do you like best? _____

(10) What barber service do you dislike most? _____

(11) Do you want a permanent job? _____

(12) Do you think a barber should emphasize cultivating a shop clientele or a personal following? _____

(13) Do you have to take off work to pay bills? _____

(14) Do you have a bank account? _____

(15) How long have you lived at your present address? _____

(16) With what religious faith do you identify yourself? _____

(17) Do you belong to any fraternal organizations? _____

(If so, ask the name or names) _____

(18) Would you be willing to follow established standard shop service procedures? _____

2. Questions not to ask applicant:
   (1) Do you like barbering?
   (2) Do you like to deal with people?
   (3) Are you temperamental?
   (4) Have you ever been fired?
   (5) Are you hard-headed?

3. If you hire anyone to work in the shop, barber, receptionist, janitor, manicurist, have him fill out a W-4 Form stating the number of his withholding exemptions and social security number. These forms are furnished by the Internal Revenue Service.

Personal appearance: Barbers should dress neatly and immaculately, be clean shaven, and keep shoes shined. Choose personal attire that is modest and in good taste.

ORGANIZATIONS

(Refer to Chapter on History of Barbering)

Barber organizations: There are two national barber organizations (1) The Journeyman Barbers, Hairdressers, Cosmetologists, and Proprietors International Union of America, whose headquarters is 1141 N. Deleware, Indianapolis, Indiana and (2) The Associated Master Barbers and Beauticians of America, whose headquarters is 537 S. Dearborn Street, Chicago 5, Illinois. The membership of each organization consists of both employers and employees. The general purpose of these organizations are to **improve working conditions, to promote favorable hours** and **prices, public** and **trade relations,** and barbering in general; provide **health** and **death benefits, group insurance, employment assistance,** and to **sponsor legislation.** The **National** officers of the union are elected for five years and those of the Master Barbers for three years. State and local officers of each organization are elected annually. The state organizations are largely devoted to legislation and the local units to local problems. The local organizations of the Union are called "locals" and those of the Master Barber's "chapters". Each local or chapter has an identifying number. Officers of the "locals" consist of president, vice-president, secretary-treasurer,, recorder, guide and guardian. Officers of the "chapters" consist of president, vice-president, secretary-treasurer, recorder, sergeant-at-arms, and chaplain. It is the duty of the president to preside at meetings and to keep a watchful eye on all affairs of the organization. The secretary-treasurer shall keep a written record of the proceedings of meetings, a written record of the membership, and collect and disburse all money paid to the organization in accordance with its constitution and as directed by the proper authority. The method of election of both national and local officers is by ballot, known as the Australian ballot system.

Barber School organizations: There are two National barber school associations. These are the National Association of Barber Schools, Inc., which has an open membership to all barber schools who meet minimum requirements, and the International Association of Barber Schools, whose membership is open only to Union affiliated schools. There are some independent state school associations. The general purposes of barber school associations are: (1) to train students properly, (2) to improve the curriculum, (3) to improve teaching methods, (4) to promote good instructor-student relations, (5) to promote trade and public relations, (6) to sponsor legislation, and (7) to help promote barbering in general.

National Association of Barber Examiners: This association is especially concerned with improved ways of conducting state examinations and the administration of barber laws. It is a source of many good general recommendations to barbers and barber schools.

The combined purposes of all these organizations spell out in what ways barbering can be promoted. A vivid example is our state laws which would have been almost impossible without organizations.

Some advantages of belonging to barber organizations:
1. Opportunity for **united effort** to promote barbering.
2. Opportunity to unite with other barbers to maintain our past accomplishments.
3. Group insurance.
4. Friendship of other barbers.
5. Knowledge of what is going on in the industry.
6. Help in establishing uniform prices and hours.
7. "United we stand; divided we fall."

Some disadvantages of not belonging to barber organization:
1. You are handicapped in helping to promote barbering.
2. You are removed from an important source of information about barbering.
3. You are limited in forming friendships among barbers.
4. You are handicapped in sponsoring new legislation.
5. You are deprived of all the advantages of belonging.

Barber shop regulations: The manager should post a set of shop regulations and see that the barbers comply with them. Most of the chapter on "How to be a Successful Barber Student" is applicable to barbers. The following are a few high points:

1. Wear immaculately clean uniform and clothes.
2. Be punctual.
3. Keep finger nails short and clean.
4. Follow sanitation code rigorously.

5. Be courteous and obliging.
6. Maintain a cheerful countenance.
7. Practice friendliness constantly.
8. Keep chair and station clean.
9. Do not speed up or slow down to choose customers.
10. Give every customer uniform service and attention.
11. Cultivate shop customers rather than a personal following.
12. Become known through community activities.
13. Do not deviate from shop established standard service procedures.
14. Avoid controversial and bad taste subjects.
15. Do not discuss your family troubles.
16. Prevent body odor and bad breath.
17. Keep clean shaven and have your hair cut at least every ten days.
18. Do not smoke while serving a customer.
19. Practice good salesmanship principles daily.
20. Be cooperative.

Money: Change—coins—currency—checks—banking.

1. **Making change:** Coins above a quarter and all currency are put on the register's slab until change is counted out to patron. Start counting from sale price, placing change in patron's hand or other suitable place.
2. **Coins come in rolls:** Pennies, $0.50; nickels, $2.00; dimes, $5.00; quarters and halves, $10.00; halves, some banks, $20.00.
3. **Obtaining coins from bank:** Obtain according to rolls.
4. **Banking:** Obtain labelled coin rolls and greenback bands from bank. Roll coins and band greenback according to labels. Inscribe your name on rolls and bands. Put 100 one dollar bills in $100.00 bands; and in separate $500.00 bands, 100 $5's; 50 $10's; or 25 $20's. Left-over uneven amounts in coin or currency are bankable. List each check by bank number. Obtain deposit forms from bank.

Magnet business policy: From Edgar A. Guest's poem, "Courtesy."

"The reason people pass one door,
To patronize another store,
Is not because the busier place
Has better silks or gloves or lace,
Or cheaper prices; the reason lies
In pleasant words and smiling eyes.
The real trade magnet, I believe.
Is just the treatment folks receive."

COMMISSIONS COMPUTATION SCALE

AMOUNT	50%	55%	60%	65%	70%	75%	80%
1.00	.50	.55	.60	.65	.70	.75	.80
2.00	1.00	1.10	1.20	1.30	1.40	1.50	1.60
3.00	1.50	1.65	1.80	1.95	2.10	2.25	2.40
4.00	2.00	2.20	2.40	2.60	2.80	3.00	3.20
5.00	2.50	2.75	3.00	3.25	3.50	3.75	4.00
6.00	3.00	3.30	3.60	3.90	4.20	4.50	4.80
7.00	3.50	3.85	4.20	4.55	4.90	5.25	5.60
8.00	4.00	4.40	4.80	5.20	5.60	6.00	6.40
9.00	4.50	4.95	5.40	5.85	6.30	6.75	7.20
10.00	5.00	5.50	6.00	6.50	7.00	7.50	8.00
11.00	5.50	6.05	6.60	7.15	7.70	8.25	8.80
12.00	6.00	6.60	7.20	7.80	8.40	9.00	9.60
13.00	6.50	7.15	7.80	8.45	9.10	9.75	10.40
14.00	7.00	7.70	8.40	9.10	9.80	10.50	11.20
15.00	7.50	8.25	9.00	9.75	10.50	11.25	12.00
16.00	8.00	8.80	9.60	10.40	11.20	12.00	12.80
17.00	8.50	9.35	10.20	11.05	11.90	12.75	13.60
18.00	9.00	9.90	10.80	11.70	12.60	13.50	14.40
19.00	9.50	10.45	11.40	12.35	13.30	14.25	15.20
20.00	10.00	11.00	12.00	13.00	14.00	15.00	16.00
21.00	10.50	11.55	12.60	13.65	14.70	15.75	16.80
22.00	11.00	12.10	13.20	14.30	15.40	16.50	17.60
23.00	11.50	12.65	13.80	14.95	16.10	17.25	18.40
24.00	12.00	13.20	14.40	15.60	16.80	18.00	19.20
25.00	12.50	13.75	15.00	16.25	17.50	18.75	20.00
26.00	13.00	14.30	15.60	16.90	18.20	19.50	20.80
27.00	13.50	14.85	16.20	17.55	18.90	20.25	21.60
28.00	14.00	15.40	16.80	18.20	19.60	21.00	22.40
29.00	14.50	15.95	17.40	18.85	20.30	21.75	23.20
30.00	15.00	16.50	18.00	19.50	21.00	22.50	24.00
31.00	15.50	17.05	18.60	20.15	21.70	23.25	24.80
32.00	16.00	17.60	19.20	20.80	22.40	24.00	25.60
33.00	16.50	18.15	19.80	21.45	23.10	24.75	26.40
34.00	17.00	18.70	20.40	22.10	23.80	25.50	27.20
35.00	17.50	19.25	21.00	22.75	24.50	26.25	28.00
36.00	18.00	19.80	21.60	23.40	25.20	27.00	28.80
37.00	18.50	20.35	22.20	24.05	25.90	27.75	29.60
38.00	19.00	20.90	22.80	24.70	26.60	28.50	30.40
39.00	19.50	21.45	23.40	25.35	27.30	29.25	31.20
40.00	20.00	22.00	24.00	26.00	28.00	30.00	32.00
41.00	20.50	22.55	24.60	26.65	28.70	30.75	32.80

AMOUNT	50%	55%	60%	65%	70%	75%	80%
42.00	21.00	23.10	25.20	27.30	29.40	31.50	33.60
43.00	21.50	23.65	25.80	27.95	30.10	32.25	34.40
44.00	22.00	24.20	26.40	28.60	30.80	33.00	35.20
45.00	22.50	24.75	27.00	29.25	31.50	33.75	36.00
46.00	23.00	25.30	27.60	29.90	32.20	34.50	36.80
47.00	23.50	25.85	28.20	30.55	32.90	35.25	37.60
48.00	24.00	26.40	28.80	31.20	33.60	36.00	38.40
49.00	24.50	26.95	29.40	31.85	34.30	36.75	39.20
50.00	25.00	27.50	30.00	32.50	35.00	37.50	40.00
51.00	25.50	28.05	30.60	33.15	35.70	38.25	40.80
52.00	26.00	28.60	31.20	33.80	36.40	39.00	41.60
53.00	26.50	29.15	31.80	34.45	37.10	39.75	42.40
54.00	27.00	29.70	32.40	35.10	37.80	40.50	43.20
55.00	27.50	30.25	33.00	35.75	38.50	41.25	44.00
56.00	28.00	30.80	33.60	36.40	39.20	42.00	44.80
57.00	28.50	31.35	34.20	37.05	39.90	42.75	45.60
58.00	29.00	31.90	34.80	37.70	40.60	43.50	46.40
59.00	29.50	32.45	35.40	38.35	41.30	44.25	47.20
60.00	30.00	33.00	36.00	39.00	42.00	45.00	48.00
61.00	30.50	33.55	36.60	39.65	42.70	45.75	48.80
62.00	31.00	34.10	37.20	40.30	43.40	46.50	49.60
63.00	31.50	34.65	37.80	40.95	44.10	47.25	50.40
64.00	32.00	35.20	38.40	41.60	44.80	48.00	51.20
65.00	32.50	35.75	39.00	42.25	45.50	48.75	52.00
66.00	33.00	36.30	39.60	42.90	46.20	49.50	52.80
67.00	33.50	36.85	40.20	43.55	46.90	50.25	53.60
68.00	34.00	37.40	40.80	44.20	47.60	51.00	54.40
69.00	34.50	37.95	41.40	44.85	48.30	51.75	55.20
70.00	35.00	38.50	42.00	45.50	49.00	52.50	56.00
71.00	35.50	39.05	42.60	46.15	49.70	53.25	56.80
72.00	36.00	39.60	43.20	46.80	50.40	54.00	57.60
73.00	36.50	40.15	43.80	47.45	51.10	54.75	58.40
74.00	37.00	40.70	44.40	48.10	51.80	55.50	59.20
75.00	37.50	41.25	45.00	48.75	52.50	56.25	60.00
76.00	38.00	41.80	45.60	49.40	53.20	57.00	60.80
77.00	38.50	42.35	46.20	50.05	53.90	57.75	61.60
78.00	39.00	42.90	46.80	50.70	54.60	58.50	62.40
79.00	39.50	43.45	47.40	51.35	55.30	59.25	63.20
80.00	40.00	44.00	48.00	52.00	56.00	60.00	64.00
81.00	40.50	44.55	48.60	52.65	56.70	60.75	64.80
82.00	41.00	45.10	49.20	53.30	57.40	61.50	65.60

AMOUNT	50%	55%	60%	65%	70%	75%	80%
83.00	41.50	45.65	49.80	53.95	58.10	62.25	66.40
84.00	42.00	46.20	50.40	54.60	58.80	63.00	67.20
85.00	42.50	46.75	51.00	55.25	59.50	63.75	68.00
86.00	43.00	47.30	51.60	55.90	60.20	64.50	68.80
87.00	43.50	47.85	52.20	56.55	60.90	65.25	69.60
88.00	44.00	48.40	52.80	57.20	61.60	66.00	70.40
89.00	44.50	48.95	53.40	57.85	62.30	66.75	71.20
90.00	45.00	49.50	54.00	58.50	63.00	67.50	72.00
91.00	45.50	50.05	54.60	59.15	63.70	68.25	72.80
92.00	46.00	50.60	55.20	59.80	64.40	69.00	73.60
93.00	46.50	51.15	55.80	60.45	65.10	69.75	74.40
94.00	47.00	51.70	56.40	61.10	65.80	70.50	75.20
95.00	47.50	52.25	57.00	61.75	66.50	71.25	76.00
96.00	48.00	52.80	57.60	62.40	67.20	72.00	76.80
97.00	48.50	53.35	58.20	63.05	67.90	72.75	77.60
98.00	49.00	53.90	58.80	63.70	68.60	73.50	78.40
99.00	49.50	54.45	59.40	64.35	69.30	74.25	79.20
100.00	50.00	55.00	60.00	65.00	70.00	75.00	80.00

AMOUNT	50%	55%	60%	65%	70%	75%	80%
5 CENTS	.02½	.02¾	.03	.03¼	.03½	.03¾	.04
10 CENTS	.05	.05½	.06	.06½	.07	.07½	.08
15 CENTS	.07½	.08¼	.09	.09¾	.10½	.11¼	.12
20 CENTS	.10	.11	.12	.13	.14	.15	.16
25 CENTS	.12½	.13¾	.15	.16¼	.17½	.18¾	.20
30 CENTS	.15	.16½	.18	.19½	.21	.22½	.24
35 CENTS	.17½	.19¼	.21	.22¾	.24½	.26¼	.28
40 CENTS	.20	.22	.24	.26	.28	.30	.32
45 CENTS	.22½	.24¾	.27	.29¼	.31½	.33¾	.36
50 CENTS	.25	.27½	.30	.32½	.35	.37½	.40
55 CENTS	.27½	.30¼	.33	.35¾	.38½	.41¼	.44
60 CENTS	.30	.33	.36	.39	.42	.45	.48
65 CENTS	.32½	.35¾	.39	.42¼	.45½	.48¾	.52
70 CENTS	.35	.38½	.42	.45½	.49	.52½	.56
75 CENTS	.37½	.41¼	.45	.48¾	.52½	.56¼	.60
80 CENTS	.40	.44	.48	.52	.56	.60	.64
85 CENTS	.42½	.46¾	.51	.55¼	.59½	.63¾	.68
90 CENTS	.45	.49½	.54	.58½	.63	.67½	.72
95 CENTS	.47½	.52¼	.57	.61¾	.66½	.71¼	.76

Fig. 652

Courtesy of the New Easy-To-Use Clayton Barber & Beauty Ledger

First Aid

Emergencies requiring first aid arise in every business. Barbers should have knowledge of first aid measures. In all severe cases a physician should be called. The telephone operator will assist you in making such a call.

How to give artificial breathing: Artificial breathing is executed by taking a position either beside or astride a patient and placing the palms of your hands on the small of his back with your fingers resting on the ribs, and repeating twelve to fifteen times a minute the double movements of pressing and letting go. Make a complete respiration—drawing in and letting out the breath—in four or five seconds. Continue such movements until the patient breathes normally.

Fainting:
1. Causes of fainting:
   (1) Mental excitement, such as fear, sight of blood, or emotional shock.
   (2) Unfavorable physical conditions, such as bad air, heat, indigestion, extreme weakness, or bad odors.
   (3) Temporary suspension of respiration and circulation.
   (4) In brief, a lack of sufficient blood in the head.
2. Signs of fainting: Dizziness, weakness, paleness, loss of muscular control; and the patient either sinks into a chair or falls unconscious.
3. Helpful steps to take:
   (1) Lay the patient flat on his back, preferably with his head slightly lower than the remaining part of the body.
   (2) Loosen all tight clothing around neck and waist.
   (3) Change the air in the room, if necessary. Anyway, see that he gets plenty of fresh air, even if fanning is advised.
   (4) Sprinkle cold water on his face and neck. (Cold towels dashed on and off may serve this purpose.)
   (5) Hold a handkerchief containing a few drops of aromatic spirits of ammonia to his nose from one to three seconds every minute or two.
   (6) When the patient becomes conscious, he should continue to lie quiet from five to ten minutes.

Epilepsy: It is a chronic nervous affliction characterized by continuous or irregular jerking of all muscles, sudden loss of consciousness, saliva run-

ning from the mouth, lasting but a short time. Literally and briefly, a fit.
1. Do not try to restrain the victim's movements any more than necessary to prevent him from hurting himself.
2. Loosen tight clothing.
3. Lay him on his side.
4. Do not force a hard object between his teeth.
5. Stand by until the person has fully recovered. Confusion sometimes follows a convulsion, but it usually is only momentary.
6. As soon as a person fully recovers, he is usually able to go about his regular activities.

Heat exhaustion:
1. Signs of heat exhaustion: Cool, moist, perspiring skin; rapid and shallow breathing; paleness, feeble and rapid pulse; but the patient is generally conscious.
2. First aid steps in heat exhaustion:
   (1) Remove patient to a cool, dark, quiet place.
   (2) Lay him down flat.
   (3) Loosen all tight clothing.
   (4) If the patient is conscious, use aromatic spirits of ammonia.
   (5) Keep the patient quiet for an hour or so, if comfort is secured.

Apoplexy:
1. Means strike down or stun. Most common in old age.
2. Victim usually becomes unconscious and snores.
3. Lay him flat on his back; apply cold towels; no stimulants.

Nose Bleed:
1. Slight nose bleed is not dangerous.
2. How to give first aid:
   (1) Pinch the soft part of the nose.
   (2) If bleeding becomes worse, seat the patient in a chair with his head slightly forward or in a barber chair only slightly reclined, loosen his collar and apply cold towels well wrung out to the back of his neck.
   (3) Or, make a cotton plug and gently push it into the nostril out of which the blood is coming. A pencil may be used for the placing of the cotton.

First aid kit available: It is recommended that the manager provide and have immediately available a first aid kit. These are purchasable as a complete unit. It must necessarily contain aromatic spirits of ammonia or smelling salts, individually packaged band aids of 1 inch compress on adhesive tape, sterile gauze squares (3 in. by 3 in.), one square yard of sterile gauze, assorted sterile bandage compresses, a roll of adhesive, 1 inch and 2 inch roller bandage, tincture metaphen or 2% tincture of iodine, burn ointment, scissors, paper cups, applicators and forceps.

Barber Chair

The barber chair is the home base of the barber's income. Around it is the area of his performances. Some barbers become sentimentally attached to a particular chair. It is sometimes necessary to refer to a certain structural part of the mechanism of a chair. The barber should be able to refer accurately to the various major structural parts of a barber chair (Fig. 593).

Ten Pointers in the Use of a Barber Chair:

1. Have the chair locked when a patron gets in or out and during a shave.

2. Lower the chair for a patron to get in or out.

3. Operate the chair noiselessly. Pump it up skillfully and gently.

4. Rotate the chair at proper times and thus minimize foot movement.

5. Press the control button to remove the headrest, and thus avoid unnecessary noise.

6. Use only regular chair oil in the casting.

7. Keep the chair in good mechanical condition.

8. The standard spacing of chairs is from four and a half to five feet from center to center.

9. To make a chair higher than it will pump up, remove the seat rail and place it over four plumbing pipes used as "sleeves" for bolts. Use bolts with a diameter the same as that of the bolt shanks of the chair. Use bolts long enough to accommodate a lock washer and nut on each protruding end. Make the length of the pipes according to the increased height desired; their diameter should match that of the bolts.

10. Make customers desirous of returning to your chair by rendering cheerful, efficient, and satisfactory services.

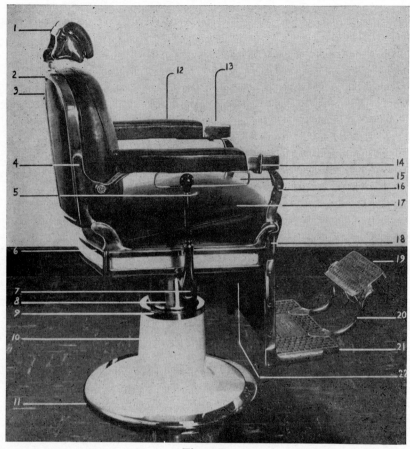

Fig. 653

1. Headrest
2. Back frame
3. Headrest control button
4. Rear side casting
5. Reclining trigger
6. Seat rail
7. Hydraulic pump handle
8. Sleeve
9. Collar
10. Enameled base (Hydraulic pump inside enameled base casting)
11. Base rim
12. Upholstered arm
13. Arm tip
14. Manicure socket
15. Towel bar
16. Front side casting
17. Upholstered seat
18. Gooseneck
19. Foot rest
20. Foot rest arm
21. Platform
22. Apron

Ethics In Barbering

Ethics is the science of conduct. As applied to barbering it means the manner in which a barber conducts his business. This is reflected in his relationship with other barbers and with the public. The ethical barber conducts his business honestly and with due consideration to all concerned. He is a man of principle.

The **truly ethical barber** applies the Golden Rule in business, and thus treats others as he himself would like to be treated. This commendable philosophy has been uniquely expressed in another way—the really ethical barber is one who carries in his mind a picture of himself as a customer.

Code of ethics: Barbers should observe a code of ethics. Such a code should be imbedded in the heart. Ethics should play a vital role in conducting a barber shop. There are innumerable ways of reflecting ethics in all business dealings and in meeting the responsibility of the shop to the customers. Here are **examples of ethical practices:**

1. Strict adherence to the sanitation requirements.
2. Give every patron the same courteous and conscientious service.
3. Treat all patrons fairly.
4. Render only quality service.
5. Recommend only services the patron needs.
6. Comply with shop rules, board rules, and the barber law.
7. Label all cosmetics correctly.
8. Refrain from "quackery treatments".
9. Practice honesty.
10. Keep all promises.
11. Cooperate with other barbers.
12. Strive to do the right things.

A dozen unethical don'ts:
1. Do not use false and misleading advertising. If the price of children's hair cuts is lower than that of adults, do not post a large predominating price for children and a small tiny one for adults.
2. Do not use undue influence to direct customer to your chair.
3. Do not add any service or product not authorized by the customer.
4. Do not use tricks to induce customers to have additional services.
5. Do not misrepresent products.

6. Do not degrade other barbers, especially to patrons.
7. Do not slow down or speed up to pick patrons.
8. Do not knowingly short change patrons.
9. Do not slight children's hair cuts.
10. Do not use profanity in the presence of customers.
11. Do not become impatient and sarcastic with unpleasant customers.
12. Do not over-serve for the sake of tips.

Cooperation with barbers: Cooperation is an ethical obligation. The ethical barber is willing to sit down with his fellow barbers and talk things over, especially regarding hours and days of operation, charges for services, advertising, commissions, and legislation.

Courtesy to license and sanitation inspectors: These inspectors are entitled to courteous treatment. They are acting in the line of duty and they contribute to the promotion of barbering.

Obligation to Laws and Regulations: The barber is ethically obligated to know the laws and regulations governing barbering and to comply with them faithfully, particularly those pertaining to sanitation. By compliance with these he is contributing to the public health and welfare of his country.

Some unethical practices:
1. Using tricks to induce customers to have extras.
2. Misrepresenting products.
3. Using false and misleading advertising. If the price of children's hair cuts is lower than that of adults, do not post a larger price sign for children.
4. Adding a service not authorized by patron.
5. Smoking while serving a patron.
6. Knowingly short-changing a patron.
7. Knocking other barbers .
8. Using undue influence to direct customers to your own chair.
9. Rushing or slowing up to pick customers.
10. Competing with other shops on the basis of longer hours of operation and lower prices than the prevailing hours and prices in your vicinity.

History Of Barbering

The practice of barbering in some form can be traced back about 6,000 years. It is therefore one of the oldest trades. Excavated implements of polished stone and horn indicate that man may have shaved his face in the Stone Age. The pyramids of Egypt have disclosed crude implements used in ancient times to cut the hair and beard and to shave. Such relics as combs, razors, hair dye formulas, and written records have been discovered. The razors were made from bits of flint, oyster shell fragments, sharks' teeth, or tempered copper and bronze. Egyptian ladies enhanced their beauty with perfumed oil, eye paint, and hennaed hair. Barbering in those ancient days, surprisingly, included shaving, haircutting, beard trimming, haircoloring, massaging, facial make-up, hairwaving, and hair adornments. Early barbers were actually hairdressers. They discovered that hair could be made temporarily wavy by encasing twisted strands in clay and baking then in the sun. There is a preponderance of evidence that shaving was practiced in ancient times. There are many allusions to shaving in Chinese history. The ancient monuments and papyrus reveal that the Egyptians shaved their heads as well as their beards. The wandering barbers carried their tools in baskets. Pictures show Egyptians kneeling in the streets having their heads shaved in accordance with custom. According to the Bible, Moses commanded that all who had recovered from leprosy should be shaved, and Joseph had his face shaved by a barber to prevent his bearded face from offending the Pharoah before whom he was summoned to appear. The word "razor" is mentioned in the Bible in Ezekiel, 5:1 (595 B.C.): "And thou, son of man, take thee a sharp knife, take thee a barber's razor, and cause it to pass upon thine head and upon thy beard: then take thee balances to weigh, and divide the hair." Moses must have taken this action as a health precaution, since the Jews then regarded a beard as the badge of manhood.

Alexander the Great (356-323 B.C.) stimulated interest in shaving. He commanded all his soldiers to be clean-shaven. This command was given after losing several battles with the Persians who caught his soldiers, the Macedonians, by the beard and threw them to the ground and slaughtered them. As the civilians followed suit, beards lost their vogue in Greece. About 325 B.C. the practice of shaving was common with the Macedonians.

In 296 B.C. Ticinius Mena arrived from Sicily, introduced and popularized shaving in Rome. The Sicilian barbers came from Messina and taught the Romans hair culture and the use of shears. The Romans, however, had been introduced to the razor several centuries before by Tarquin, King of Rome, as a campaign against unhygienic beards.

Barbers gained so much prestige that a statue was erected to the memory of the first barber of Rome. The Romans seemed to take to barbering naturally. It is only fitting therefore that the word "barber" is derived from the Latin word **Barba.** This word translated simply means "beard." But the custom changed when Hadrian was Emperor (117-138 A.D.). He grew a beard to cover his warts and scars, and long beards again became the fashion of Roman subjects.

Bucking religious differences and customs during the first centuries after Christ, barbers continued to shave the face and trim the beard wherever they were privileged to do so. The vogue changed many times in various centuries. Charlemagne (742-814) set the fashion of long hair in his country. And in the 11th century in France, William, Archbishop of Raven, prohibited the wearing of beards. Today shaving is almost universally the custom.

Superstition stimulated barbering in certain areas. Some early tribes believed that bad spirits entered the body through hairs on the head and that the only way to eradicate bad spirits was cutting off the hair. The barbers were the doctors of those days and even officiated at religious ceremonies, arranging marriages and baptizing children.

Early barbers were assistants to the clergy during the first centuries of the Christian era. These barbers were the only professional surgeons. Barbers started the practice of surgery as far back as 110 A.D., and became known as barber-surgeons. The clergy sought to heal the sick by faith and the barber-surgeons performed blood-letting. Blood-letting was considered "cure all" of all diseases. The barber-surgeon-clergy teams worked together in this way until 1163 when a new edict of the Catholic Church held it was sacriligious for the clergy to draw or to assist in drawing blood from the human body. Separated from the clergy, the barber-surgeons continued to practice their own and some relinquished duties of the clergy. They continued to so practice for several centuries, expanding their scope of practice somewhat, but their surgery gradually became regarded as quackery and they gave it up entirely. The rise of the medical profession pushed the barber aside, and laws were passed prohibiting barbers from practicing surgery, dentistry, and cauterization. The barbers were then limited to beard trimming, except they were allowed to make wigs, cut hair, and shave. The declining date for early barbers is 1745 when the alliance between the surgeons and the barbers was entirely dissolved.

Significant developments led up to the dissolution of the barber-surgeons. The clergy severed connections with the barbers in 1163. In the middle of the 13th century the first school to instruct barbers in surgery was founded in Paris. It was the school of St. Cosmos and St. Domain. In 1450, the Guild of Surgeons was instituted by an act of Parliament. The dissolution of the alliance between the barbers and surgeons in 1745. From about 1100 to 1750, barbers gave more attention to surgery and were known as barber-surgeons. Some of them resorted to down-right quackery and the public complained that they did more harm than good. During these "Black out" years for barbers, the more progressive ones became professional wig makers. Wigs were the vogue in many countries, especially in France, Prussia, and England, from about 1750 to about 1850. There was of course some beard-trimming during those years. Comparatively little is known about barbers from 1750 to about 1875 when haircutting and shaving slowly became the vogue. The advance of medical science, emphasis upon sanitation, and education helped to pave the way for haircutting and shaving. Separated from medicine, surgery, and dentistry, barbers struggled for existence until this modern era found a place for them that is indispensable. In this connection it is noteworthy that the early barber shops were "hang outs" where low characters assembled to gossip, tell smutty stories, and to scandalize people. Women dared not enter these shops. Today the picture is very different. Many shops are lavish salons where the atmosphere is respectable and suitable places for the patronage of women and children.

About 1,000 years before Christ there were known to be fairly well established barber shops in Greece. Prominent citizens frequented these shops to have their beards trimmed and curled, and their toenails and fingernails cleaned. It was there too that the news of the day was discussed and political opinions expressed. But it was not until about 500 B.C. that beard-trimming became the vogue in Greece. While most of the phases of modern barbering were practiced by the early barbers at various times in some measure, the fact remains that their practice consisted primarily of four services:

1. Beard-trimming.
2. Blood-letting (used as a cure all of diseases).
3. Tooth-pulling.
4. Cauterization.

SCOPE OF BARBERING IN AMERICA

In the history of barbering the scope was sometimes broad and narrow. By "scope" is meant not only the multiplicity of services the barber has to offer the public, but the whole net-work of the barber industry. The Barbers' Journeymen Union has a national headquarters and national line of officers; a state association with a line of state officers; locals in the states with a local line of officers; and district organizers. Likewise, the

Associated Master Barbers has a national headquarters and a national line of officers; a state association with a line of state officers; local chapters with a local line of officers; and district organizers. There is National Association of Barber Schools and an International Association of Barber Schools, and each has a line of officers. There are state barber school associations with a line of state officers. And then there are association of supply dealers, of manufacturers, and of distributors, with various officers. To be added to all this are the barber trade magazines, Barber Shows and clinics, publishers of textbooks on barbering, established barber school curriculums, State Barber Board regulations, and state barber laws governing the practice of barbering. All this is a magnificent picture and is indicative of a great future for barbers.

BARBER POLE

There are several accounts of the origin of the barber pole. Probably the most reliable story is that the pole originated when blood-letting was the most typical service of the barber. The two spiral ribbons painted around the pole were symbolic of the two bandages used in blood-letting. One ribbon represented the bandage bound around the arm before the surgery was performed, and the other one afterwards. The true colors of the barber emblem are white and red. Red, white and blue are widely used in America. This is due partly to the fact that the national flag has these colors. But red and white are regarded by most authorities as the true colors of the barber pole.

Another interpretation of the colors of the barber pole is that red is symbolic of arterial blood, blue of venous blood, and white of the bandage. The sure thing that can be said about the modern barber pole is that it is very beautiful. The barbers are fortunate to have such a marvelous emblem of their trade.

All three of these colors were used in England. A statute required the barbers to use blue and white and the surgeons to use red. A statute was enacted to this effect after the barbers and surgeons were incorporated. At that time each group was restricted to their own specified practice. It is noteworthy that there was a 14th Century barbers' Guild that had strict supervision over barbers. Violators of its regulations were guilty of a misdemeanor and punishable by prison terms. The guild was known as the Worshipful Company of Barbers, and was formed in London in 1308. This is the oldest barber organization that is still in existence. (The first barber-surgeons organization formed earlier in France did not survive).

The important role that the early barber had in community life—serving as surgeon-doctor and dentist—entitled him to be one of the principal characters in several famous operas, such as Rossini's "Barber of Seville" and Peter Cornelius' "Barber of Bagdad." "Figaro," the name of a witty, jocular barber, has been immortalized in these operas. A barber named Figaro actually lived and practiced in Spain.

STATE LAWS IN AMERICA

Forty-eight of the fifty states have enacted state barber laws. These were sponsored by the organized barbers. These various state laws are very similar. Their source is the so-called Model Law of Minnesota: it served as a pattern for the other state barber laws. It was passed in 1897. The chief purpose of laws is to promote the general welfare and health of the public. The basis of the argument for barber laws is the need for sanitation in barber shops. The various state laws have many similar provisions. Some of these are as follows:

1. A Sanitation code shall be followed.
2. Barbers shall be licensed.
3. Apprenticeships shall be completed.
4. Minimum number of hours shall be completed in a barber school.
5. Minimum educational requirement shall be met.
6. Barber shops shall be inspected.
7. Barber shops shall be licensed.
8. State boards shall be appointed by the governor.

Factors influencing barbering: The history of barbering reflects many factors that have influenced barbering.

1. International factors:
   (1) Historical characters. These individuals either by popularity or mandate set the fashions of beards, shaving, haircutting, and mustaches. Some of these historical characters were Moses, Alexander the Great, Hadrian, Charlemagne, and William, Archbishop of Roven.
   (2) Climatic conditions:
      a. In cold climates, people are inclined to wear longer hair.
      b. In warm climates, people are more inclined to wear shorter hair.
   (3) Race or nationality. The hair of the various races responds differently.
   (4) Religion. Certain creeds specify rules for the beard.
   (5) Education. The educated man is more likely to be interested in his appearance.
   (6) Customs. Compliance with the customs is almost imperative if one is to live without friction.
   (7) Passing vogues.
   (8) Discovery of electricity.

   (9) Invention and improvement of electric implements.

 (10) Scientific research.

 (11) Modern cosmetics.

 (12) Organizations.

 (13) Barber colleges.

 (14) Textbooks.

 (15) Trade publications.

 (16) Manufacturer of modern implements.

2. National factors in America:

  (1) The Journeymen Barbers' International Union of America was formed in Buffalo, New York, in 1887. (Its forerunner, The Barbers' Protective Association was organized in 1886.) The present full name of this Union is Journeymen Barbers', Hairdressers', Cosmetologists' and Proprietors' International Union of America. Its headquarters is in Indianapolis, Indiana. The Union is affiliated with AFL-CIO.

  (2) Founding of barber colleges. The first one was founded by A. B. Moler in Chicago, in 1893.

  (3) Passage of state barber laws. Minnesota led the way in 1897.

  (4) The Terminal System, New York City, was started in 1916. Emphasis was placed upon sanitation in a way to attract the attention of patrons, and to give them uniform and superior service. The system was originated by Mr. Schuster, an Austrian by birth, who came to New York City.

  (5) The revival of women's haircutting, about 1920. This resulted in making men more conscious of their hair.

  (6) A higher caliber of men began to be attracted to barbering, and they emphasized professionalization. They re-set the atmosphere of the barber shop. Parents now allow their children to visit a shop unaccompanied.

  (7) The Associated Master Barbers of America was organized on November 19, 1924, in Chicago, Illinois. (At their convention in Cleveland, Ohio, in October, 1941, the organization changed its name to the National Association of Master Barbers and Beauticians of America.)

  (8) Publication of textbooks on barbering.

  (9) Publication of trade magazine.

 (10) In 1925, Associated Master Barbers and Beauticians of America established the National Educational Council to improve and standardize the curriculums of barber schools, and to conduct research in the field of barber science.

 (11) The National Association of Barber Schools, Inc., was organ-

ized on October 19, 1927, in Cleveland, Ohio. (It's original name was the National Association of Standardized Barber Schools.)

(12) The National Association of Barber Examiners was organized on October 21, 1929, in St. Paul, Minnesota.

(13) The Journeymen Barbers' Union established their Educational Department in 1933. This department has sponsored improvements in the educational program for barbers and barber schools. It also conducts research in barber science.

(14) The International Barber Schools Association was organized on September 11, 1948, in Indianapolis, Indiana.

(15) State Barber College Associations were organized.

(16) The National Barber Show, New York City, 1958.

International dates and developments.

1. Barbering in some form has been practiced for about 6000 years.

2. In ancient times barbers were highly respected and patronized by the nobility, such as the poets and philosophers.

3. Barbering was introduced in Rome in 296 B.C.

4. Rome became known for its fine baths and splendid barbers. All free men in Rome could then be clean shaven, whereas slaves were forced to wear beards.

5. The first barber-surgeons organization was formed in France in 1096. Soon thereafter the barber-surgeons founded a school of surgery in Paris.

6. The clergy and barbers severed relations in 1163. This was occasioned by an edict issued by Pope Alexander III forbidding the clergy to practice surgery on the grounds that it was sacreligious to draw blood from the human body. Prior to that time, the barbers and clergymen worked together to heal the sick—the barbers performed the surgical operations and the clergymen administered prayer.

7. In 1450, by an act of Parliament in England, the barbers and surgeons were incorporated. The work of barbers was greatly restricted. A law was enacted to provide that anyone practicing surgery should not practice barbering, and that no barber should practice any part of surgery except tooth-pulling. The action of the Parliament was taken because the barber-surgeons had been practicing so much quackery. For the next two hundred years the barbers had less and less to do, but they continued, especially in small outlying towns, to practice blood-letting, tooth-pulling, beard-trimming, and simple cauterizing. There was considerable jealousy and dissatisfaction among these two united groups. Finally, a law was enacted for the complete separation of these barbers from the surgeons.

8. The year 1745 marks the decline of early barbers. This is the date when the alliance between the surgeons and barbers was entirely dissolved. This left the barbers out on a limb.

Noteworthy monuments to Barbers:

1. A statue, erected to the memory of the first barber in Rome.
2. The Barber-Surgeons Hall in London.
3. Coat of Arms, issued at London.

First Barber-Surgeons in America: The Dutch and Swedish settlers in America brought the First barber-surgeons to America. They performed common medical and surgical practices.

Foreign influence on barbering in America: German and Italian barbers migrated to America and established barber shops. They, along with the French, English, Dutch, and Swedish had a strong influence on American barbering.

HIGH POINTS IN HISTORY OF BARBERING

1. Beard-trimming became an art in Greece about 500 B.C.
2. Barbering was introduced in Rome in 296 B.C.
3. The first barber-surgeons organization was formed in France in 1096.
4. The barber-surgeons and clergy severed relations in 1163.
5. The year of 1745 marks the decline of early barbering.
6. The J.B.I.U. of A. was organized in 1887.
7. The first barber college was founded in 1893.
8. Minnesota passed the first state law in America in 1897.
9. The A.M.B.B. of A. was organized in 1924.
10. The National Association of Barber Schools was organized in 1927.
11. The National Association of Barber Examiners was organized in 1929.
12. The International Association of Barber Schools was organized in 1948.

Cells

A knowledge of cells contributes to a barber's understanding of facials and scalp treatments. The human body is composed of millions of cells and the barber should know in what ways he can encourage the normal function of these tiny living bodies as he performs services on the face and scalp.

Cells are the foundation of all living structure. They are even **responsible for the varied activities of the body.** The proper function of cells, therefore, determine very largely the health of the skin.

The importance of the study of cells may be indicated by the fact that low down in the scale of life there are simple animals which consist of only one cell. These are called unicellular animals. Human beings are described as multicellular beings. (The ameba is a typical one-cell animal.) Every part of the body is composed of cells, including of course the skin of the face and scalp.

PART I

Aspects of Cells Closely Related to Barbering

Purposes of study:
1. To learn the importance of the function of cells.
2. To learn how the barber can promote the functions of cells.

Definition of cell: A cell is a structural unit of living substance.

Cellular activity: Cellular activity may take place normally in the skin of the face and scalp that are healthy, but such activity may be increased by scientific treatments within the scope of barbering.

Ways of stimulating cellular activity:
1. By massaging. The best scientific means by which a barber can stimulate cells is massaging. This is because cells are exceedingly sensitive and responsive to external stimulus.
2. By heat-applications, such as steam-towels, dermal lights, infra-red lamps.
3. By high frequency.

Cell growth requirements: For a cell to grow normally, it must have sufficient food, water, oxygen, eliminate waste and be free from poisons, pressure, and improper temperature. **Except nerve cells,** almost all body cells are capable of self repair after injury.

Metabolism: This is the building up and breaking down process within the cell. These processes are normal and necessary to the health of all tissue. Unless these changes take place, an unhealthy condition will result. Such changes may occur normally, but how to stimulate sluggish cells is the principal concern of the barber. Metabolism is a complex process whereby cells are nourished and supplied with energy to discharge their activities.

Metabolism illustrated: The cells of the body might be likened to a pool of water. The water will be stagnant and unusable unless there is a constant replacement of the water—there must be an inlet and an outlet for it to keep healthful. This same principle applies to human tissue. The cells which compose tissue must be constantly reproduced and the waste matter must be carried away.

Function of cells: In general, the function of cells is to maintain and produce life; that is, a cell **repairs** and **produces** tissue. By massaging the barber encourages the function of the cells. An existing cell is the only means of producing another cell. (Nerve cells, however, do not reproduce themselves.)

Structural parts of cell: Inside the cell membrane or wall, a cell consists of two major parts.

1. **Nucleus.** This is **the functional center of a cell,** that is, the **life producing part of a cell.** This active portion of a cell regulates cellular activities and participates in cell reproduction.
2. **Cytoplasm:** This is the substance that surrounds the nucleus. It is the passive portion of a cell, but it contains the food materials essential for self-repair, growth, and reproduction.

Mitosis: Mitosis is the process of **human** cell reproduction. As soon as a cell reaches maturity, it reproduces a like cell by **indirect cell division.** Two nuclei and two daughter cells are formed, and then the **cell divides** in half and forms two cells. A constant **reproduction of cells** is required to keep tissues healthy.

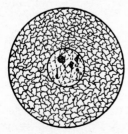

Fig. 654
Diagram of Cell

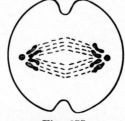

Fig. 655
Cell Beginning to
Divide

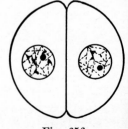

Fig. 656
Cell Division Completed

Essential Steps of Mitosis

How cells grow: Cells grow from food stuff. They absorb food from the surrounding tissue fluid and lymph.

Elements in body: There are sixteen elements in the body. The symbols of five of them may be recalled by the name COHNS. Each letter of this name stand for an element—Carbon, Oxygen, Hydrogen, Nitrogen, Sulphur. Incidentally, these are the same five elements found in the hair.

Cell respiration: The lungs occupy most of the chest cavity. The functions of the lungs are carried on by "air cells." As we breathe we fill these air cells with oxygen that is taken in by the blood which gives up its impurities through exhaling. Two pulmonary veins carry the purified blood from each lung to the heart from whence it is sent throughout the body.

Purposes of cell respiration:
1. To furnish oxygen to cells.
2. To produce heat and energy.
3. To remove waste matter (carbon dioxide).

Definition of tissue: An organized mass of similar cells.

Examples of tissue: Muscles, nerves and blood.

Protoplasm: This is the living substance that is the physical basis of life.

PART II

Other Aspects of Cells

1. **Mitosis:** This is an **indirect type of cell division.** Human cells multiply by the process of mitosis. After a cell divides in half and becomes two separate cells a series of **complex** changes occurs.

2. **Amitosis:** This is a process of **direct** cell division which occurs among plant life and bacteria (and rarely in human tissues.) After **simple** changes occur, the cell elongates and then divides in half, forming two separate cells.

Two parts of metabolism:

1. **Anabolism:** This is the **building up process within cells.** During this process a cell absorbs food, water, and oxygen for repair, growth, and reproduction. These food materials are transformed into tissue elements. A thin cell membrane permits such soluble substances to enter and leave the protoplasm.

2. **Catabolism:** This is the **breaking down process within cells.** During this process, a cell **consumes** what it has absorbed to use for secretion, digestion, and muscular activity. That is, complex chemical changes—muscle cells burn up sugars—and produce energy, as well as to eliminate waste products.

Various shapes of cells: Cells are round, flat, elongated, and cubical.

General composition of protoplasm:
1. Protoplasm consists of cytoplasm, a nucleus, and a cell membrane.
2. Protoplasm is a colorless jelly-like substance consisting of fat, protein, carbohydrate, mineral salts and water.

Size of cells: The size ranges from 1/3000 to 1/300 of an inch in diameter.

Tissues: A tissue is a group of similar cells, having its own function or functions. While there are only **four** distinct kinds of tissues, "liquid tissue" referred to by some authorities is added to complete the traditional number of FIVE.

1. Epithelial tissue. This tissue forms a **protective covering** for the outer surface, and for the linings of many internal parts, of the body. (It is devoid of blood vessels. Besides protection, this tissue absorbs, as in the lungs and intestines; secretes, as in the glands; excretes, as in the kidneys and liver; and receives stimuli.)

2. **Connective** tissue: This is the **most widely spread tissue** of the body. It supports, protects and binds together other tissues of the body. Examples of this tissue are ligaments, tendons, bones, and adipose tissue. The fatty (adipose) tissue surrounds the vital organs, gives support to the blood vessels and nerves, and provides a protective layer underneath the skin. (Muscles are "wrapped" in connective tissue).

3. **Muscular** tissue: This kind of tissue provides bodily movement. There are **three** types of muscular tissue:
   (1) Voluntary muscle tissue: The striated muscles that make up this tissue and the movement of the muscles under their control, such as those of the face, arms and legs, are **directed by the will** of each individual.
   by the will of each individual.
   (2) Involuntary muscle tissue: The non-striated muscles **make** up this tissue, and the movement of the muscles under **their** control are directed by the nerve centers that permit the function of the stomach, blood vessels, and intestines without the will.
   (3) Cardiac muscular tissue: This tissue directs the movement of the heart—pumps blood through the heart.

4. **Liquid tissue:** (Also called Vascular) Blood and lymph are liquid tissue. It transports food, hormones, and waste matter.

5. **Nerve** tissue. This tissue responds to stimuli and transmits impulses to other cells, such as those pertaining to seeing, feeling, and hearing. It coordinates body functions. Its cells are called neurons.

Organs: Organs are a group of tissues, performing a specific function. Examples of important organs are the liver, kidneys, heart, brain, and

ungs. (The liver is the **largest** organ **in** the body). Each organ has a specific function.

Systems: A system is a group of organs, performing a unified series of
vital functions. The human body consists of **nine systems:**

Circulatory system	Excretory system	Skeleton system
Digestive system	Muscular system	Reproductive system
Endocrine system	Nervous system	Respiratory system

1. Circulatory system: This system is composed of the blood vessels
   and lymphatics, blood, lymph, and heart. It carries food and **oxygen**
   to the cells and takes away waste matter.

2. Digestive system: This system is composed of the mouth, stomach,
   and intestines. Its function is to prepare foods for absorption by
   cells.

3. Endocrine system: This system is composed of the pituitary and
   thyroid glands. Its hormone secretions regulate growth and metabolism.

4. Excretory system: This system is composed of the skin, lungs,
   liver, kidneys, and large intestines. Its function is to eliminate
   waste products from the body.

5. Muscular system: This system is composed of muscles that cover
   and shape the skeleton. All muscular activity, such as facial expressions, contraction of the heart and stomach, movements of the
   arms and hands, and general locomotion of the body, are regulated
   by the muscular system.

6. Nervous system: This system is composed of nerve tissues. Its
   function is to transmit messages to and from all parts of the body.

7. Skeletal system: This system is composed of bones, ligaments, and
   cartilages. Its function is to form the framework of the body, to
   protect organs, to provide solid attachments for muscles, and to
   serve as levers for bodily motion.

8. Reproductive system: (also urogenital). This system is composed
   of the reproductive or genital organs. Its function is to continue the
   human race.

9. Respiratory system: This system is composed mainly of the lungs.
   Its function is to purify blood by the intake of oxygen and to
   remove carbon dioxide.

Elements in body: These are the sixteen elements in the body:

1. Calcium	9. Manganese
2. Carbon	10. Nitrogen
3. Chlorine	11. Oxygen
4. Fluorine	12. Phosphorus
5. Hydrogen	13. Potassium
6. Iodine	14. Silicon
7. Iron	15. Sodium
8. Magnesium	16. Sulphur

Definition of elements: An element is a substance which cannot be decomposed by ordinary chemical means.

Most abundant element: Oxygen is the most abundant element.

Bones

This study of bones is confined to the head, face and neck. A barber does not treat bones in any way, but knowing the names and locations of them serves as a "map" of the sections of the anatomy over which he works and thus enables him to refer accurately to these various areas.

PART I
Aspects of Bones Closely Related to Barbering

Chief purpose of study: To learn the names of the principal anatomical sections of the head, face and neck.

Divisions of head: The head consists of two divisions: the cranium is the brain case and the face is called the anterior region of the head.

1. The face—the front part of the head.
2. The cranium—the top, sides, and back of the head.

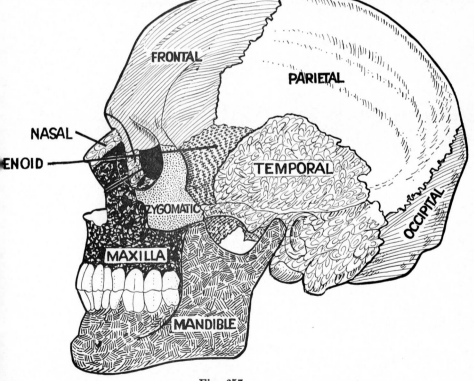

Fig. 657
Principal Bones of Head

Skull: The skull is the entire framework of the head. In other words, the **skull is the skeleton of the head.** (The skull has been referred to as the oval bony case that encloses and protects the brain.)

Paired bones:
1. The only paired cranial bones are the temporals and parietals.
2. All bones of the face are paired except the mandible and vomer

Locations of principal bones of cranium and face:
1. Cranial bones: The frontal bone is located at the forehead; the two parietal bones at the sides of the skull, between the frontal and occipital and above the temporals; the two temporal bones at the sides of the skull beneath the parietals; the sphenoid bone at the anterior base of the skull, joining other cranial bones together the occipital bone at the back and base of the skull.
2. Facial bones: The mandible bone is the lower jaw; the two maxilla bones are the upper jaw bones; the two zygomatic bones are the cheek bones; the two nasal bones are the nose bones.

Some alternate names of some bones: The mandible is also known as the inferior maxillary or lower jaw bone; the maxilla as superior maxillary or upper-jaw bones; and the zygomatic as malar or check bone.

PART II

Other Aspects of Bones

Purposes of bones:
1. To form the framework of the body.
2. To protect organs and other systems of the body.
3. To provide a solid attachment for muscles.
4. To serve as levers for bodily movements.

Number of bones: The adult skeleton consists of 206 bones.
1. The face consists of 14 bones.
2. The cranium consists of 8 bones.
3. The skull consists of 22 bones.
4. The neck consists of the Hyoid and seven cervical vertebrae bones

Color of bones: Externally bones appear to be light pink, and, internally deep red.

Bone defined: A bone is the hard tissue which forms the framework of the body.

Osteology: This is the study of bones.

Composition of bones: Bones are composed of about one-third organic matter and about two-thirds inorganic matter.

1. **Organic** (animal) **matter** is composed of blood vessels, bone cells, marrow, and connective tissue.
2. **Inorganic** (mineral) **matter** is composed of calcium, phosphorous, but mainly of **lime.**

Function of lime in bones: Lime (Carbonate of lime) gives bones their stiffness and hardness. It composes about two-thirds the weight of the bones.

Blood vessels in bones: Capillaries are the kind of active blood vessels in the bones. (In the covering of bones there are capillaries, lymphatics, and nerves.)

Marrow of bones: This is a soft fatty substance that fills the cavities the bones. Red corpuscles and some white corpuscles are formed in the red marrow.

Covering of bones: Bones are covered by a tough fibrous membrane, called **periosteum.** The periosteum serves as an attachment for ligaments, tendons, nerves, and blood vessels. Its main **function** is to protect the bones.

Maturity of bones: Bones do not reach their full size before the age of 25.

Elasticity of bones: A bone has a slight degree of elasticity. A bone will usually bend before it breaks.

Nourishment of bones: Bones receive their nourishment through blood vessels (capillaries).

Joints: A joint is the junction of two or more bones. Some are movable as in the fingers, and some immovable as in the skull.

Ligaments: Ligaments are flexible bands of tissue that help to hold bones together at their joints.

Tendons: Tendons are bands of connective tissue that attach muscles to bones.

Cartilage: Cartilage means gristle. (It is a firm elastic structure.) Its function is to cushion the bones at the joints.

Classification of bones according to shapes:
1. Flat bones. (Bones of the cranium.)
2. Long bones. (Bones of the arms and legs.)
3. Short bones. (Bones of the fingers and toes.)
4. Irregular bones. (Bones of the spine.)

Weight of all bones: The 206 bones comprise about 16% of the weight of the body.

One bone disease: "Rickets" is the name of the bone disease which results from the lack of vitamin D.

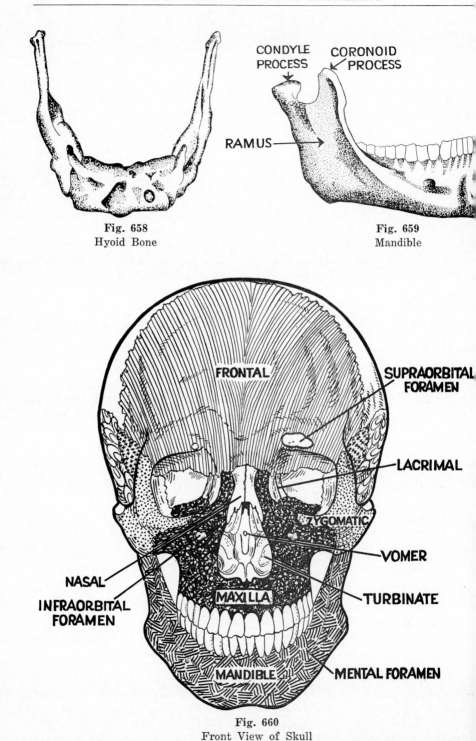

Fig. 658
Hyoid Bone

CONDYLE
PROCESS

CORONOID
PROCESS

RAMUS

Fig. 659
Mandible

FRONTAL

SUPRAORBITAL
FORAMEN

LACRIMAL

ZYGOMATIC

VOMER

NASAL

TURBINATE

INFRAORBITAL
FORAMEN

MAXILLA

MANDIBLE

MENTAL FORAMEN

Fig. 660
Front View of Skull

CRANIAL BONES

rontal bone: This bone forms the forehead and assists in the formation f the roof of the orbits (eye-sockets) and of the nasal cavity. This bone ontains the supra-orbital foramen.

arietal bones: These bones form the sides and major portion of the roof f the cranium.

ccipital bone: This bone is situated at the back and base of the cranium. t has an oval opening at the base known as the foramen magnum.

emporal bones: These bones are situated on either side of the cranium elow the parietals.

phenoid bone: This bone is situated at the anterior base of the cranium. ince it joins other cranial bones, it is known as the "interlocking" bone.

thmoid bone: This is a spongy bone situated between the orbits at the oot of the nose. It provides an opening for the passage of the nerve of mell.

Facial Bones

All the facial bones are in pairs except the vomer and mandible bones. he facial bones provide mastication, shape to the face, supporting struc-ures for the sense organs (eyes, nose, tongue) and a vestibule for the espiratory and vocal organs.

Iandible: This is the lower jawbone and is also called inferior maxillary. t is the largest, strongest and only movable bone of the face. It contains he lower teeth and the mental foramen through which the mental blood essels and mental nerves pass.

uperior Maxillary bones: These bones are situated on either side of the ace and by their union form the upper jawbone. These bones are also nown as "Maxilla." They contain the upper teeth and infra-orbital fora-nen. Besides forming a greater part of the mouth, they form the floor of he orbits, and the floor and part of the outer walls of the nasal cavity.

Iasal bones: These two bones are placed side by side and form the bridges f the nose.

omer: This bone is situated at the back of the nasal fossae, and forms art of the partition (Septum) of the nose.

acrimal bones: These bones are situated at the anterior of the inner vall of the orbits (eye sockets). These are the smallest and most fragile ones of the face. They contain part of the canal through which the tear ucts pass.

Palatine bones: These bones are situated at the back part of the nasal avity. They form the floor and outer wall of the nose and the back portion f the roof of the mouth.

Inferior turbinate bones (Turbinal bones): These bones are situated o either side of the outer wall of the nasal cavity. They are thin layers o spongy bone curled upon themselves.

Zygomatic bones: These are four-sided bones situated at the upper an outer part of the face and are commonly known as cheek bones. They ar also called "Malar" bones. They give prominence to the cheeks and forr part of the outer wall and floor of the orbits.

Bones of Neck

Hyoid bone: This bone is situated in front of the throat—between the roo of the tongue and the "Adam's Apple." It is an isolated bone without at tachment to any other bone. It supports the tongue.

Cervical vertebrae: These seven bones are situated in the neck region a the top of the vertebral column.

Interesting shapes of some bones:
1. Frontal—resembles a cockleshell.
2. Sphenoid—resembles bat with wings extended.
3. Palatine—resembles the letter "L."
4. Lacrimal—resembles the finger nail.
5. Hyoid—resembles the letter "U."
6. Vomer—resembles a plowshare.

Sutures of the cranium: A suture is the line of junction between bones
1. The **Coronal** suture is between the frontal and parietal bones.
2. The **Squamosal** suture is between the temporal and parietal bones
3. The **Lambdoidal** suture is between the occipital and parietal bones

Miscellaneous Details on Bones:
1. A **foramen** of a bone is an opening for the passage of nerves and blood vessels.
2. Four **foramens:**
   (1) The **foramen magnum** is a large opening of the occipital bone. It is oval shaped. The spinal cord passes through the foramer magnum.
   (2) The **mental foramen** serves as a passageway for the menta blood vessels and mental nerves.
   (3) The **infra-orbital foramen** serves as a passageway for infra orbital blood vessels and infra-orbital nerves.
   (4) The **supra-orbital foramen** gives passage to the supra-orbita artery, veins, and nerve.
3. The **ramus** is the perpendicular portion of the mandible. It has two processes—the coronoid and the condyle.
4. The skeletal system is composed of bones, ligaments, and cartilages
5. A fossa is a depression or pit in the bones. (The plural is fossae.)
6. The Zygomatic arch is formed by the zygomatic and temporal bones

Bones of Cranium, Face, and Neck

Bones of Cranium		Bones of Face	
Frontal	1	Mandible	1
Parietal	2	Superior Maxillary	2
Occipital	1	Zygomatic	2
Temporal	2	Vomer	1
Sphenoid	1	Nasal	2
Ethmoid	1	Lacrimal	2
Total	8	Inferior turbinate	2
Bone of Neck		Palatine	2
Hyoid	1	Total	14

Circulatory System

The circulatory system has a vital relation to the skin and hair. This is why the barber should know something about the subject. The skin and hair must have nourishment and waste matter must be removed from the skin. The barber can assist this system with those particular functions by stimulating circulation in the areas he serves. This the barber can do by facials and scalp treatments. But he can best perform these services if he understands the operation of the circulatory system—the relation of its functions to the skin and hair, the direction in which the blood flows, how blood circulation can be stimulated, and the location of the principal arteries of the scalp, face and neck.

PART 1

Aspects of Circulatory System Closely Related to Barbering

Purposes of study:

1. To learn how the functions of the circulatory system vitally affect the skin and hair.
2. To learn how to stimulate circulation in the scalp, face and neck.

Transportation system: The circulatory system is known as the "transportation system" of the body. It is so designated because it carries substances to and from all parts of the body.

Divisions of circulatory system: The circulatory system is divided into two parts. These are as follows:

1. **Lymphatic system.** This system consists of tiny vessels that are called **lymphatics.** These vessels transport lymph. (**Refer to** definition of lymph.)
2. **Blood Vascular System.** This system consists of vessels that transport blood ("vascular" signifies vessels). These vessels **are the arteries, veins** and **capillaries.** (Refer to definition of blood).

Lymph defined: Lymph is filtered blood. That is, that portion of blood plasma that has been forced through the walls of the capillaries by blood (lymph vessels) is called lymph. In other words, lymph is derived from plasma that has been forced through the walls of the capillaries by blood and has entered the vessels of lymph by osmosis. (This fluid gradually re-enters the blood stream.)

Functions of lymph: Lymph continues and completes the functions of blood. Body cells located outside the blood stream are served only by lymph. Lymph has been called the **middleman** between the blood and these cells. Oxygen and food in the blood vessels enter lymph through the walls of capillaries by osmosis. The two-fold functions of lymph are:

1. To transport oxygen and nourishment from the blood to body cells.
2. To transport waste matter from body cells to the veins.

Amount of blood and lymph compared:

1. Blood comprises about 1/20 or 5% of the weight of the body. The amount of the blood in the average body is **four quarts.**
2. The amount of lymph is estimated at three times the amount of blood.

Blood defined: Blood is the nutritive fluid that circulates in the blood vessels.

Functions of blood: Some of the functions of blood are as follows:

(1) To transport nourishment to the tissues.
(2) To transport oxygen to the tissues.
(3) To transport waste matter from the tissues.
(4) To help protect the body from disease germs.
(5) To help regulate the temperature of the body.
(6) To coagulate. (This means that the body has the ability to jellify or solidify and thus **form a clot** which closes an injured vessel. Coagulation prevents the excessive loss of blood from minor cuts.)

Source of nourishment in blood: The food we eat is the source of nourishment in the blood, however, such food does not acutally become such nourishment until it is fully **digested.**

How nourishment enters blood stream: Nourishment enters the blood stream through the walls of the small intestines.

How lungs assist blood:

1. The lungs relieve the blood of waste matter.
2. The lungs purify blood.
3. The lungs supply blood with oxygen.

How waste matter is excreted from blood: The blood transports waste matter to the lungs. In the lungs waste matter passes through tiny air-sacs and is excreted by exhalation. Waste matter is **carbon dioxide.**

What causes waste matter in blood: The cells make use of food by oxidation. This is nature's process of burning up food by oxygen. As food is oxidized, it throws off waste matter. Such waste matter may be likened to ashes from burned wood. Waste products also result from metabolism. (For meaning of metabolism refer to chapter on cells.)

How waste matter is excreted from body: Waste matter (carbon dioxide) is transported to the organs of excretion by the **blood.** These excretory organs are the lungs, kidneys, liver, large intestines, and skin. This function in the **skin** of the scalp, face, and neck can be stimulated by **facials** and **scalp treatments.**

How blood is purified: The lungs purify blood by the use of oxygen. Breathing is the process of inhaling oxygen and exhaling carbon dioxide. This process takes place in the air passages and lungs. **The bronchial tubes that take air** to the lungs become tiny air-sacs called **alveoli.** The walls of these air-sacs are well supplied with blood. It is in these alveoli that the exchange of oxygen and carbon dioxide takes place. Oxygen is absorbed by the blood in these air-sacs and carbon dioxide is thrown off.

How blood obtains oxygen: The blood obtains oxygen from the lungs. It is then transported to the blood vessels.

Composition of blood: The blood in general is composed of the following:

1. Red corpuscles.   3. Plasma.
2. White corpuscles.   4. Platelets.

Functions of red and white corpuscles, plasma and platelets:

1. Red corpuscles carry oxygen to tissues and carbon dioxide from them.
2. White corpuscles help to protect the body from disease germs.
3. Plasma carries nourishment to the cells and waste matter from them.
4. Platelets enable blood to coagulate.

Definitions of corpuscles, plasma, platelets.

1. Corpuscles are blood cells. They have been referred to as "tiny boats" floating in the blood stream.
2. Plasma is the fluid part of the blood. (It is a yellowish fluid and about 9/10 of it is water.)
3. Platelets are small, irregular bodies in the blood. (Refer to "functions of blood".)

Alternate names of red and white corpuscles:

1. Erythrocytes is the other name for red corpuscles.
2. Leucocytes is the other name for white corpuscles. They are also known as the "policemen" of the body, because they guard the body against disease germs.

Blood vessels: Blood vessels may be thought of as vehicles that transport blood. There are three blood vessels. These are arteries, capillaries and veins.

1. **Arteries.** These vessels convey blood **from the heart** to the tissues. The arterial walls are **strong, thick** and **elastic,** and they expand and contract easily. The **final extensions** of arteries are the **tiny capillaries.**
2. **Capillaries.** These are tiny vessels that **operate between the ar-**

teries and veins. These hair-like tubes have extremely thin walls and thus permit the passage of nourishment and oxygen to the tissues. The capillaries also transport waste matter to the veins. The capillaries are the most important blood vessels, since it is through their walls that all the exchange between the blood and tissue fluids take place. For example, these vessels transport food and oxygen to the lymphatics which deliver these essentials to the body cells and remove waste matter from them. It is noteworthy that the **scalp contains a profuse network of capillaries,** and that all cells and tissues, with the exception of hair, nails, cuticles, and cartilages are transversed by a network of capillaries.

3. **Veins.** These vessels convey blood **to the heart.** Venous walls are thinner and less elastic than those of arteries.

Natural circulation: The body's own ways of circulating blood constitute natural circulation. They are as follows:

1. By the **heart.** The heart is a "blood pump". It pumps blood throughout the body (The heart is a muscular organ.)
2. By **respiration.** Breathing promotes circulation. The movements of breathing make a suction affect that encourages circulation.
3. By **muscular activity.** As muscles contract they push blood onward and as they relax they draw in fresh blood. In this way, muscles exert a sort of pumping action that increases circulation.
4. By the **sympathetic nervous system.** This nervous system controls circulation. (Refer to chapter on nerves.)

Artificial circulation: The external ways of promoting circulation constitutes artificial circulation. Here are some of these ways:

1. Massaging.
2. Heat applications, such as steam-towels, red dermal lights and infra-red lamps.
3. High frequency.
4. Alcoholic solutions.

How to stimulate circulation by massaging.

1. Learn the locations of the arteries of the scalp, face and neck, and apply pressure directly over them.
2. Apply pressure only in the upward direction of the movement or manipulation. In the scalp, face and neck, blood flows upward.
3. Apply enough pressure to force blood through the arteries. Too much pressure, however, irritates and breaks down tissue.

Value of stimulating circulation: Stimulating circulation hastens the delivery of nourishment and oxygen to the scalp, face, and neck and the removal of waste matter. Such functions are necessary for healthy skin and hair. (Refer to section 'artificial stimulation".)

Why scalp may need artificial circulation: If there is any break down in the circulatory system, the scalp is likely to suffer first from insufficient blood, **because it is the highest point from the heart.**

Other reasons for need of artificial circulation are:
1. Lack of normal muscular activity.
2. Lack of normal circulatory function.
3. Stiffness and hardness of arterial walls, caused by advancing age.

Two systems of blood circulation: Technically, these two systems could be referred to as the sub-systems of the blood vascular system. **They are general** and **pulmonary** systems.

1. The **general** circulation system transports blood from the heart to all parts of the body and back to the heart, except to the lungs. **Alternate** names of this system **are central and systemic** circulation.
2. The **pulmonary** circulation system transports blood from the heart to the lungs and back to the heart.

Vessels of pure and impure blood:
1. In the **general** circulation system, arteries transport pure blood and veins impure blood.
2. In the **pulmonary** system, the pulmonary arteries transport impure blood and the pulmonary veins pure blood.

Color of blood:
1. Pure blood is bright red. Arterial blood, being pure, is bright red, except in the pulmonary arteries where it is impure and dark red.
2. Impure blood is dark red. Venous blood, being impure, is dark red, except in the pulmonary veins where it is pure and bright red.

How blood reaches scalp, face and neck: Blood reaches these areas through the external carotid arteries and their branches. These carotids originate at the aorta, a large artery, from which all blood leaves the heart. (There are **external** and **internal** carotids. The external serve the skin of the scalp, face and neck, except that the supra-orbital arteries which are branches of the internal carotids. The carotids are the principal large arteries on each side of the neck.)

Locations and names of arteries of scalp and face: Unless the barber knows the locations of the arteries in the areas he serves, massaging would be a hit and miss deal. When he knows the locations of the arteries, he can proceed with assurance that he can stimulate circulation. Knowing the names of arteries is also necessary for accurate reference. (Refer to Figs. 661-662).

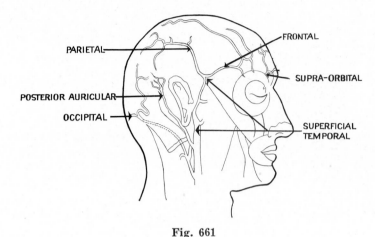

Fig. 661

Six Important Arteries of Scalp

Selected list of arteries: (Fig. 662)

1. Superficial temporal arteries. These are a continuation of the external common carotids. The **branches** of these arteries transport blood to the muscles and skin of the scalp, face, and neck.
2. Facial arteries. These arteries transport blood to the lower **regions** of the face and to the mouth and nose. (The alternate name is external maxillary arteries.)
3. Transverse facial arteries. These arteries transport blood to the parotid glands and masseter muscles.
4. Orbital arteries. These arteries transport blood to the obicularis oculi.
5. Parietal arteries. These arteries transport blood to the crown and sides of the scalp. (The alternate name is Posterior Temporal Arteries.)
6. Supra-orbital arteries. These arteries transport blood to the forehead.
7. Angular arteries. These arteries transport blood to the eye muscles and lacrimal sacs.
8. Superior labial arteries. These arteries transport blood to the upper lip.
9. Posterior auricular arteries. These arteries transport blood to the areas immediately behind the ears.
10. Occipital arteries. These arteries transport blood to the back of the scalp, between the crown and nape.

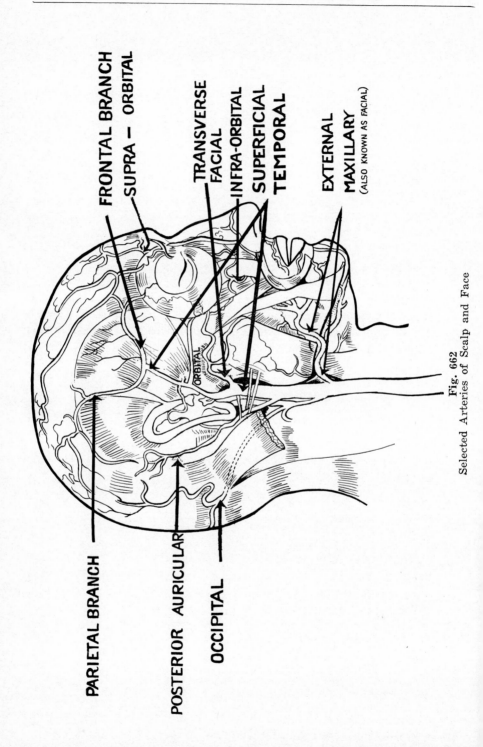

FRONTAL BRANCH
SUPRA – ORBITAL
TRANSVERSE FACIAL
INFRA-ORBITAL
SUPERFICIAL TEMPORAL
EXTERNAL MAXILLARY
(ALSO KNOWN AS FACIAL)
PARIETAL BRANCH
POSTERIOR AURICULAR
OCCIPITAL
ORBITAL

Fig. 662
Selected Arteries of Scalp and Face

PART II

Other Aspects of Circulatory System

Hemoglobin: This is an iron-containing compound which enables red corpuscles to combine and release oxygen. Thus combined, they turn the corpuscles bright red, a color which they retain until they enter venous blood. Hemoglobin has been called (1) **the coloring matter of the red corpuscles** and, (2) the **oxygen carrier** in the blood. In short, **hemoglobin enables the red corpuscles to function;** that is, to carry oxygen to the tissues and waste matter from them.

Shape of red corpuscles: These corpuscles are coin-shaped.

Corpuscle count: There are about 700 red corpuscles to one white.

Origin of corpuscles and platelets: The red corpuscles and platelets, along with a majority of the white corpuscles, originate in the marrow of the bones.

How blood is returned to heart in general circulation system:
1. The **Superior** Vena Cava returns the blood from the upper portions of the body to the heart. Other veins in these portions transport blood to this large vein.
2. The **Inferior** Vena Cava returns the blood from the lower portions of the body to the heart. Other veins in this portion transport blood into this large vein.
3. Blood leaves the scalp, face, and neck by the **jugular veins** which transport it to the superior Vena Cava.

Venous Valves: These valves prevent the backward flow of blood in the veins.

Structure and definition of heart:
1. The heart is the strong muscular organ which pumps blood throughout the body.
2. The heart is about the size of a closed fist and is shaped like a blunt cone or like a pear.
3. It is divided into four cavities or chambers. The two upper cavities are known as auricles.
4. Normal heart beats run 72 to 80 times a minute.
5. The valves in the heart control the flow of blood so that it will flow in only one direction, and they also prevent the blood from flowing backward. These four valves are:
   (1) The Tricuspid valve is between the right auricle and the right ventricle.
   (2) The Pulmonary valve opens from the right ventricle into the pulmonary artery.
   (3) The Bicuspid valve is between the left auricle and the left ventricle.
   (4) The Aortic valve opens from the left ventricle into the aorta.
6. The heart is enclosed in a membrane called the pericardium.

7. The heart is located slightly to the left of the center of the chest, between the lungs, and underneath the breast bone.

8. This muscular organ belongs to the involuntary muscle class.

9. No chamber has an opening into any other chamber (except through the heart valves).

10. All openings are guarded by valves.

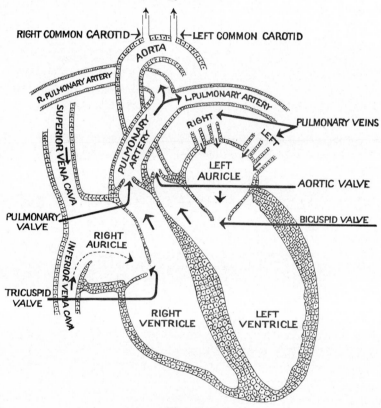

Fig. 663
Structure of Heart

The cycle of blood circulation:

General or Systemic circulation	left auricle to left ventricle to aorta and its branches to organs of the body to veins which form the vena cava to right auricle to right ventricle
Pulmonary circulation	right ventricle to pulmonary artery to lungs to pulmonary veins

Largest arteries in body: The aortic and pulmonary arteries are the largest arteries in the body. The aorta is the arch-shaped artery through which all blood leaves the heart for general circulation.

Three protective powers of blood:
1. Germicidal. (White blood cells have power to kill bacteria.)
2. Coagulative. (The blood has the ability to clot and seal wounds to prevent infection and to prevent bleeding.)
3. Phagocytic. (The blood has the power to engulf and digest foreign bodies.)

Miscellaneous details:
1. William Harvey: Dr. Harvey discovered that the blood has a continuous circulation, in 1628. The blood circulates through the entire body in 23 seconds.
2. Angiology is the study of the circulatory system.
3. The normal temperature of the body is 98.6 degrees Fahrenheit.
4. Erythroblasts are forerunners of red corpuscles.
5. Phagocytes are the white corpuscles found in lymph glands.
6. Blood has a salty taste; it is sticky; and has an alkaline reaction.
7. All tissue, except the hair, nails, cartilages, and cuticle are transversed by capillaries.
8. Portions of the aorta and pulmonary arteries are about one inch in diameter.

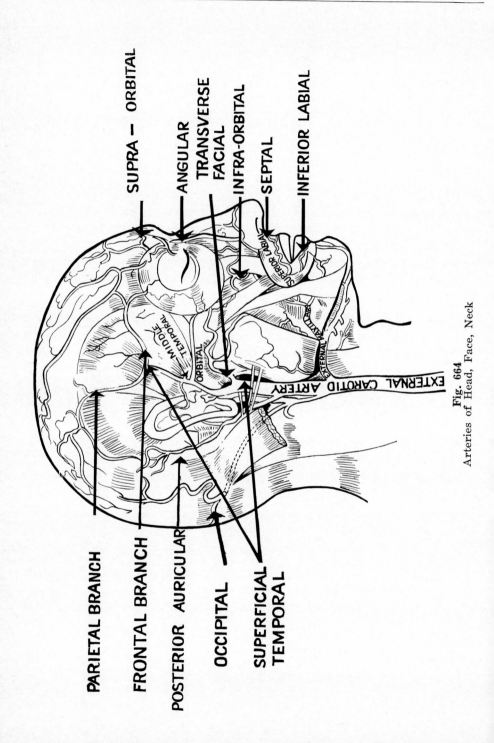

Fig. 664
Arteries of Head, Face, Neck

Hygiene

Hygiene deals with the rules of health. The barber should be familiar with these rules, because health is necessary for his success.

Definition of hygiene: Hygiene is the science of healthful living.

Major purpose of hygiene: The major purpose of hygiene is to preserve health. (Hygenic living helps prevent diseases and restore health.)

Phases of hygiene:

1. Cleanliness.
2. Ventilation.
3. Sunshine.
4. Balanced diet.
5. Exercise and recreation.
6. Posture.
7. Relaxation.
8. Mental attitude.
9. Digestion (See chapter on "Digestion.")

Kinds of hygiene: There are several kinds of hygiene, external, internal, preventive, etc. Only four types will be mentioned.

1. Personal Hygiene. Personal hygiene pertains to the individual. Using a clean towel on one's self is a rule of personal hygiene.
2. Community or Public Hygiene. Community hygiene pertains to a group, or the community at large. Using clean towels on customers is a rule of community hygiene, because this act affects other people.
3. Domestic Hygiene. Domestic hygiene pertains to the household. Keeping the house well ventilated is a rule of domestic hygiene.
4. Mental Hygiene. Mental hygiene deals with attitudes and thoughts that promote good health.

Relation of health to skin and hair: The health of the body is vitally related to the skin and hair. The skin has been called the "mirror of health". While the skin of a perfectly healthy body may become infected, the fact still remains that health is a good safeguard against skin disorder. The protective layer of skin and the function of the white corpuscles can be relied on only when the body is healthy. Hair and skin bear the same general relations to health, for what affects one affects the other.

Functions of food:

1. To furnish energy.
2. To supply the materials required for growth and repair.
3. To help regulate the functions of the body.

Balanced diet: A balanced diet consists of the proper assortment of foods. Eat plenty of vegetables. The balanced diet includes the six constituents of food.

Six constituents of food: Each constituent has a definite function.

1. Carbohydrates. These supply energy and include such sugar and starchy foods as corn, wheat, potatoes, grapes, cane and malt sugars.
2. Proteins. These build tissues and include such foods as milk, cheese, eggs, beans and lean meat.
3. Fats. These help regulate the body heat. (They also assist in supplying energy and form tissue.)
4. Water. Next to air, water is the most necessary substance to life. (Two thirds of the body's weight is water.)
5. Mineral salts. These help keep the proper acid base of tissues. (The tissues and fluids of all living things contain these salts. They are found in vegetables and fruits.)
6. **Vitamins:** Vitamins are food substance necessary for proper body functions. Some of these vitamins are known as A, B Complex, C, and D. These, as well as other vitamins, can be purchased in tablet, capsule and liquid forms.

    (1) Vitamin A is known as the skin vitamin. This vitamin is abundant in green leaves, cheese, eggs, milk, and vegetables such as carrots, yellow corn, and sweet potatoes. Prolonged deficiency of vitamin A can cause dryness and scaling of skin. (Such a deficiency can also cause sensitiveness to light known as night blindness.)

    (2) Vitamin B Complex in abundant in bran, germs of cereals, lean meat, spinach, eggs,beans, milk and fruits. Effects from lack of B Complex are nervous weakness, lack of appetite, neuritis, and **general malnutrition.**

    (3) Vitamin C is abundant in the juice of oranges and lemons, fresh fruits and vegetables generally. Effects from lack of C are scurvey and possible hemorrhage in the skin and mucous membranes.

    (4) Vitamin D is abundant in fish, eggs, and raw milk. D is the anti-ricket vitamin.

Elements in body: There are sixteeen elements in the body. (Refer to chapter on "Cells.) The six constituents of food contain all these elements. (Oxygen, carbon and hydrogen are found in carbohydrates; oxygen, carbon, hydrogen, sulphur and phosphorus in proteins; oxygen, carbon and hydrogen in fats; and silicon, sodium, sulphur, calcium, cholrine, iodine, iron, phosphorus, potassium, and flourine in mineral salts.

Calories: A calorie is a unit of heat. In a more practical sense, a calorie is a unit of energy, since **calorie** is the term used to designate the value of food. The body needs approximately 2500 calories daily.

Exercise: Exercise develops and helps maintain muscle tone and stimulates all the organs of the body to healthful activity. Deep breathing and plenty of fresh air are indispensable to help utilize the body fuel provided by daily food.

Posture: Good posture is partly a matter of habit. The barber should avoid unnecessary humped positions in his work. He should not habitually take the same stance and standing position too long at one time. This will help him guard against a droopy posture. Healthy muscles are necessary for good posture. In order for a person to walk and stand erect, keep his shoulders back, and keep his abdomen flat, all without strain, his body weight must be properly distributed, else he cannot attain this body balance.

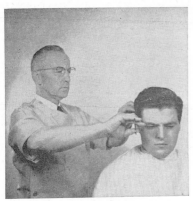

Fig. 665
Hair Cutting Posture

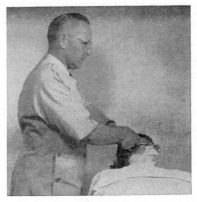

Fig. 666
Shaving Posture

Cleanliness: The barber should not only keep the shop immaculately clean, but he should give ample consideration to his own personal habits. Here are some details:

1. Clean teeth.
2. Clean finger nails.
3. Clean smock.
4. Clean shirt.
5. Clean trousers.
6. Clean shaven.
7. Well groomed hair.
8. Absence of body odor.

Other details of hygenic living:
1. Stand with equal weight on both feet most of the time.
2. Have recreational interest.
3. Drink enough water daily.

4. Do not over-eat.
5. Walk erectly.
6. Get plenty of fresh air.
7. Do not exert yourself.
8. See your doctor as he recommends.

Mental hygeine: Mental hygiene teaches the healthful mental attitudes. These are healthy mental habits. It is significant that these habits are under the control of the will and therefore they can be adopted and developed. A cheerful attitude is an asset to health, whereas a morose, despondent spirit is a liability and a handicap. Over-work and monotony breed despondency; rest and recreation are preventives of despondency. Healthful mental attitudes are partly a matter of resolve. A person must desire them and willingly strive to develop them.

Is not one as cheerful as one he has DECIDED to be. Remember "smile and the world smiles with you."

Importance of hygiene:

We should be keenly aware of the importance of hygiene. If the body is not exercised, rested, and adequately fed, its organs and appendages, including the skin and hair will not function properly. Such neglect can cause disorders of the skin or hair as well as organic diseases.

Digestion

Digestion is necessary for the general health of the body and for the skin and hair. Food cannot nourish the cells and tissues until it is digested. Digestion prepares food for absorption and use by the body. When digestion is impaired, the skin and hair suffer from lack of nourishment. Knowing this about digestion gives the barber a better understanding of the needs of the skin and hair.

PART I

Aspects of Digestion Closely Related to Barbering

Objective of Study: To determine the general relation of digestion to the skin and hair. When digestion is impaired blood circulation cannot properly deliver nourishment to the skin and take away waste matter. Consequently, the skin becomes over-burdened and sluggish in its excretion function and its pores become clogged. And its resistance to germs and disease is weakened.

Definition: Digestion is the process by which food is made suitable to be used by body tissues.

Chief Function: The chief function of digestion is to manufacture nutriment for the cells throughout the body.

Aids to Digestion:

1. Saliva.
2. Gastric juice.
3. Intestinal juice.
4. Balanced diet.
5. Mastication.
6. Exercise.

Glands that produce aids to digestion:

1. Salivary glands. (These are located in or near the mouth, and they secrete saliva.)
2. Gastric glands. (These are located on the walls of the stomach and they produce gastric juices.)

Importance of mastication: Thorough chewing of the food enables the digestive fluids to act upon the food quickly and completely. Good mastication prevents the stomach from being over-worked by having to assimilate food not properly chewed, and helps to prevent indigestion.

Some causes of indigestion:

1. Insufficient mastication.
2. Nervousness.
3. Excitement.
4. Pain.
5. Over-eating.
6. Worry.
7. Anger.
8. Fear.
9. Lack of balanced diet.
10. Vigorous exercise right after a heavy meal.

Some possible effects of indigestion:
1. Anemia.
2. Blood stream becomes filled with impurities.
3. Skin becomes over-worked in its duty of carrying off waste matter.
4. Acidity.

Indigestion, a possible contributory cause of some skin disorders:
1. Acne Vulgaris.
2. Acne Comedo.
3. Urticaria.
4. Acne Rosacea.
5. Whiteheads.
6. Eczema.

Relation of digestion to skin and hair: The blood stream cannot deliver the proper ingredients to the skin and hair unless the foods consumed are properly digested. When there is indigestion, the functions of the blood is impaired. The eliminative function of the skin is also retarded, paving the way for rash or other abnormal signs.

PART II
Other Aspects of Digestion

Salivary glands: There are three pairs of salivary glands. They secrete about two pounds of saliva daily. Saliva aids digestion.

1. The parotid, the largest pair. These are located below and in front of the ears, one on each side.
2. The submaxillary, located beneath the lower jaw toward the back, one on each side.
3. The sublingual, located underneath the tongue.

General course of digestion:
1. Digestion **starts** in the mouth.
2. Digestion is **completed** in the small intestines.

Stages of digestion:
1. Prehension—putting food into the mouth.
2. Mastication—chewing the food.
3. Swallowing—passing of food from the mouth down the pharynx and into the food pipe into the stomach.
4. Stomach action.
5. Intestinal action.
6. Defecation (exit).

Stomach action: Stomach action is like that of a washing machine.

Bolus: Food chewed and ready for swallowing is bolus.

Organs of digestive system: Lips, teeth, tongue, salivary glands, stomach, liver, pharynx, esophagus, intestines and pancreas.

Beriberi: This is the term for extreme physical weakness.

How nourishment passes from small intestine into blood stream: Digested food is drawn through thousands of finger-like projections. These projections are called VILLI. They are small pumpers that draw digested nutriments from the small intestines into the blood stream.

Bacteriology

Knowledge of bacteria is of importance to anyone rendering a personal service to the public. Since the very nature of barbering brings the barber in direct contact with customers, he should understand the relation of bacteria to the principles of shop sanitation and sterilization in order to guard the health of patrons and insure his own protection. Such understanding alerts the barber to the necessity of strict adherence to the sanitation code of the board of health and the barber board. Contagious diseases, particularly skin infections, are caused by the conveyance of disease germs from one person to another or by the use of contaminated implements, such as combs, shears, clippers, tweezers, and brushes.

PART I
Aspects of Bacteriology Closely Related to Barbering

Purposes of study:
1. To learn how bacteria can cause infection and disease.
2. To learn how to combat bacteria—to prevent the spread of disease.
3. To cultivate alertness as to the danger of bacteria.
4. To learn the importance of sanitation and the precautions against the spread of diseases.

Bacteriology: Bacteriology is the study of bacteria.

Two-fold reason for precaution against bacteria:
1. Bacteria definitely cause infection and disease.
2. In size bacteria are too small to be seen with the naked eye. They range in size from 1/100,000th to 1/3000th of an inch in diameter. They are the smallest living organism yet revealed by science.

Definition of bacteria: Bacteria are minute one-celled organisms of the vegetable kingdom. "Bacteria" as a term is used inter-changeably with "germs" or "microbes" when referring to harmful bacteria. They are called "micro-organisms" because they are microscopic in size—seeable only by a microscope.

Types of bacteria: There are both helpful and harmful bacteria, although in common usage, the unqualified use of the term "bacteria" implies the harmful type. The **two general types of bacteria** are:
1. **Pathogenic.** This is the term for disease producing bacteria.
2. **Non-pathogenic.** This is the term for helpful bacteria. (These bacteria do not produce disease.)

Meaning of pathogenic: Patho comes from the Greek and signifies pathos, but more especially disease. Genic has the force of genesis, meaning beginning or origination. Thus, **pathogenic** means disease producing.

Why bacteria are undersirable:
1. They breed and spread disease.
2. They produce poisons and toxins.
3. They consume body foods needed by the body for normal health.
4. They cause infection. There can be no infection without the presence of Pathogenic bacteria.

Transmitters of bacteria in barber shops:
1. Soiled linen.
2. Dirty finger nails.
3. Feet of flies.
4. Breathing.
5. Dirty hands.
6. Air.
7. Dust.
8. Dirty implements.

Routes bacteria can enter the body: The body has internal and external defenses against the invasion of bacteria, such as the leucocytes within the body and the skin on the outside of the body. But there are **vulnerable points** at which disease-hungry bacteria can enter, such as surface openings of the sweat glands and hair follicles, but more particularly the mouth, nose and eyes. Three routes by which bacteria can enter the body are:

1. By a break or an opening in the skin, such as a pore, a scratch, a cut or a pimple.
2. By breathing (inhaling).
3. By swallowing.

Where bacteria exist: Bacteria exist wherever there is Life. They are the most universal form of life in nature. They exist in decaying matter, in all bodies of water, on the surface of our body, on our clothing, in every crevice and pore of the skin, in the secretion of body openings, and even under our nails.

Conditions necessary for bacterial growth: These conditions are (1) warmth, (2) moisture, (3) filth, and (4) food.

How often bacteria multiply: Bacteria can multiply about every half hour.

Agencies for destroying bacteria: The agencies for the destruction of disease germs fall under two catagories:
1. Natural agencies. These are sunshine and the lack of sustenance. The human body defense mechanisms consist of leucocytes, unbroken skin, acids in the digestive system, and certain anti-toxins in the blood stream.
2. Artificial agencies. These are sterilization and all septic precautions. Pathogenic bacteria can be destroyed by chemical disinfectants, but basically by **strong acids, strong alkalies,** and **boiling water.**

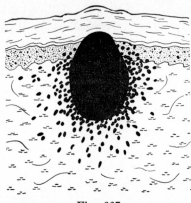

Fig. 667
Swollen Infected Area

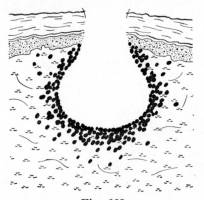

Fig. 668
Cavity from Rupeured Infected Area

Effect of heat and cold on bacteria:
1. Germs can be destroyed by intense heat or sunlight.
2. Bacteria cannot be killed by freezing. They survive a freezing temperature, but remain inactive in that state.

How bacteria can be destroyed:
1. By strong alkalies and strong acids.
2. By sterilization.

Formation of pus: Pus consists of decayed tissue, dead and living corpuscles and bacteria, and waste matter. **Pus is a sign of infection.** Staphylococcus is the most common pus forming bacterium. If pathogenic bacteria should enter the skin through a puncture or some other opening, and become deposited there, their toxins would destroy cells and cause infection. Immediately, however, leucocytes wage a battle with the disease producing germs, and dead corpuscles and dead bacteria result, and redness, swelling, and pain are discernable, and pus is formed. As a result of the invasion of pathogenic bacteria, pimples, boils, carbuncles or other infections may develop. **(A pimple containing pus is a pustule.)**

Infection: Infection is a condition in which pathogenic bacteria have taken control. There can be no infection without bacteria.

Indications of infection: (1) Redness, (2) swelling, (3) burning, (4) pus, and (5) sometimes itching.

Some skin diseases caused by pathogenic bacteria: Such skin diseases as sycosis barbae, favus, impetigo, ringworm, and erysipelas are caused by the direct entrance of pathogenic bacteria through the skin permitted by some break or opening due to a scratch, cut or pimple.

How bacteria multiply: A bacterium divides into two halves or two daughter cells and thus becomes two bacteria. Each new bacterium reproduces in the same manner.

PART II
Other Aspects of Bacteriology

General shapes of bacteria: The hundreds of species of bacteria have three general characteristic shapes:

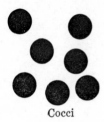 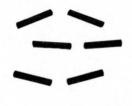 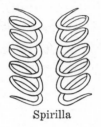

Cocci   Bacilli   Spirilla
Fig. 669
General Shapes of Bacteria

1. Round (technically, **Coccus**, singular; **Cocci**, plural).
2. Rod-shaped (technically, **bacillus**, singular; **bacilli**, plural).
3. Corkscrew-shaped (technically, **spirillum**, singular; **spirilla**, plural).

Local and general infection:
1. Local infection is confined to a certain portion of the body. It may be localized to a boil.
2. General infection means that bacteria have entered the blood stream and spread their poisons to all parts of the body.

Formations of cocci: Cocci arrange themselves differently. When they grow in grape-like clusters or bunches they are called staphylococci; when they grow in chain-like or bead-like strings they are called streptococci; and when the grow in pairs they are called diplococci. (Figs. 670-71).

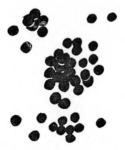 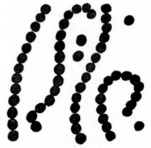

Fig. 670
Bunches of Clusters
(Staphylococci)

Fig. 671
Chain-like formations
(Streptococci)

Species of bacteria: There are hundreds of different species; however, their minuteness defies anatomical description except three general forms. Each of these species has a name, but only four will be discussed.

1. **Staphylococcus.** This kind of bacteria causes such ailments as pimples, boils, carbuncles, and pus forming infections. It is the mos common pus forming bacterium.
2. **Streptococcus.** This kind of bacteria causes such ailments as bloo poisoning, septic sore throat, lung diseases, erysipelas, and ap pendicitis.
3. **Spirocheta pallidum.** This kind of bacteria causes syphilis.
4. **Anthrax Bacillus.** This kind of bacteria is sometimes found in the bristles of new lather brushes. Manufacturers now process bristle to guard against anthrax. (Anthrax is a rare infection of the ski —a malignant pustule.)

Immunity: Immunity means a resistance that over-comes bacteria—t be safe from infectious disease.
1. Natural immunity may be partial or full, and it results from heredity that gives the body the ability to resist microbes.
2. Acquired immunity is obtained by successfully recovering from a given disease which leaves ample antibodies in the blood to counter act another attack, by building up a healthy body, or by injections

Phases of bacterial life cycle: Bacteria may be active or inactive.
1. Bacteria are **active** when they are growing and reproducing.
2. Bacteria are **inactive** when they are dormant and not growing or reproducing.

Parasites and saprophytes: These are classes of bacteria.
1. **Parasites** are harmful bacteria that live on living organic matter.
2. **Saprophytes** are helpful bacteria that live on dead organic matter

Toxins (poisons) and Ptomaines: These are by-products of bacterial activ ity in the body. By contaminating food, they are a menace to health.

Spore: A spore is formed when bacteria protect themselves by a dense membrane and become temporarily inactive. In this form a bacterium may survive freezing or other adverse conditions, and, if the cell remains dry its power of germination may be preserved in this inactive stage for months and even years. **When bacteria are thus inactive they form a spore** Many bacilli produce spores.

Diseases of lungs caused by pathogenic bacteria: Disease germs inhaled can cause certain diseases such as influenza, common cold, tuberculosis bronchitis, and pneumonia.

Benefits from non-pathogenic bacteria: The beneficial type of bacteria are indispensable to the continuance of life. We derive many benefits from their activities. Such bacteria produce helpful chemical changes:
1. In the tanning of leather.
2. In the curing of tobacco.

3. In the making of cheese. (Lactic acids formed by milk bacteria are active in cheese making—they cause milk to sour.)
4. In improving the fertility of the soil. (These bacteria cause fallen leaves, dead plants, and dead animals to decay, and the decayed matter goes into the soil and enriches it.)
5. In the making of vinegar and alcoholic liquors.

Leeuwenhoek: This man, a lens grinder in Holland, **discovered bacteria** in 1683. Under lenses he observed living creatures on some tartar which he had scraped from his teeth.

Pasteur: Louis Pasteur, about the middle of the nineteenth century, saw the value of Leeuwenhoek's discovery and designated the minute living cells as pathogenic bacteria. Pasteurization of milk resulted from Pasteur's contribution.

Type of majority of bacteria: There are more non-pathogenic than pathogenic bacteria.

Electricity

Electricity plays an important role in barbering. Such equipment as electric clippers, vibrators, dermal lights, infra-red lamps, electric steamers, electric dryers, heating caps, electric barber poles, and electric lather-making machines, and illumination, are made possible by electricity.

PART I

Aspects of Electricity Closely Related to Barbering

Purposes of study:
1. To learn applicable safety precautions.
2. To learn what a barber should know about electricity.
3. To learn about electrical appliances used in barbering.

Safety practices:
1. Changing a fuse: Have a flashlight available when removing a burned out fuse, touch only its rim. Never put a coin in the fuse box "behind" a fuse. Avoid contact with wet floor while changing fuse. Hands should be dry.
2. Electric cords: Do not walk on cords or expose them to excessive heat. If a cord of an appliance becomes extremely hot, the cord is overloaded.
3. Touching pipes and metal surfaces: When you have an electrical implement or appliance in your hand, do not touch plumbing pipes or other metal objects or surfaces.
4. Examine cords regularly. Repair or replace badly worn cords to prevent short circuit, fire or shock.
5. Remove plug without pulling cord. Grasp the plug itself.
6. Preferably use only one plug to each outlet.
7. In an emergency, such as a fire, turn off main switch. This will shut off electricity for the entire shop.

Purpose of fuses: A fuse is a safety device to prevent the overheating of electric wires.

Electrical appliances and machines used in barbering:

1. Electric clippers	5. Infra-red lamps
2. Electric vibrators	6. Electric steamers
3. High frequency machine	7. Electric hair dryers
4. Dermal lights	8. Heating caps

Types of lighting fixtures:
1. Incandescent. This is the ordinary type of bulb filaments used for intense illumination. They generate heat.
2. Fluorescent. This type of fixture illuminates by gas in tubes without heat.

Footcandles for barbering: The proper number of footcandles at the barber chair height is 100. (Refer to chapter on Shop Management for details.)

110 Volt circuits: Barber shop equipment is designed for use on 110 volt circuits. Equipment is stamped accordingly.

Types of current:
1. Direct current. (Symbols D.C.) This is a constant even current flowing in **one** direction. (Battery current.)
2. Alternating current. (Symbols A.C.) This current changes its direction of flow at regular intervals.

Cycle: A cycle is one complete revolution of an A.C. current. A sixty cycle implement completes 60 cycles and a 50 cycle 50 cycles per second. Magnetic clippers are designated according to cycle, and will run satisfactorily only on the cycle indicated.

Volt: A volt is a unit of electrical force. Barber shop equipment is designed for 110 volt. An implement so constructed will not work off a six or twelve volt battery current.

Converter: A converter is a device for changing an electric current from one form to another, such as an A.C. to a D.C. It is also called **Rectifier.**

Rheostat: A rheostat is a device for regulating the degree or flow of electricity. A strong vibrator can be toned down by this device.

Conductor: A conductor is any substance that transmits an electric current.
1. Conductors are such items as metal, carbon and watery solutions of acids, bases and salts.
2. Non-conductors are such items as rubber, drywood, and silk. Non-conductors are also called insulators.

High frequency: This is a current of high voltage and low amperage having 10,000 or more cycles per second. The current is made to pass through a glass electrode which becomes violet in color. This is why it is also called violet ray.

Purposes of high frequency: The high frequency is used in both facials and scalp treatments.
1. Effects of high frequency.
   (1) Relaxes or stimulates according to its intensity and the degree used.

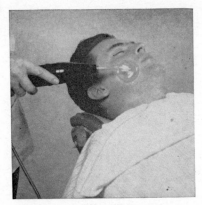

Fig. 672
High Frequency on Face

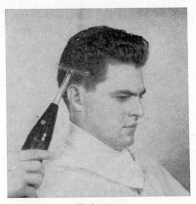

Fgi. 673
High Frequency on Scalp

    (2) Acts as germicide.

    (3) Promotes metabolism.

    (4) Helps to dry up simple pustular conditions.

    (5) Normalizes function of oil glands.

2. It should not be used on any area longer than five minutes.

3. This current should not be used over alcoholic preparations since it can ignite.

4. The high frequency accomplishes its purposes by the emission of ozone. Ozone is germicidal.

5. Upon **making** or **breaking contact** on the face or scalp, place the second and third fingers of the free hand on the electrode. (Fig. 674.).

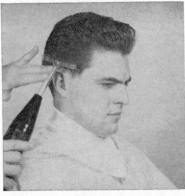

Fig. 674
Making or Breaking Contact

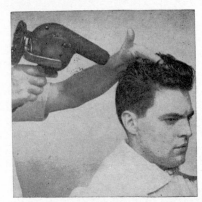

Fig. 675
Hand Hair Dryer

Methods of using high frequency: (Also other special currents):

    1. **Direct method:** The electrode comes in direct contact with the skin

of the patron. (This is the preferred method.) Some electrodes are designed for the face and some for the scalp.

2. **Indirect method.** The patron holds a special electrode while the barber massages with his hands. The current passes from the patron's scalp to the barber's finger tips.

3. **General electrification.** The machine is so designed that the patron receives the current direct while holding the electrode in his hands.

Electric Steamer. An electric scalp steamer is an electric appliance which produces steam. The steam pours onto the scalp from a composition hood. The advantages of an electric steamer over steam towels are:

1. It provides a continuous and uninterrupted flow of steam.
2. It is more effective—the steam is more potent and therefore penetrates more surely and deeper.
3. It allows for scalp manipulations during the process of steaming.
4. It is psychologically better, for it impresses the customer.

Heating caps: Heating caps are electric devices, applied over the head, to heat the scalp. They stimulate circulation and prepare the scalp for the absorption of preparations.

Additional electrical appliances: By visiting your local supply house and reading trade magazines, you will find many electrical appliances designed for use in barbering.

PART II

Other Aspects of Electricity

Types of special currents used for cosmetic and therapeutic purposes:

1. High frequency
2. Galvanic
3. Faradic
4. Sinusoidal

Effects of special currents classified:

1. High frequency effects are **thermal.**
2. Galvanic effects are **chemical.**
3. Faradic effects are **physical.**

Use of special currents in barbering: The use of some of the special currents, particularly galvanic and faradic, has dwindled considerably. Many barber and beauty schools do not teach them anymore. This same thing applies to phoresis. The high frequency, however, has increased in popularity.

Duration of application of special currents: The prescribed time runs from three to five minutes over any given area, except sinusoidal.

Galvanic current: It is a constant direct current generated by a direct current (D.C.) or by battery cells.

Purposes of galvanic current: The galvanic current is released through two poles, the positive and negative. The effects of each pole are different, but each produces chemical effects when it passes through the tissues and fluids of the body.

1. Effects of positive pole on tissues:
   (1) Constricts the tissues and closes pores.
   (2) Forces astringent solutions into the skin.
   (3) Charges the tissues with an acid reaction that is germicidal.
   (4) Decreases circulation and thereby reduces redness as in Rosacea.
   (5) Helps to make flabby skin and tissues firmer.
   (6) Soothes the nerves.
   (7) Recommended for an oily condition.

2. Effects of negative pole:
   (1) Relaxes and softens the tissues and opens pores.
   (2) Forces bleaching solutions into the skin.
   (3) Charges the tissues with an alkaline reaction.
   (4) Increases circulation.
   (5) Removes superfluous hair by electrolysis.
   (6) Irritates the nerves.
   (7) Recommended for a dry, pale conditon of face and scalp.

Faradic current: It is an alternating interrupted current with a strong mechanical action.

Purposes of Faradic current: Do not use on a patron with high blood pressure.
1. Increases stimulation.
2. Stimulates nerves, muscles and blood circulation.
3. Activates metabolism.

Theoretical effects of High Frequency, Galvanism, Faradism: From Faradism they are only physical; from the other two they are both physical and chemical. An effect of a current is chemical when it acts as an astringent or germicide; an affect of a current is physical when it stimulates such functions as circulation and metabolism or induces relaxation.

Sinusoidal current: This is an alternating current that produces contractions in muscles. This current has deeper penetration, greater stimulation, and less nerve irritation than the faradic. Its effects are as follows:
1. Adjustable so as to soothe the nerves.
2. Improves circulation.
3. Enhances nerve tone.
4. Accelerates glandular activity.
5. Builds up flabby tissue.

Wall Plates: The use of wall plates has been almost discontinued in barber shops. Any merit they have may advisably be left to medical therapists. A wall plate is a device designed to deliver the high frequency, galvanic, faradic, and sinusoidal currents.

Electricity defined: Electricity is an invisible force capable of producing heat, light, power, chemical and magnetic effects.

Circuit: A circuit is the path of an electric current. A short circuit means the flow of electricity has been interrupted by leakage across the lines.

Watt: A watt is a unit of electrical power.

Phoresis: This is the process of forcing chemical solutions into unbroken skin by means of a galvanic current.

Cataphoresis: This is the process of charging tissues with an acid reaction by use of the positive galvanic current. (Acids are positive chemical reacting solutions such as astringent solutions.)

Anaphoresis: This is a process of charging tissues with alkaline solutions by use of the negative galvanic current.

Electrolysis. This is the process of destroying tissues by an electric needle. A negative galvanic current is used. Electrolysis is used to remove superfluous hairs and some skin outgrowths. It should **not** be practiced by the barber.

Fulguration: This is a process of cauterizing warts and other such growths by high frequency. This practice is not within the scope of barbering.

HOW TO DETERMINE POLARITY

Polarity is either positive or negative. There are two methods of determining which each electrode is.

1. **Bubble test:** (also known as water method): Upon immersing both terminals in a container of clear water, bubbles will occur at each terminal in a short time. The bubbles gathering at the **negative pole** will be more numerous and larger.

2. **Litmus test:** With a water moistened piece of blue litmus paper contact one of the electrodes. If the terminal is positive, the litmus will turn red; if it remains blue the terminal is negative.

$\mathcal{L}$ight $\mathcal{J}$herapy

Light therapy is the treatment of diseases by light rays. Such use is therapeutic. In barbering, however, lights or light rays are used for **cosmetic** purposes in facials and scalpials.

PART I
Aspects of Light Therapy Closely Related to Barbering

Purposes of study:
1. To learn about light therapy appliances which may be used in facial and scalp treatments.
2. To learn how to use these appliances.
3. To find out the purpose of each appliance.

Dermal lights: A dermal light is a special type bulb in a reflector for use on the skin. This is why they are called **dermal** lights. The bulbs of such lights are of different colors—red, white or blue. The effects of each color of light are essentially the same and to some extent the difference has been regarded as psychological. Their effects are usually differentiated as follows:

1. Effects of red light. (Red signifies heat.)
   (1) Penetrates the skin (more deeply than blue light).
   (2) Aids absorption of oily substances.
   (3) Stimulates circulation.
   (4) Activates oil glands.

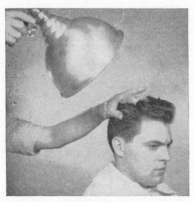

Fig. 676
Dermal Light on Scalp

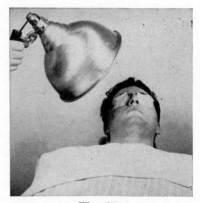

Fig. 677
Dermal Light on Face

414

2. Effects of blue light.
    (1) Soothes the nerves.   (3) Antiseptic.
    (2) Produces almost no heat.   (4) Penetrative.
3. White light is used mainly to relieve pain in such congested areas as the back of the neck. (Penetrative.)

Use of dermal light:

1. Dermal lights are used to aid the penetration of oils, ointments, and emollients. Do not use them to aid the penetration of an alcoholic or aqueous solution such as a hair tonic, since they would evaporate the solution and cause stinging.
2. Dermal lights are also used to dry facial packs, such as clay, egg and milk, and egg and honey packs.
3. When such lights are used in facials, protect the eyes with cotton pads saturated with warm water or witch hazel, or by some other suitable means.
4. In scalp work, hold the light about 12 inches from the scalp and in facials, 12 to 18 inches from the face.

Infra-red lamp: The infra-red lamp is a simple heat appliance made from metal generators or special glass bulbs. Infra-red rays come from almost all heat sources, but more especially from non-luminous infra-red elements. **Infra** means below or beneath and going into. The infra-red lamp produces the **most penetrating** of any of the invisible rays.

Major characteristics in infra-red lamp:

1. Long wave length.
2. Low frequency.
3. Deep penetrating power.
4. Heat a given area without raising body temperature.

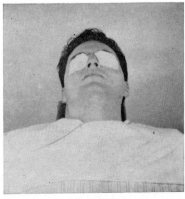

Fig. 678
Protcet Eyes from Heat Lamps

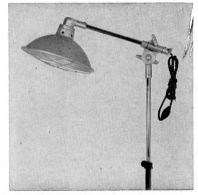

Fig. 679
Infra-red Lamp

Some effects of infra-red lamp:
1. It alleviates pain.
2. It stimulates circulation.
3. It activates the oil glands.
4. It opens the pores.
5. It aids absorption.
6. It increases metabolism.

Use of infra-red lamp: Use it much in the same way as instructed for the dermal lights, only it should be about 24 to 30 inches away from the face. This type of lamp is usually attached to a pedestal.

PART II
Other Aspects of Light Therapy

General effects of light rays on skin:
1. Dermal lights have a **physiological** effect by the emission of heat.
2. Ultra-violet rays have a **chemical** effect by the emission of ozone, vitamin D, etc.

Ultra-Violet lamp: The ultra-violet lamp produces "actinic" rays. These rays are invisible and their effects similar to those of the sun. Improvements in ultra-violet lamps make them less hazardous and some are designed even for home use; they are low voltage lamps. The fact still remains that over-exposure of the lamp can permanently injure tissue and conceivably result in malignant effects. For this reason, its use should be restricted to the hands of a physician, theraptist, or a person with thorough training. Its use in a barber shop is questionable.

Effects of ultra-violet rays:
1. Increases iron in the blood.
2. Puts Vitamin D in the blood.
3. Increases number of red and white corpuscles in the blood.
4. Eliminates waste products.
5. Stimulates circulation.
6. Produces tanning.
7. Can cause erythema (sunburn).
8. Penetrates the skin 1/250 to 1/25 of an inch.
9. Irritates the eyes under direct exposure.

General types of ultra-violet ray lamps:
1. The glass bulb.
2. The cold quartz.
3. The hot quartz.

The glass bulb: This is the type of ultra-violet ray lamp used for tanning and cosmetic purposes.

Three kinds of rays produced by sun:
1. Ultra-violet rays.
2. Infra-red rays.
3. Color rays.

Composition of sun rays: Sun rays are composed of 80% infra-red rays, 12% visible rays and 8% pure ultra-violet rays. The ultra-violet rays are the shortest light rays of the spectrum.

Erythema: This is a redness of the skin caused by exposure to ultra-violet rays. It occurs in patches of variable sizes and shapes. Erythema can mean the same as sunburn, depending upon its degree. The ultra-violet rays can produce erythema, depending upon their intensity and duration and the sensitivity of the skin.

Erythema in four degrees:

First degree produces a slight reddening without itching, burning or peeling. **No more than a first degree erythema** should be administered for cosmetic purposes.

Second degree produces marked reddening and slight peeling.

Third degree produces excessive reddening, swelling and thickening of skin, and pronounced peeling.

Fourth degree produces intensive reaction, blistering, itching, burning, peeling, and occasionally fever.

Visible and invisible rays:
1. The rays of the sun are both visible and invisible. The visibles ones can be divided into the colors of the spectrum. They are red, orange, yellow, green, blue, indigo and violet. (Light rays travel at the rate of 186,000 miles per second.)
2. Infra-red or heat rays are long, invisible rays.
3. Ultra-violet or chemical rays are short invisible rays.
4. **A. U. Symbols:** A. U. means Angstrom Unit, after A. J. Angstrom, Swedish physicist. A. U. is a unit of measurement of the length of light rays. One A. U. equals 1/250,000,000 of an inch.
5. The visible light rays are the color rays of the spectrum of the sun. They range in length from 3900 to 7800 A. U.
6. Dermal lights produce visible rays and also invisible HEAT rays.

Muscles

Muscles are a fundamental part of the scalp, face, and neck. The barber should have sufficient knowledge of muscles to understand their relation to skin and hair.

PART I

Aspects of Muscles Closely Related to Barbering

Purposes of study:
1. To learn the relation of muscles to skin and hair.
2. To learn how muscles should be massaged.
3. To learn how muscles are benefitted by massaging.
4. To learn how sagging muscles cause wrinkles.

Definition of muscle: A muscle is a fleshy band of contractile tissue. (This means in part that a muscle is rubber-like in its ability to contract.)

Myology: Myology is the study of muscles.

Purposes of muscles:
1. **Chief purpose of muscles:** To produce body motion.
2. **Other purposes of muscles:**
   1. To give exterior shape to the body.
   2. To provide attachments for some muscles.
   3. To protect the bones and organs.

Muscles affect health of hair and skin: Sagging and unhealthy muscles are antagonistic to the skin and hair, because such muscles interfere with proper blood circulation by tightening the skin, because they throw poison into the blood stream, and because they hinder the function of the glands. The function of the muscles of the neck, face and scalp assist in bringing blood or lymph to those areas and the skin and hair are thereby benefitted.

Importance of massaging muscles: The manipulation or kneading of muscles stimulates the circulation of blood, activates metabolism, encourages glandular activity, and assists in the elimination of waste material. Lack of exercise, fatigue, malnutrition, illness, or late maturity can cause muscular tissue gradually to become weak and flabby. This condition opens the door to the need of scientific massaging. This kind of massaging is impossible without familiarity with the structure and location of the muscles of the head, face, and neck, and with their blood and nerve supply. This knowledge removes the barber from the "hit and miss" procedure to a scientific basis of massaging.

Attachments of muscles:

1. Muscles are attached to other muscles, bones, skin, ligaments, tendons, and cartilage; and typically they are attached at each end.
2. Names and nature of attachments.
   (1) The "less movable" end attachment is called the **origin.**
   (2) The "more movable" end attachment is called **insertion.**

Direction of pressure in massaging:

1. As a general rule, manipulate from the insertion to the origin. Exceptions to the afore-mentioned rule are negligible. Some of the more fixed attachments, however, have sufficient flexibility to permit massaging over, crosswise or towards origins without irritating the muscles. EXAMPLES: Nasalis and Triangularis.
2. Light massaging over muscles may be done without respect to the origin and insertion, such as is involved in spreading lotions, creams and powders.
3. A muscle may be gently manipulated crosswise its structure.

Favorable attachments of facial muscles: The insertions of nearly all face muscles extend downward from their origins. Therefore, apply pressure in the upward direction.

Reasons for massaging from insertion to origin:

1. To massage in harmony with the structure of muscles.
2. To massage in harmony with the flow of blood.
3. To prevent irritating muscles.
4. To facilitate muscular contraction. A muscle responds more readily when exercised from its more movable to its less movable attachment.

Correct pressure in massaging muscles:

1. Firm pressure is suitably applied over muscles of the scalp (including the forehead), and over those of the nose, cheeks, sides and back of the neck.
2. Light pressure over muscles around the eye, those around the chin and along the mandible, and those around the Adam's apple.

Ways of stimulating muscles:

1. By massaging.
2. By heat-applications, such as steam-towels.
3. By solutions (alcohol, salts, acids).

4. By electrical agencies (violet ray).

5. By pleasantness (nerve impulses).

Characteristics of healthy muscles:

1. Suppleness.   3. Normal contraction.

2. Elasticity.   4. Good muscle tone.

Characteristics of unhealthy muscles:

1. Flabbiness.   4. Roughness.

2. Sallowness.   5. Sluggishness.

3. Sagginess.   6. Wrinkles.

How muscles are nourished: Muscles are nourished by food elements in the blood. They are also supplied with oxygen in the blood. Lymph carries nourishment and oxygen to the cells of muscles and takes away waste matter.

Composition of muscles: Muscles are composed of reddish fibres which form the red flesh of the body, hence they are likened to lean meat. Muscles are well supplied with **capillaries, lymphatics,** and **nerves.** In short muscles are composed of bundles of muscle fibres wrapped together.

The capillaries do not come in contact with muscle cells, but lymph does.

Contraction: This is the process by which a muscle becomes shorter and thicker. A muscle performs its functions through contraction. Contraction is a **normal function** of a muscle. (Fig. 680-681).

Value of contraction:

1. By contraction a muscle gives motion to the body.

2. The vacuum or suction effect of contraction ushers in blood which feeds the muscles.

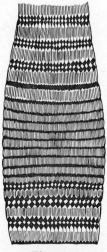

Fig. 680
Relaxed State of Muscle

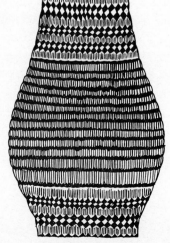

Fig. 681
Muscle at Apex of Contraction

3. By contraction the nerves are relaxed, metabolism is increased, and glandular activity is promoted.

Artificial contraction: A healthy muscle contracts normally, but contraction can be artificially induced by exercising muscular tissue. Massaging exercises muscles and accomplishes contraction. Such exercise, if executed properly, stimulates circulation, pushing blood through the arteries to the tissues and the blood in the veins back to the heart. In other words, **massaging assists nature.**

Muscle tone: Muscle tone means muscle tension. A muscle with normal tension is tuned up and warmed up and ready to perform its function; that is, it has the ability to respond readily to stimuli. Muscles without proper muscle tone are flabby, sluggish, and irresponsive. Massaging is one way to help maintain or restore muscle tone. The barber therefore has a scientific service to render via massage. Massaging helps to build up firmness, tension, and the readiness of muscles to function. "Premature wrinkles don't like muscle tone."

How muscles perform function of motion:
1. By muscle tone. (Just explained.)
2. Contractibility. (Just explained.)
3. Excitability. This means the ability of muscles to respond to stimulation. A muscle with normal tension has this ability.
4. Extensibility. This means the elastic ability of a muscle to stretch. This is the opposite of contractibility.

Arrector muscles: (also called arrectores pilorum) : These tiny, involuntary muscles are attached to hair follicles. Their insertion is near the bottom of the follicle and their origin is in the papillary layer or surface of the dermis. When these muscles contract they help draw blood to the papilla, and activate the oil glands. These muscles are stimulated by cold and fright and by massaging. (See chapter on Study of Hair.)

Locations of selected muscles of neck, face and scalp: (Study Fig. 682 and Part I of muscle chart at end of chapter.)

1. Buccinator. Located in the cheek near the corner of the mouth.
2. Caninus. Located upward from the upper lip and close to the corner of the mouth.
3. Corrugator. Located in the eyebrow underneath the orbicularis oculi and frontalis muscles and near the root of the nose.
4. Frontalis. Located at the forehead.
5. Masseter. Located between the cheek bone and lower jaw and about half way between the corner of the mouth and the ear.
6. Mentalis. Located on the side near the tip of the chin.
7. Nasalis. Located across the nose near the nostrils.
8. Occipitalis. Located at the back part of the scalp.

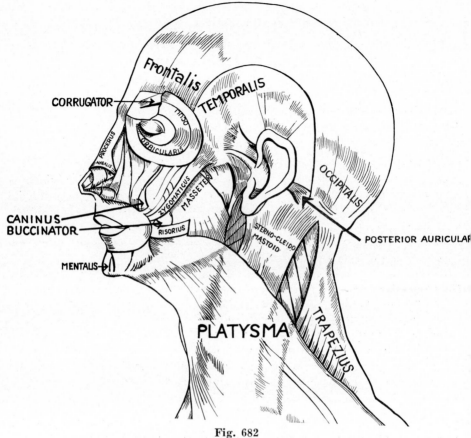

Fig. 682
Selected Muscles of Neck, Face, Scalp

9. Orbicularis Oculi. Located around the eye.
10. Platysma. Located on the side of the neck.
11. Posterior Auricular. Located behind and about midway of the ear.
12. Procerus. Located on the nose above the nazalis.
13. Risorus. Located from the corner of the mouth and underneath the buccinator.
14. Sterno-cleido-mastoid. Located between the chest bone and collar bone, across the neck and behind the ear.
15. Temporalis. Located at the temple and partially around the ear.
16. Trapezius. Located at the upper and back part of the neck and shoulders.
17. Zygomaticus. Located between the corner of the mouth and cheek bone.

Origins and insertions of six muscles: (See summary chart at end of this chapter.) Give special attention to Part I. It is not necessary to learn everything on the chart.

PART II
Other Aspects of Muscles

Types of muscles: There are three types.
1. Voluntary.
2. Involuntary.
3. Cardiac.

Functions of muscles according to type:
1. Voluntary muscles are controlled by the will. They are designated as "striated" because they consist of long threadlike striped cells. These muscles function in speech, facial expressions, and movements of the arms and legs.
2. Involuntary muscles function without the conscious use of the will. They are non-striated and are composed of small spindle-shaped cells. The function of these muscles involves the blood vessels, walls of the stomach, and intestines.
3. Cardiac muscles are found only in the heart. They are a special involuntary type. They are quadrangular in shape and composed of indistinctly striped cells.

Number—arrangement—weight of muscles:
1. There are about 500 muscles in the body.
2. There are about 50 muscles of the head, face, and neck.
3. Nearly all muscles are in pairs, and thus counterbalance each other.
4. Muscles comprise from 40% to 50% of the body weight.

Special classifications of facial muscles:
1. Expression. By contraction these muscles indicate gladness, anger, pain, attention, etc.
2. Mastication. These muscles assist in raising and retracting the lower jaw, as in talking and chewing.

Muscles of mastication: Muscles of mastication are the muscles which are primarily used in chewing and masticating food.
1. **Two** major mastication muscles.
   (1) Masseter (raises lower jaw against the upper jaw).
   (2) Temporalis (brings the incisor teeth together and closes the mouth).
2. **Two** minor muscles of mastication. These muscles are located between the mandible and cheekbone. They draw lower jaw forward and from side to side.
   (1) Internal pterygoid.   (2) External pterygoid.

Shapes of muscles: Muscles are of various shapes—flat, broad, roundish, elongated, fan-shaped, triangular, cockleshell, etc.

Some muscles with interesting shapes:
1. Fan-shaped: Temporalis, Anterior and Superior Auricular.
2. Triangular: Triangularis and Trapezius.
3. Pyramidal: Corrugator and Procerus.

Muscles of expression: Some muscles convey certain facial expressions, such as laughing and frowning. This fact illustrates how important it is to massage muscles with knowledge and understanding. Some examples of muscles of expression are:
1. Zygomaticus, the muscle of laughing.
2. Risorius, the muscle of grinning.
3. Corrugator, the muscle of frowning or pain.
4. Frontalis, the muscle of attention.
5. Procerus, the muscle of anger.

Innervation of muscles: Muscles receive their nerve supply from particular nerves. **This nerve supply is called innervation.**
1. Nearly all muscles of the **scalp, face and neck** are innervated by the facial nerve (seventh cranial).
2. The masseter and temporalis, muscles of mastication, receive their nerve supply from the mandibular branch of the **tri-facial nerve (fifth cranial).**
3. Other nerve supplies to the head, face, and neck are the tri-facial, mandibular branch, cervical, spinal accessory, and the accessory and third and fourth cervicals. Refer to the chart on the names, origins, insertions, functions, and innervation.

Ligaments are flexible bands of tissue that help hold bones together at their joints.

Tendons are bands or cords of tissue that attach muscles to bones. (Also called sinews.)

Aponeuroses are flat, wide bands of tissue that connect a muscle with another muscle or with the covering of bones.

Grouping of muscles: The muscles of the head, face, and neck are divided into seven groups. Learn some of these muscles and be able to classify them according to the following groups:

Muscle of the scalp.	Muscles of the mouth.
Muscles of the ear.	Muscles of the jaw.
Muscles of the nose.	Muscles of the neck.
Muscles of the eyebrow and eyelid.	

MUSCLE OF THE SCALP

The **epicranius** is the broad muscle that covers the top of the skull. It consists of two parts: the **frontalis**, the frontal portion, and the **occipitalis,**

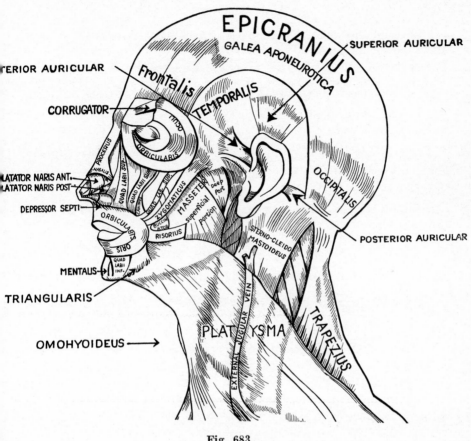

Fig. 683
Mucles of the Head, Face, and Neck

the rear portion. It is also known as the occipito-frontalis. It is connected by an aponeurosis called galea aponeurotica. This muscle controls the movements of the scalp—forward and backward—and the frontalis causes transverse wrinkles across the forehead.

MUSCLES OF THE EYEBROW AND EYELID

The **corrugator.** This muscle draws the eyebrows downward and inward, causing vertical wrinkles that give an expression of frowning.

The **orbicularis oculi.** This muscle closes the eyelids and causes wrinkles or squinting known as "crowsfeet" at the outer corners of the eyes. Since it is a ringlike muscle able to control or close the eyelids, it is called a "sphincter muscle". (Massage gently over and around this delicate muscle.)

MUSCLES OF THE EAR

The **anterior auricular.** This muscle draws the ear forward.
The **superior auricular.** This muscle draws the ear upward.
The **posterior auricular.** This muscle draws the ear backward.

MUSCLES OF THE NOSE

The **nasalis.** This muscle compresses the nostrils.
The **procerus.** This muscle draws the eyebrows downward, causing wrinkles across the bridge of the nose, giving the expression of anger.

The **depressor septi.** This muscle draws the wing of the nose downward and contracts the nostrils.

The **dilator naris.** This muscle helps to expand the opening of the nostrils.

MUSCLES OF THE MOUTH

The **quadratus labii superioris.** This muscle raises the upper lip and gives the expression of sadness.

The **quadratus labii inferioris.** This muscle depresses the lower lip, and gives the expression of sarcasm.

The **zygomaticus.** This muscle draws the upper lip upward and backward, and gives the expression of laughing.

The **caninus.** This muscle raises the angle of the mouth.

The **buccinator.** This muscle compresses and deflates the cheeks in blowing or whistling—forces air out between the lips. It is used in wind playing instruments. (This muscle also prevents food from accumulating between the teeth and cheek.)

The **risorius.** This muscle draws the corner of the mouth out and back, giving an expression of grinning.

The **mentalis.** This muscle wrinkles the skin of the chin and causes the lower lip to protrude, and gives an expression of doubt or dislike.

The **triangularis.** This muscle pulls the corner of the mouth downward, and gives an expression of contempt.

The **orbicularis oris.** With the assistance of the muscles inserted in this muscle, it holds the mouth closed and protrudes the lips as in kissing or whistling. (This muscle has its anchorage in the muscles that surround it, but is regarded to be without an insertion—It provides insertions for nine muscles.)

MUSCLES OF THE JAW

The muscles of the jaw are also known as the muscles of mastication. Only the two major ones will be mentioned here.

The **masseter.** This muscle assists in raising the lower jaw against the upper jaw.

The **temporalis.** This muscle assists in raising and retracting the lower jaw.

MUSCLES OF THE NECK

The **platysma** is a broad sheet muscle. It depresses the corner of the mouth. It produces wrinkles on the side of the neck, and gives an expression of melancholy. It is the **most widely spread muscle.**

The **sterno-cleido-mastoideus** draws the head obliquely downward to one side; and when this muscle on each side of the neck functions simultaneously, the head is drawn forward and downward. This is the **most prominent muscle of the neck.**

The **trapezius.** This muscle draws the head directly backward and sideways and rotates the shoulder blade.

Miscellaneous details on muscles:

1. Muscles are well supplied with capillaries and nerves but lymph supplies individual cells with nutriment and oxygen and removes waste.

2. **Fascia:** This is the connective tissue that covers and separates the various layers and fibrous bundles that form muscles.

3. Aponeurosis is the tissue connecting frontalis and occipitalis.

4. "Orbicular" means circular. "Oculi" pertains to the eye and "oris" pertains to the mouth.

5. The orbicularis oculi is also known as orbicularis palpebrarum.

6. The corrugator is also known as the corrugator supercilii.

7. The procerus is also known as the pyramidalis nasi.

8. The nasalis is also known as the compressor naris.

9. The depressor septi is also known as the depressor ala nasi.

10. The septum is the partition of the nose.

11. The caninus is also known as the levator anguli oris.

12. The mentalis is also known as the levator menti.

13. The quadratus labii inferiors is also known as the depressor labii inferioris.

14. Triangularis is also known as the depressor anguli oris.

15. "Labii" pertains to the lip.

ORIGINS, INSERTIONS, FUNCTIONS, INNERVATIONS OF MUSCLES
PART I

Name	Origin	Insertion	Function	Innervation
1. Buccinator	Alveolar process of lower and upper jaw	Angle of mouth	Flattens and deflates cheeks	Facial
2. Caninus	Below infra-orbital foramen	Angle of mouth	Raises angle of mouth	Facial
3. Corrugator	Inner margin of orbit	Eyebrow	Draws eyebrows inward and downward, causing wrinkes between eyebrows	Facial
4. Frontalis	Galea Aponeurotica	Skin of forehead near eyebrows	Elevates eyebrows, pulls scalp forward, causes transverse wrinkles on forehead	Facial
5. Masseter	Zygomatic bone	Ramus of mandible	Closes jaw	Mandibular branch
6. Mentalis	Incisive fossa of mandible	Skin of chin	Raises chin and pushes up lower lip, wrinkles skin of chin	Facial
7. Nasalis	Upper jaw near wing of nose	Skin over bridge of nose	Compresses nostrils	Facial
8. Occipitalis	Superior ridge of occipital	Galea Aponeurotica	Draws scalp backwards	Facial
9. Orbicularis oculi	Inner margin of orbit	Skin about eyelids	Compresses eyelids, draws medially the skin of forehead, temple, and cheek	Facial
10. Platysma	Pectoral (chest) and Deltoid (shoulders) muscles	Mandible and angle of mouth	Wrinkles skin of neck, aids depression of lower jaw	Cervical branch of facial
11. Posterior Auricular	Temporal bone	Ear	Pulls ear backward	Facial
12. Procerus	Tissues at bridge of nose	Skin of forehead	Draws inner angle of eyebrow downward, causes wrinkles at root of nose	Facial
13. Risorius	Fascia of masseter	Skin at angle of mouth	Draws out angle of mouth	Facial
14. Sterno-cleido-mastoid	Sternum and clavicle	Mastoid process of temporal bone	Turns head obliquely and pulls it forward	Spinal accessory

Name	Origin	Insertion	Function	Innervation
15. Temporalis	Temporal bone	Coronoid process of mandible	Closes jaw	Mandibular branch
16. Trapezius	Occiput and vertebral spines	Clavicle and shoulder	Draws head backward and sideways	Accessory & 3rd & 4th cervicals
17. Zygomaticus	Zygomatic bone	Angle of mouth	Raises angle of mouth upward and outward	Facial

PART II

Name	Origin	Insertion	Function	Innervation
1. Anterior Auricular	Scalp in front of ear	Ear	Pulls ear forward	Facial
2. Depressor Septi	Incisive fossa	Septum and ala of nose	Contracts nostril	Facial
3. Dilator Naris anterior	Cartilage of nose	Near tip of nose	Enlarges opening of nose	Facial
4. Dilator Naris posterior	Upper jaw near wing of nose	Skin of nostrils	Enlarges opening of nose	Facial
5. Omohyoid	Upper margin of shoulder blade	Hyoid bone	Depresses hyoid bone in swallowing	Cervical of facial
6. Orbicularis oris	Fibres of muscles about mouth	Serves as insertion for other muscles	Closes and protrudes lips	Facial
7. Pterygoid exterior	Wing of sphenoid	Condyle of mandible	Chewing	Trifacial
8. Pterygoid interior	Fossa of sphenoid	Angle of mandible	Chewing	Trifacial
9. Quadratus labii inferioris	Lower jaw	Skin of mouth and lower lip	Depresses lower lip	Facial
10. Quadratus labii superioris	Maxilla and zygomatic bones	Skin of mouth and upper lip	Raises upper lip	Facial
11. Superior Auricular	Scalp above ear	Ear	Pulls ear upward	Facial
12. Triangularis	Oblique line of lower jaw	Angle of mouth	Pulls corners of mouth downward	Facial

Cosmetic Preparations

This study of cosmetic preparations is confined to barbering. The barber should have knowledge of the **ingredients** and **uses** of the various cosmetic preparations that he uses. Acquaintance with the names and purposes are hardly sufficient. He should know the effects that certain ingredients have on the skin and hair. With this understanding, he is better prepared to serve the public, by making proper cosmetic selections, by knowing their correct uses, by knowing "why" certain ingredients are used. The principal cosmetic preparations used in barbering are soaps, creams, oils, tonics, shampoos, ointments, powders, and antiseptic and astringent lotions.

PART I

Aspects of Cosmetic Preparations Closely Related to Barbering

Cosmetics defined: Cosmetics are preparations used to improve or beautify the skin and hair.

Purposes of study:
1. To learn to select the proper cosmetic preparations.
2. To find out the principal ingredients of the cosmetic preparations used in barbering.
3. To learn the effects of certain cosmetic ingredients.
4. To learn the correct uses of certain cosmetic preparations.

Major uses of cosmetic preparations in barbering:
1. To cleanse the skin and hair.
2. To beautify the skin and hair.
3. To help preserve the health of the skin and hair.
4. To provide skin antiseptics.
5. To alleviate or correct certain skin conditions.

Classification of cosmetics used in barbering:
1. Cleansing cosmetics, such as soaps, shampoos, and cleansing creams.
2. Beautifying cosmetics, such as face powder, packs, hairdressing preparations, oils, and hair creams.
3. Corrective cosmetics, such as tonics, astringents, oils, medicated liquids, and ointments.

SOAPS

Hand soaps: Soap is the **most widely used cosmetic.** Solid soap is made from sodium hydroxide (lye) and an oil or fatty substance. Cocoanut oil added to soap improves its lathering ability. Hand soaps are usually prepared in solid (cake) or powdered form. **Medicated** soaps contain sulphur or some other antiseptic; **Castile** soap contains **olive** oil; **superfatted** soap contains **lanolin** or some other emollient; and **green** soap contains **linseed oil** and potash. Since an alkali can irritate sensitive skin, it is neutralized as much as possible in the best soaps, while in poor quality soaps it is less refined. Regular hand soaps are not intended for use on the scalp and hair, because they often contain an excess of alkali.

Soap defined: Soap is a compound of an alkali and a fatty acid. The standard alkalies are potassium and sodium. Potassium produces a soft soap; sodium a hard soap. Fatty acids come from oils and fats. Good soaps contain pure oils and fats and a minimum of alkali.

Some kinds of soaps:
1. **Castile soap** is made from **olive oil** and sodium.
2. **Green soap** is made with **linseed oil** and potash, and alcohol.
3. **Medicated soaps** contain ingredients added to the basic mixture, such as sulphur, boric acid, witch hazel, phenol or any antiseptic or medicinal compound suitable for the skin.
4. **Shaving soap** is usually a cocoanut oil base. Steric acid is a common ingredient. This kind of soap contains animal and vegetable oils, water, and alkaline substances. Steric acid occurs in many solid animal fats. Palmitic acid, also used, occurs in the glycerides of many fats and oils. Shaving soap is an antiseptic.

Fatty acids in soaps: There are different kinds of fatty acids, such as stearic acid (found in tallow), lauric acid (found in cocoanut oil), oleic acid (found in many fats and oils), and palmitic acid (found in palm oil).

Fats in soaps: These fats are animal fat (lard oil) and vegetable oils, such as olive oil, castor oil, palm oil, and cotton seed oil.

Lather producing substance: Resin, a vegetable substance, is used in many soaps to produce lather. (It also has strong detergent ability.)

SHAMPOOS

Soap shampoos: Potassium hydroxide (potash) is used to make soft or liquid soaps. Soap shampoos are liquid cleansing preparations for the scalp and hair. Castile soap is the standard soap used to make liquid soap shampoos and it is of superior quality. This soap is named after Castile, a province in Spain, where it was first made five or six centuries ago. Soap shampoos include tar shampoo which contains oil of tar or oil of cade.

and the so-called "dandruff-removing" shampoos usually contain tinctures of green soap. Soap shampoos come in jelly, cream, or liquid form.

Soapless Oil Shampoos: Soapless oil shampoos are chemical compound of sulphuric acid or other sulphonated agents, oils and fatty acids. In short, they are a compound of sulphonated oils and fatty acids. Such shampoos rinse out equally well with hard or soft water. There are two kinds of soapless oil shampoos:

1. Non-foamy soapless oil shampoo.
2. Foamy soapless oil shampoo.

The **non-lathering type** is **high in oil** content—castor oil and olive oil. Castor oil alone is apt to be too sticky and olive oil lacks body. Sulphonated together they are a perfect blend. The standard ingredients of this type of soapless shampoo are sulphonated castor oil, sulphonated olive oil, water, color, and perfume. Since this foamless shampoo contains sulphuric acid and a high oil content, it is best for oily scalp and hair; but its blend of pure oils make it also usable for dry scalp and hair. The **foamy soapless oil shampoo** is of low oil content and is made for normal, dry or oily scalp and hair.

Castile Shampoo Formula:

Crumble or slice into tiny strips a one-pound bar of castile soap.
1 gallon of soft water
1 teaspoonful of borax
1 teaspoonful of baking soda
Heat gently until soap is dissolved.

Caution: Do not boil, since boiling would separate the oils and alkalies in the soap and nullify its cleansing proclivities.

FACE CREAMS

Several kinds of face creams are used in barbering. A **face cream** is principally an emulsion of **oils, waxes,** and **water.** An emulsion is the conversion of an oil, wax and water into a permanent mixture. Some of these creams are:

1. Cold cream.
2. Cleansing cream.
3. Tissue cream.
4. Astringent cream.
5. Vanishing cream.
6. Rolling cream.
7. Medicated cream.
8. Emollient cream.

1. **Cold cream:**
   (1) It consists of oil, borax, wax, perfume and water.
   (2) It has been called an "all purpose" cream. It is used as a base for massaging, to cleanse and protect, and to lubricate the skin.

2. **Cleansing cream:**
   (1) It consists of a cold cream base but has a high content of mineral oil.
   (2) It is intended mainly for cleansing the skin. Some cleansing creams are liquid. A good cleansing cream should leave the face smooth, not sticky or greasy, perfectly clean and relaxed.

3. **Tissue cream:** Theoretically, tissue cream is skin food cream, but this claim should be accepted with definite reservation.
   (1) It contains such ingredients as oil, water, wax, lanolin, perfume, and cocoa butter.
   (2) It is softening and helps replace natural oil.
   (3) It is ideal as a base for face massaging.

4. **Vanishing cream:** It is also called a finishing cream or a foundation cream.
   (1) It is an oil-in-water greaseless emulsion. The basic formula is modified by cocoa butter, lanolin, glycerine, mineral oil, stearic acid, borax, and alcohol.
   (2) It is properly a finishing cream and a powder base.

5. **Rolling cream:**
   (1) This is a casein base cream with a solid filler. It is usually pink.
   (2) It cleanses the skin by a crumbling frictionite action.

6. **Medicated cream:** This term too should be accepted with reservation. It contains some ingredient to give it an astringent effect or some drug that is medicinal.

7. **Astringent cream:** A cold cream becomes an astringent cream when an astringent, such as alum or tannic acid, is added. It is recommended for an oily skin with large pores.

8. **Emollient cream:** Emollient cream contains lubricating ingredients that smooth and soften the skin. Such ingredients as honey, olive oil, cocoa butter, lanolin, sweet almond oil, and glycerine are found in good emollients.

Creams deteriorate unless kept sealed tightly, but not quickly. The terms "cold cream" and "cleansing cream" are used interchangeably. Vanishing creams are also known as finishing or powder foundation creams. Vanishing creams do not actually vanish—they reduce down to a thin film effect that conceals slight skin roughness, and become dry enough for powder. Soap and water and cleansing cream are considered more cleansing than rolling cream. While creams consist essentially of waxes, oils, and water, manufacturers add various ingredients.

Emollient: An emollient is a soothing and softening substance. Examples are lanolin, cocoa butter, and honey for external use.

Tonics: Some of the **ingredients** used for making hair tonics are quinine, alcohol, borax, bay rum, resorcin, sulphur, pilocarpine, tannic acid, tincture of mullein, tincture of copsicum, tincture of jaborandi, distilled water, and various vegetable extracts.

1. Pilocarpine activates the oil glands.
2. Resorcin is very cleansing.
3. Alcohol adds antiseptic properties and acts as a preservative.
4. Distilled water mixes more readily and keeps solution from discoloring.

Tonic defined: A tonic is a cosmetic liquid for the hair and scalp.

Types of tonics: (Refer to chapter on Tonics.)

1. Hydro-alcohol
2. Non-alcoholic
3. Oil Mixtures
4. Cream oils

Brilliantines. A brilliantine is an oil compound used to add brilliance or sheen to the hair. The plain brilliantines consist of a mixture of oils; the **combination** brilliantine consists of oils and either an alcoholic or hydro-alcoholic solution; and a **paste** brilliantine consists of petrolatum jellies, and other oils or waxes.

Ointments: Ointments are medical preparations intended for the scalp. They are a mixture of such organic substances as lard, petrolatum, or wax, and a medicinal agent. An example is sulphur ointment which may contain ingredients as laolin, quinine, drops of carbolic acid, vaseline, and sulphur. Only the barber with much knowledge of chemistry should make up his own ointments. There are good scalp ointments on the market.

Face lotions: Face lotions usually have antiseptic and astrigent properties. They are used as part of the finish of a shave or facial. Common ingredients in face lotions are alcohol, tannic acid, zinc sulphate, rose or perfumed water, menthol, and glycerine. **Three popular** finishing lotions are:

1. **Witch hazel:** This solution contains alcohol, water, and an extract of witch hazel bark Usual per cent of alcohol is about 15%.
2 **Bay rum:** This solution contains alcohol, oil of bay or other fragrant oils
3 **Lilac vegetal.**

Witch Hazel was discovered by the Indians It is a product distilled from the twigs of the Hamamelis Bush. It is soothing, healing, and acts as an antiseptic and deodorant.

Bay rum is a fragrant distillation of the leaves of the West Indian bay berry mixed with rum.

Astringents: Astringents have a constricting effect on the skin. Three examples are: (1) Tannic Acid, (2) Zinc Sulphate, and (3) Powdered or Liquid Alum. Some face lotions are astringents.

Face Powders: Face powders are used to beautify, to give the face a smooth good finish. A good quality powder spreads easily and adheres to the skin. Face powders are composed of such harmless ingredients as orris roots, starches, bismuth salts, French chalk, zinc oxide, perfumes, stearates, etc.

There are many tints of powder. Flesh tints are favored by blondes, and cream color by medium dark or brunette types.

Oils: There are several kinds of oils used in barber shop cosmetics. The two general classifications of these oils are vegetable and mineral.

1. **Vegetable oils:** Such oils include olive oil, castor oil, and almond oil. These oils are used in scalp treatments, because they are absorbent and soothing, and facilitate the removal of scales and crusts from the scalp. The oils of this category are recommended for hot oil scalp treatments and shampoos.

2. **Mineral oils:** They are refined petroleum. Their poor absorbent ability makes them less suitable for scalp treatments than vegetable oils, but they are excellent for hair grooming, since they do not rancidify on exposure to the air as do some of the vegetable oils, and they add glossiness to the hair. **Crude oil** is a mineral oil, and while in its raw form it is a parasiticide (kills parasitic germs) it is irritating to the skin.

There are other kinds of oils. **Oil of tar** is produced from the distillation of pine wood. While it has an offensive odor, it is parasiticidal and stimulates tissues. Because they are less offensive in odor and accomplish the same results, **oil of cade** or **oil of rusci** are preferred to oil of tar. These oils are found in preparations for oily scalp conditions, psoriasis, eczema, and some seborrheic conditions.

Fatty substances:
1. **Cocoa butter** is a yellowish white fat obtained from roasted cocoa beans that grow on a South American chocolate tree. It is used as a base for some creams and ointments, because of its soothing, softening, and absorbent properties.

2. **Lanolin** is the purified fat from the wool of sheep. In composition it is very **similar to sebum,** the oil from the oil glands. It is an excellent base for ointments and is used in more than 50% of all cosmetic preparations. Lanolin serves to replace the natural oil of the skin, scalp, and hair. It is a **soothing** and **softening** emollient.

3. **Lard** is used as the base of some ointments. One disadvantage is that it melts at body temperature.

4. **Glycerine** is a skin **emollient,** a thick syrupy liquid. It is a by-product from saponification of natural fats and oils in soap making. Because it aids **penetration,** it is a constituent in many lotions and creams.

Use glycerine on the skin in not more than 50% solutions; in concentrated form it is irritating. Glycerine is a skin softener. It is added to chemical solutions to prevent them from corroding implements.

5. **Cholesterol** is a fatty substance extracted from animal and vegetable oils and fats. It is regarded as a skin food, and as having the ability to provide nourishment for hair and skin. It is a favorite ingredient of creams. It is a product of the piliferous glands, also known as sebaceous (oil) glands.

Water: Water is the most abundant substance. Two kinds are:
1. **Soft water.** It is almost free from minerals. It is ideal for shampooing and coloring. Examples are rain and distilled water.
2. **Hard** water contains minerals—calcium and magnesium salts. It curdles soap and tends to prevent the forming of lather. It may leave curd which dulls the hair and causes the scalp to itch.

Ways to soften hard water:
1. By distillation. 2. By use of borax.
3. By water softening equipment.

Solvents: A solvent is a liquid that dissolves a substance. **Water** is the most universal solvent used in cosmetic preparations. Denatured alcohol in another usable solvent in such preparations. Isopropyl alcohol is also a solvent but has an objectionable odor.

Alcohol: Next to water and soap, alcohol is probably the most common ingredient used in cosmetic preparations. The kinds used in cosmetics are grain and ethyl. Corn, cane, and molasses are sources. Isopropyl alcohol is also used but very little. It is made from oils and the distillation of certain wood. It has the objection of unpleasant odor and it is poisonous, and is therefore inferior to grain or ethyl alcohol.

At 50%, alcohol is an antiseptic; and at 70%, it is a disinfectant. Alcohol is a good **preservative** of solutions. Its effects on the skin are due largely to the degree of concentration.
1. In small concentration it is soothing, it takes up moisture from skin; it tends to harden the cuticle; it is antiseptic. Up to 50% it is a small concentration.
2. In greater or strong concentration it is irritating; it causes burning and itching; it causes inflammation.

Detergent: A detergent is a cleansing agent. Soap is a universally used detergent. Sulphonated oils are detergents. The term "detergent" connotes positive **cleansing ability**, although water was the first known detergent. For practical purposes, detergents may be classified as (1) Soap detergents, and (2) Soapless detergents (Sulphonated Oils).

Some common symbols:
1. H_2O stands for water. Two parts hydrogen and one part oxygen.
2. HCL, stands for hydrochloric acid.
3. NACL, stands for sodium chloride (table salt).
4. O, stands for oxygen.
5. H, stands for hydrogen.

Ammonia: Ammonia hastens the action of peroxide, but do not use it unless a reddish cast is desired. Use 28% ammonia. Do not use ammonia if ash or drab shades are desired.

Chemistry and pharmacology: Cosmetics include both of these sciences:
1. Chemistry deals primarily with the **composition** of matter. (It includes the characteristics and changes of matter.)
2. Pharmacology is the study of drugs, their action and reaction.

Facial masks: These are usually clay packs or wrinkle pastes. They are composed of inorganic substances such as Fuller's earth, Kaoline or colloidal clay. Glycerine and a mild astringent are added to form a paste. Yeast and egg masks are other examples.

Some common cosmetic ingredients:
1. **Sulphur** has several uses and is found in some ointments. It is melted from crystals and condensed into a yellow powder.
   (1) It has antiseptic power.
   (2) It helps allay itching.
   (3) It is used to treat eczema and sycosis barbae.
2. **Honey** is an emollient. It soothes, heals, softens and helps relieve dryness.
3. **Salicylic** acid is a colorless, crystalline acid.
   (1) If used too strong it peels off the skin.
   (2) It helps diminish perspiration.
   (3) It is a powerful antiseptic.
4. **Iodine** is an antiseptic.
   (1) It comes from seaweed.
   (2) It is used in the treatment for alopecia areata.
   (3) Iodine stains can be removed with alcohol.
5. **Resorcin** is a strong antiseptic. It dissolves skin debris (dandruff).
   (1) It is used in many dandruff remedies.
   (2) It is used in many scalp ointments.
   (3) It can discolor gray and blond hair if an overdose is used.
6. **Camphor** is a mild skin stimulant. It can dilate blood vessels sufficiently to cause redness and warmth. It slightly numbs nerve endings and gives a cooling after-effect. Camphor is obtained from the camphor tree in Formosa and Japan.

7. **Alum** is an astringent and comes in two forms, powder and liquid. It is used to stop bleeding from a minor nick. Alum is potassium aluminum sulphate.

8. **Quinine** is extracted from the bark of a tree.
   (1) It is a mild antiseptic.
   (2) It is used in many hair tonics.
   (3) It is irritating in strong solutions.

9. **Menthol** is a greasy alcohol having the odor and cooling taste of peppermint. It has a decided cooling effect and helps to allay itching.

10. **Lard** comes from the fat of swine. It is used as the basis for some ointments.

11. **Mineral oils** are used as the base of some face creams.

12. **Water** and **soap are the most universal base of cosmetics.**

PART II
Other Aspects of Cosmetic Preparation

1. **Matter** is anything that occupies space and has weight. There are three forms of matter—**solids, liquids,** and **gases.**
   (1) A solid has a definite shape.
   (2) A liquid has volume but no definite shape.
   (3) A gaseous substance has neither volume nor definite shape.

2. **Three principal types of chemical compounds:**
   (1) **Bases** are bitter substances that contain hydrogen, oxygen and some metallic element such as sodium or potassium. A base that has disinfectant power turns **red** litmus **blue.** (A base is better known as an alkali which forms a salt when united with acid.)
   (2) **Acids** are sour substances that contain hydrogen and some non-metallic element such as sulphur or nitrogen. Examples of acids are vinegar, hydrochloric, and sulphuric. An acid solution has disinfectant power if it turns **blue** litmus **red. An acid** is present in any substance that has a sour taste.
   (3) **Salts** are formed when a base is combined with acids. Sodium chloride is a salt.

3. An **element** is a substance that cannot be broken up into simpler substances. There are about 100 known elements. Examples are oxygen, hydrogen, nitrogen, sulphur, and carbon.

4. A **compound** is a substance formed by two or more elements in a specific proportion.

5. **Distillation** is the process of boiling a liquid to a vapor and then cooling and condensing it back to a liquid. Its purpose is to remove impurities.

6. A **depilatory** is a substance used to dissolve or remove superfluous hair. Depilatories come in two forms, namely, wax and cream.

7. **U.S.P.** means United States Pharmacopoeia. These initials on any product means that it is listed in the book defining and standardizing drugs.

8. **Boiling** means heating to a temperature of 212° Fahrenheit.

9. **Freezing** starts at 32° Fahrenheit.

10. **Solutions:**
    (1) An **aqueous** solution consists of water and another substance.
    (2) A **diluted** solution is one that has been weakened by a solvent.
    (3) A **concentrated** solution is one that has been purified by reduction of solvent.
    (4) A **tincture** is a solution with alcohol as a solvent.

11. **Benzoin** is an astringent. Mixed with glycerine, it soothes chapped lips and hands.

12. **Sodium bicarbonate** is baking soda. Mixed with water, it helps allay itching.

13. **Ferric subsulphate** is Monsel's styptic, and comes in powdered or liquid form. It is used to retard bleeding from minor cuts.

14. **Hormone** is an organic product of the cells. Hormones are used in many face creams.

15. **Thymol** is a white crystalline phenol, an anti-parasitic drug. It is used to combat ringworm and pityriasis. It is used in some ointments for eczema, psoriasis, and acne.

16. **Sodium theosulphate** is white or colorless salt often used in ointments.

17. **Capsicum** is a stimulating ingredient in many hair lotions.

18. **Zinc sulphate** is a strong astringent, but a mild bleach. It is used as a preservative for creams and lotions.

19. A **calamine lotion** is a soothing agent recommended for sunburn, dermatitis, acne artificialis, and eczema.

20. The term **"cosmetic"** comes from the Greek word **kosmos,** meaning ornament.

21. **Water** consists of two parts hydrogen and one part oxygen (H_2O).

22. The term **organic** indicates living organs or living substances of the vegetable kingdom.

23. **A soluble substance** is one capable of dissolving and mixing with another substance.

24. **Zinc oxide** is a mild antiseptic. It protects the skin from sunburn and also protects inflamed tissue.

25. **PH** is the symbol for the Hydrian paper used to test the per cent of alkali in a liquid soap shampoo. The correct per cent of alkali is PH-8. If above this per cent, the shampoo would irritate the skin and if below it would not properly saponify and the shampoo would turn **foggy**.

Nerves

The function of nerves directly affects the skin and hair. In fact, the nervous system has been called the "ruler of the body." Nerves greatly influence circulation, glandular activity, digestion and other vital functions which are necessary to the health of the skin and hair.

PART I
Aspects of Nerves Closely Related to Barbering

Purposes of study:
1. To learn how nerves are relaxed or irritated.
2. To learn the value of developing the "right touch" in shaving and massaging.
3. To find out the influence of nerves on skin and hair.

Definition of a nerve: A nerve is a thread-like structure of tissue that transmits impulses.

Neurology: Neurology is the study of nerves.

Functions of nervous system: The nervous system has been called the "ruler of the body." It has been called the "telephone system" of the body, since it is largely concerned with receiving and sending messages.
1. It controls the functions of the body, such as circulation.
2. It gives the power of thinking, seeing, hearing, smelling, talking, walking, tasting, and feeling.

Ways of relaxing nerves: The nerves can, in some instances, be relaxed by the same means they can be stimulated. The degree and intensity makes the difference. Some special ways of relaxing the nerves are:
1. Moderately hot-steamers.
2. Massaging of moderate duration.
3. Light massaging.
4. Rhythmical massaging.
5. Soft music.
6. Pleasantness.

How nerves are irritated:
1. Overly heated steamers.
2. Unevenly heated steamers.
3. Dullness of razor.
4. Halitosis.
5. Loud radio.
6. Talkativeness.
7. Vigorous massaging.

Nerves in skin: The nerves in the skin terminate partly in the epidermis and in the corium. Nerves are innumerable in the covering of the body. The skin is highly endowed with sensibility; this is especially true in the

441

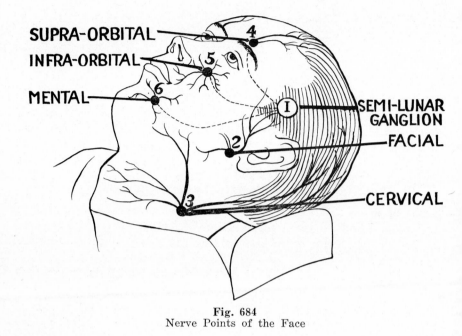

Fig. 684
Nerve Points of the Face

face and finger tips. It is therefore very important to develop just the right "touch" in massaging or in any service in which the skin is contacted. The nerves can be irritated and the patron displeased by the wrong "touch." Steam-towels, too, should be evenly heated to the proper degree.

Principal nerve points of face: (There are six pairs—six points on each side of the face. (Fig. 684).

1. **Semi-lunar ganglion** of the trifacial nerve is located slightly in front of the upper part of the ear.
2. The **facial nerve** is located in front of the lower tip of the ear.
3. The **cervical nerve** is located on the side of the neck.
4. The **supra-orbital nerve** is located just above the orbit of the eye.
5. The **infra-orbital nerve** is located just below the orbit of the eye.
6. The **mental nerve** is located downward from the corner of the mouth near the chin on the lower jaw.

Nerves the barber should know: The barber should know the names and locations of the principal nerves of the scalp, face, and neck. He can serve these areas more scientifically if he knows the exact locations of the nerves imbedded in them.

Cranial nerves serving scalp, face, and neck most: The fifth, seventh, and eleventh cranial nerves and their branches innervate the areas served most by the barber. These, therefore, are the three most important cranial nerves for the barber to know.

1. Tri-facial or Trigeminus (5th cranial).
2. Facial (7th cranial).
3. Spinal Accessory (11th cranial).

Four nerves of scalp: (Fig. 685).

1. The Greater Occipital. It is located at the back and base of the head, and extends to the vertex of the head.
2. The Posterior Auricular. It is located back of each ear.
3. The Superficial Temporal. It is located on each side of the head and it provides the nerve supply for the skin of the temporal region. (It follows the path of the superficial artery and is not the same as the temporal nerve.)
4. The Supra-orbital. It extends from the eyebrow onto the forehead and into the scalp. It serves the front and top portions of the scalp.

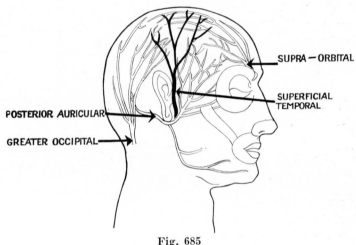

Fig. 685
Four Nerves of Scalp

Two kinds of nerves: Sensory and motor.

1. Sensory nerves carry messages from sense organs to the brain. (The alternate name of these nerves is **afferent.**) Nerves of **sight, hearing, smell,** and **taste** are sensory nerves. The sensory nerves are called the **outermost** sentinels of the body because the sensations which they receive serve as an alarm. These sensations are **heat, cold, touch, pain, and pressure.**
2. Motor nerves carry messages from the brain to the muscles. (The alternate name of these nerves is **efferent.)**

High Nerve Tension: Nerves become very tense as a result of worry, wrong diet, disease, over-work, etc. High nerve tension prevents the nerves from performing their duties, and consequently, many vital functions such as circulation and digestion are impaired. Accordingly, the skin and hai are affected. Nerve tension can be greatly relieved by the Rest Facial.

Symptoms of prolonged nervous tension:

1. Lusterless hair.
2. Falling hair.
3. Poor complexion.
4. Fatigue.
5. Irritability.
6. Staring eyes.

Tension fatigue: Means tenseness and tiredness. Recommend Res Facial.

PART II
Other Aspects of Nerves

Divisions of nervous system: The divisions of the nervous system ma; be classified in many ways. Any classification of these divisions ha: little or no significance in barbering. (Refer to end of chapter fo explanation.) For the purpose of studying this phase of the subject the two most applicable and **convenient divisions** are:

1. Cerebrospinal nervous system.
2. Sympathetic nervous system.

Functions of the cerebrospinal nervous system:

1. It controls the voluntary muscles and other functions under th control of the will, such as the senses of sight, smell, sound feeling, and taste.
2. It controls such voluntary actions as walking, talking, thinking
3. It consists of the spinal nerves and cranial nerves.

Functions of sympathetic nervous system:

1. It controls the involuntary and cardiac muscles.
2. It controls the heart, glands, digestion, breathing, and other in voluntary functions.

Nerves of blushing and paleness:

1. Vaso-dilators. These dilate blood vessels; cause blushing.
2. Vaso-constrictors. These constrict blood vessels; cause paleness

Nutrition of nerves: Nerves are nourished through blood vessels, lympha tics, and lymph spaces located in the connective tissues surrounding them

The Brain:

1. The brain is the largest and most complex nerve center. It is the headquarters of the nervous system—**the principle nerve center.** It controls voluntary muscles, sensations, and the power to think.
2. The brain includes the cerebrum, cerebellum, and medulla ob longata.
3. The **cerebrum** is the front part of the brain and comprises about three-fourths of the entire brain. It controls **thinking.**

4. The **cerebellum,** the lower part of the brain, governs muscular tone and coordination—it gives the body equilibrium.
5. The **medulla oblongata** is the part of the brain that controls such involuntary actions of the body as heart beats, breathing, reflex actions, etc.

Pons Varoli: (Pons means bridge.) This is the "bridge" that connects the cerebrum and cerebellum.

Reflex action: This is an involuntary muscular action, such as winking or closing the eyelids.

Cranial nerves:
1. These nerves are called "cranial" because they originate in the cranium.
2. There are twelve pairs of cranial nerves.
3. Some cranial nerves are only sensory, some only motor, and some are both.
4. Study the chart and diagram on cranial nerves.

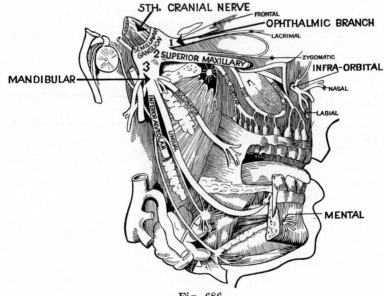

Fig. 686
Fifth Cranial Nerve

Three brances of trifacial: (Fig. 686).
1. **Ophthalmic** branch; the **smallest** branch, and it is sensory. It serves the eyeballs and eyebrows, lining of nose and eye, and the tear gland.
2. The **superior maxillary,** the middle branch, is a sensory nerve serving mainly the upper lip and upper teeth.

3. **Inferior maxillary** is the **largest** of the three branches. It is also known as the **mandibular** branch. It supplies mainly the lower lip, teeth, gums, and the muscles of mastication.
4. The ophthalmic and superior maxillary branches are **sensory,** but the inferior maxillary is both sensory and motor.

Spinal Nerves: The spinal nerves are arranged in groups named for regions of the spinal column from which they emerge. The **cervical** spinal nerves are located in the seven vertebrae at the top of the spinal column.

1. There are **31 pairs** of spinal nerves.
2. The spinal nerves extend from the spinal cord and are distributed to the muscles of the skin of the trunk and limbs.
3. The spinal nerves connect with the nerves of the sympathetic nervous system.
4. The **spinal cord originates** in the lower part of the brain.

Ganglion: A ganglion is a group of nerve cells forming a "knot" where two or more nerves join or separate. Examples are:

1. The semi-lunar ganglion, located between the corner of the eye and the ear, is the branching point of the 5th cranial nerve.
2. The otic ganglion is located in front of the lower tip of the ear.

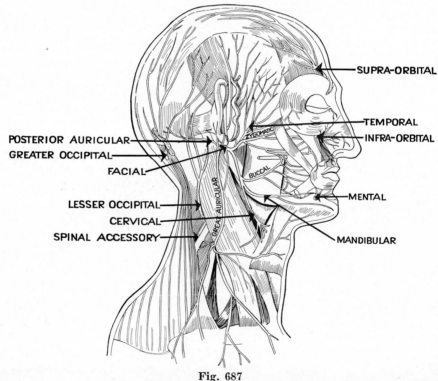

Fig. 687
Principal Nerves of Head, Face, Neck

CRANIAL NERVES

Name & No.	Type	Function	Noteworthy Points
1st Olfactory	Sensory	Sense of smell	20 branches
2nd Optic	Sensory	Sense of sight	————
3rd Oculomotor	Motor	Chief Mover of eye muscles	————
4th Trochlear	Motor	Pulls eye downward and inward	Smallest
5th Trifacial or Trigeminal	Both	Sensory nerve of head and face Motor nerve of muscles of mastication	3 branches One of three most important for barber to know Largest
6th Abducens	Motor	Pulls eyeball outward	
7th Facial	Both	(1) Sensory nerve of four salivary glands (2) Motor nerve of muscles of expression (3) One of nerves of taste	One of three most important for barber to know
8th Auditory	Sensory	Sense of hearing	————
9th Glosso-pharyngeal	Both	Sensory nerve of Parotid glands One of nerves of taste Motor nerve of Pharynx	————
10th Vagus of Pneumogastric	Both	Sensory nerve of Stomach Motor nerve of voice and heart	————
11th Spinal accessory	Motor	Motor nerve of trapezius and sterno-cleido-mastoideus	One of three most important for barber to know
12th Hypoglossal	Motor	Motor nerve of tongue	————

Keynote words may prove helpful in learning the names of the cranial nerves. The first letter of each word is the first letter of a cranial nerve in correct sequence, beginning with number one:

ON OLD OLYMPUS TOWERING TOPS A FAT AGED GERMAN PICKED SOME HOPS.

CRANIAL NERVES

There are twelve pairs of cranial nerves. These nerves originate in the cranium and each pair is connected to some part of the surface of the brain. Their fibres emerge through openings on the sides and bottom of the cranium. Refer to the chart on cranial nerves.

1. The fibers of the **first** cranial nerve, the nerve of smell, are distributed in the lining of the nasal chamber.

2. The cells of the **second** cranial nerve, the nerve of sight, are located at the rear portion of the eye.

3. The **third** cranial nerve, the motor oculi nerve, acts on most of the muscles that move the eye.

4. The **fourth** cranial nerve, the trochlear nerve, governs the muscles that raise the eye and rotate it downward and inward.

5. The **fifth** cranial nerve, the trigeminus or trifacial nerve is the **sensory** nerve of the head and face and the **motor** nerve of the muscles of mastication.

6. The **sixth** cranial nerve, the abducens, supplies the external rectus muscle that moves the eyeball outward.

7. The **seventh** cranial nerve, the facial nerve, is both sensory and motor. It serves the muscles of facial expression, some muscles of the neck and ear, and two pairs of salivary glands, the submaxillary and sublingual glands. This nerve is the nerve of taste to the anterior two-thirds portion of the tongue.

8. The **eighth** cranial nerve, the auditory nerve, is the nerve of hearing.

9. The **ninth** cranial nerve, the glossopharyngeal nerve, is both sensory and motor, and it serves the tongue, pharynx, tonsils, and one pair of salivary glands, the parotid glands. This nerve is the nerve of taste to the posterior part of the tongue.

10. The **tenth** cranial nerve, the vagus or pneumogastric nerve, is both sensory and motor. It extends to the upper part of the stomach, heart, and pharynx.

11. The **eleventh** cranial nerve, the spinal accessory nerve, supplies the trapezius and sterno-cleido-mastoid muscles.

12. The **twelfth** cranial nerve, the hypoglossal nerve, is the motor nerve of the tongue.

Neuron: A Neuron is a complete nerve cell. It is the structural unit of the nervous system. The nerve cell stores energy and food for cell processes that convey nerve impulses all through the body. Nearly all nerve cells are in the brain and spinal cord.

Largest and smallest nerves: The sciatic is the largest nerve; the smallest nerves are the tiny tendrils that enter the dental structure.

Some branches of trigeminal nerve: Supra-orbital, infra-orbital, mental, mandibular, and superior maxillary.

Some branches of facial nerve: Temporal, cervical, buccal, posterior auricular, and zygomatic.

Sizes of nerves: Nerves vary in size, from the tiny tendrils of the dental structure to the sciatic, the largest nerve in the body. In size the sciatic is a half inch in diameter and at places even larger. The ailment of this nerve causes terrific pain in the feet and legs.

ELABORATION ON DIVISIONS OF NERVOUS SYSTEM

To this point in the study of nerves, the only divisions of the nervous system discussed are the cerebrospinal and sympathetic, for two reasons: one, to avoid conflict with some other textbooks on barbering, and, two, because they are two nervous systems that govern the muscles and nerves relating to barber services. Two things certain are that "cerebro" and "spinal" pertain to he brain and spinal cord and thus are **under the will power;** and "sympathetic" signifies "self-acting" or "automatic" functions **not** under the will power.

The author is fully aware that the consensus of authorities use different terminology to classify the major divisions of the nervous system; yet they also refer to the cerebrospinal and sympathetic nervous systems, but as sub-divisions of the peripheral system.

Still, the functions of the cerebrospinal and sympathetic nervous systems as set forth in this chapter are the same functions that these authorities ascribe to them.

The prevailing consensus is that the nervous system consists of two major systems, and these are the (1) **Central Nervous System** and (2) the **Peripheral Nervous System,** although one authority divides the nervous system into three simple terms: (1) brain, (2) spinal cord, and (3) nerves. The **Central** System consists of the brain and spinal cord; and the **Peripheral** system of the cranial nerves, spinal nerves and end-organs.

Some other terms for the divisions of the nervous system are:

1. **Voluntary** for cerebrospinal.
2. **Autonomic, visceral** or **involuntary** for sympathetic.

The complexity of the nervous system lends itself to many highly technical synonymous classifications, general as well as subordinate, such as **somatic** or **craniospinal** for cerebrospinal. As contended earlier in this chapter, the various classifications of the nervous system are of little or no significance to the barber. Such matters are unfortunately present in too many textbooks on barbering and in too much of the subject matter of state board examinations.

Skin

The competence of a barber is enhanced by knowledge of the skin of the scalp, face and neck. He can scarcely have a comprehensive understanding of massaging, facials, and scalp treatments without knowledge of the structure and functions of the skin.

PART I
Aspects of Skin Closely Related to Barbering

Purposes of study: The purposes of this study are to learn the characteristics, structure, and functions of the skin of the neck, face and scalp, and the fundamental requirements for healthy skin.

Principal phases of study:

1. The physical needs of the skin.
2. The ways the barber may assist nature in meeting the needs of the skin.
3. The characteristics of healthy skin.
4. The characteristics of unhealthy skin.
5. The causes of unhealthy skin.
6. The structure of the skin.
7. The functions of the skin.

Some physical needs of the skin:

1. Skin must have adequate blood circulation. The skin's source of nourishment is the blood. (The blood receives its nourishment from the food consumed by the body.)
2. Skin requires metabolism. (See chapter on Cells.)
3. Skin requires the normal function of the oil and sweat glands.
4. Skin must be kept clean. Dirt, scales, ond oil clog the pores and hair follicles, and this condition besides creating an inviting place for germs, interferes with the action of the sweat and oil glands and further hinders the normal respiration of skin.

Services of barbering that can benefit skin:

1. Massaging.
   - (1) It stimulates circulation.
   - (2) It activates metabolism. (See chapter on Cells.)
   - (3) It soothes and relaxes the nerves.
   - (4) It increases muscular tone.
   - (5) It strengthens skin tissue.

(6) It stimulates or normalizes oil and sweat glands.
2. Cleansing (shampooing).
3. Antiseptics.
4. Heat applications. (Hot-towels; red dermal light; infra-red lamp.) These stimulate circulation and glandular activity, relax nerves.
5. High frequency.

Characteristics of healthy skin:

1. Smoothness.
2. Softness.
3. Moistness.
4. Flexible.
5. Free from disease.
6. Proper color.

Characteristics of unhealthy skin:

1. Eruptions.
2. Tightness.
3. Sallowness.
4. Roughness.
5. Premature lines.
6. Extreme paleness.
7. Extreme redness.
8. Mottled and blue.
9. Excessive dryness.
10. Excessive oiliness.

Contributing causes of unhealthy skin:

1. Poor blood circulation.
2. Sluggish glands.
3. Retarded metabolism.
4. Worry.
5. Uncleanliness.
6. Inferior cosmetics.
7. Prolonged indigestion.
8. Disease.

Definition of skin: The skin is the outer covering of the body. (It has been called the **living envelope** of the body. The skin is an organ of the body with definite physiological functions.)

Dermatology: Dermatology is the study of skin. (**Derma** refers to skin and **ology** means the study or science of.)

Dermatologist: A dermatologist is a skin specialist—a physician who specializes in the treatment of skin diseases.

Layers of skin: The skin consists of **three** major layers. Only two of these layers are clearly definable and so current authorities list only two, epidermis and dermis, but the traditional three will be listed to avoid conflict with some other textbooks.

1. **Epidermis.** This is the outside layer. (Also called **scarf skin.**)
2. **Dermis.** This is the middle layer between the epidermis and subdermis. It is also known as the **corium** or **true** skin.
3. **Subdermis.** This is the inmost layer of the skin; also called **subcutaneous** layer.

Epidermis: (Known also as **scarf skin**)
1. It is the **protective** covering of the body. This function is necessary for life—a person could not live without the epidermis.

2. It contains no blood vessels, but has many small nerve endings.

3. It consists of five sub-layers.

4. Normally, cells of the epidermis shed constantly.

Layers of the epidermis (Fig. 688): Current authorities hold there are only FOUR layers of the epidermis. Some contend the **mucous** layer is the deepest layer, but state it is sometimes called **germinating,** while others say the germinating layer is the deepest layer, but state it is also called mucous. **All list only one** of these as the **fourth** and **deepest layer.** The traditional five layers will be listed here to avoid conflict with some other textbooks.

1. **Cuticle** layer. This is the outermost layer of the epidermis. It is also called the **corneum.** This layer consists of tightly packed horny flat, scale-like cells which are continually being shed and replaced.

   (1) As the cells of this layer develop, they form **Keratin** which acts as a water-proof covering.

   (2) Its cells are almost dead and become a horny substance.

   (3) It is this layer that protects against germs, dirt, water, etc., because of its horny structure.

2. **Lucidum** layer. This is the layer just underneath the cuticle.

   (1) It is the **clear** layer through which light can pass.

   (2) It consists of small transparent cells, closely packed.

3. **Granular** layer. This layer is immediately under the lucidum.

   (1) It is filled with specks, like grains that resemble granules, and hence its name **granular.**

4. **Mucous** layer. This layer is just under the granular layer.

   (1) It consists of several tiny layers of cells.

   (2) The cells of this layer do not divide. They are pushed up by the growing and rising cells in the layer below.

   (3) It is also called Malpighian layer, after Malpighi, who first described its cells.

5. **Germinating** layer. This is the bottom layer of the epidermis.

   (1) This is the **birth** layer of the cells of the epidermis.

   (2) The cells in this layer have the power of reproduction by cell division. They reproduce through the process of mitosis.

Cells of epidermis: All cells of the epidermis are born in the germinating layer. They are the "mother" cells. They pass from the birth layer through all the other layers and finally into flat, horny scales in the cuticle layer.

Dermis: (Known also as **true skin or corium**)

1. The dermis consists of two layers:

   (1) The Papillary layer. This is the upper layer of the dermis. Its cone-shaped projections, called **papillae,** form the elevations between the epidermis and dermis.

    (2) The Recticular layer. This is the lower layer of the dermis. It contains blood and lymph vessels, fat cells, the oil and sweat glands, and the hair follicles.

2. The dermis is composed of the following:

    (1) Blood vessels.   (4) Sweat and oil glands.
    (2) Lymphatics.   (5) Arrector muscles.
    (3) Nerve endings.   (6) Hair follicles.

3. The majority of the blood vessels in the dermis are **capillaries**

Elasticity of skin: The elasticity of the skin is its rubber-like quality. It has the ability to regain its original shape immediately after being stretched. This ability gives the skin its cushion property. The **elasticity depends upon the fibers of the dermis,** determined by nature.

Subdermis: (Known also as subcutaneous layer.) It is the inmost layer of the skin, and actually the continuation of the dermis.

1. Being a little deeper it contains more of the coil-shaped bases of the sweat glands, and more adipose tissue.
2. It is from the subdermis that the principal blood vessels of the skin ascend to supply the oil and sweat glands and the papilla.

Papillae: These are **cone-shaped elevations** located between the dermis and epidermis. They fit into the depressions at the bottom of the epidermis. They contain capillaries and nerve endings which give the skin a keen sense of touch. The papillae contain some of the melanin skin pigment.

Two important glands in skin:
1. Sebaceous glands. (Oil glands.)
2. Sudoriferous glands. (Sweat glands.)

Sebaceous glands (Fig. 689): Commonly known as oil glands.
1. **Sebum** is the name of the oil produced by these glands.
2. Sebum is a semi-fluid composed of fats, salts, and water.
3. Their chief function is to lubricate the skin and hair.
4. Their structure is **spongy** and **sacular.**
5. These glands are stimulated by increased blood supply to the gland and a rise in skin temperature.
6. From one to six of these glands are attached to one hair follicle.
7. The ducts of these glands usually open into the hair follicles but some of them open directly upon the surface of the skin.
8. Sebaceous glands are found almost everywhere in the skin, espe-of the face, and they are abundant in the scalp.
9. The largest of these glands are located on the nose and other parts cially at the hair roots, but none on palms or soles of feet.

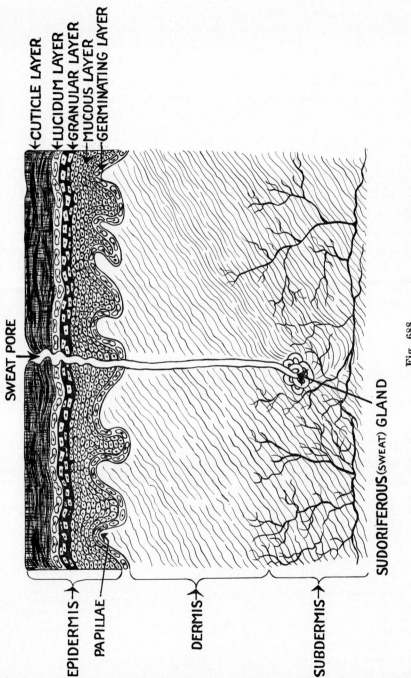

Fig. 688

Anatomy of the Skin Minus Folicle and its Closely Related Structures
PART I

10. They are **not** under the direct influence of the nervous system.

11. Being situated between the hair follicle and the arrector muscle, when this muscle contracts it exerts a squeezing effect on this sacular, spongy structure—the oil gland—and causes it to secrete oil from its duct. Here again such services as manipulation and heat applications assist nature—**these services produce artificial contractions of these tiny but important muscles.**

12. Each oil gland is supplied with a network of capillaries.

How function of Sebaceous glands influenced:
1. Massaging.
2. Heat applications.
3. High frequency.
4. Various drugs.

Functions of sebum:
1. To keep the skin flexible.
2. To keep the skin from becoming abnormally dry.
3. To protect the skin against hot wind and the sun.
4. To keep the hair from becoming abnormally dry.
5. To add glossiness to the hair.

Sudoriferous glands (Figs. 688, p.454: Commonly known as sweat glands.

1. Their principal functions are:
   (1) To elminate waste matter from the skin.
   (2) To help regulate body temperature.
2. Perspiration is 98% water and 2% organic substances.
3. These glands are most numerous in the palms of the hands, soles of the feet, arm pits, and forehead.
4. They are more deeply situated than the oil glands.
5. They are coil-shaped at their origin.
6. They are under the direct influence of the nervous system.
7. Each gland like the oil gland consists of a single tube.
8. A sweat pore is a funnel shaped opening on the surface of the skin.

How function of sweat glands are influenced:
1. Muscular exercise.
2. Heat applications.
3. Various drugs.
4. Strong emotions.

Arrector Muscles: These tiny muscles are **involuntary,** and are also known as **arrectores pilorum.** ("Arrecto" means to erect or raise up, and "pili" means hair.) These muscles **arise from** the papillary layer of the dermis and are inserted into the hair follicles below the sebaceous glands. None are attached to lanugo hair. Hairs lie slanting on the surface of the skin and the arrector muscles are situated on the side toward which the hairs slant. Fright or cold causes these muscles to function and produce a roughened effect on the surface of the skin, a condition known as "gooseflesh" (Fig. 689).

Appendages of skin:

1. Sebaceous (oil) glands.
2. Sudoriferous (sweat) glands.
3. Nails.
4. Hair.

Keratin: Keratin is the chief constituent of horny tissue, such as hair, nails, and the cuticle layer of the epidermis. While keratin is very resistant and can even withstand hydrochloride acid, it is readily dissolved by alkalies. Keratin is a protein substance.

Pigment of Skin: Pigment means coloring matter. The exact location of the pigment cells has not been determined. In general they are located between the dermis and epidermis (in the germinating and papillary layers). The number of pigment cells vary according to race: the white race has fewer; the the yellow and brown races more; the black race most. The coloring matter of skin is called melanin, and the more melanin the darker the skin. It helps to protect skin from sun rays. Because of fewer pigment grains, blond skin is more susceptible than brunet skin to the effects of sunlight. Skin pigment is of racial and hereditary origin.

Texture of skin: In the general feeling the surface of the skin is smooth and fine-grained. This "velvety" feeling is due to the fineness of scales of the corneum layer of the epidermis, to the presence of sebum, and (on the body) to the downy lanugo hairs. Actually, however, except on young children, the skin is not very smooth, but rather pitted in appearance, a condition due to the openings of its various glands, called pores. The largest pores are in the skin of the face. The **thickness of the skin** varies in different parts of the body. It is **thinnest** on the eyelids, and **thickest** on the **scalp, palms of the hands,** and **soles of the feet.**

Functions of skin: Besides serving as a general covering of the body, the skin has the following functions:

1. Protection.
2. Sensations.
3. Absorption.
4. Heat regulation.
5. Secretion and excretion.
6. Respiration.

Protective function of skin: The skin encases the body and forms a covering that protects the body from injuries, bacteria, dirt, and sun rays.

Sensations of skin: The skin is imbedded with many nerve endings of sensitivity and they register **five kinds** of sensations. These sensations are **pain, heat, cold, touch,** and **pressure.** The nerve endings that register pain are deeper seated in the tissue than the others, but the nerve endings of pressure are also deep seated. All these message-carrying nerves convey sensations from the skin to the brain.

Value of knowledge of sensations of skin:

1. It alerts the barber to the need for the "proper touch" whenever he touches the skin, especially in shaving and massaging. Hands

that are heavy, rough, clubby, or cold irritate the patron.

2. It alerts the barber to the fact that overly sharp-toothed combs, stiff bristles of a hair brush, a dull razor, an over-honed rough, scratching razor, or an unevenly heated steam towel give patrons unpleasant sensations.

Absorptive function of skin: The skin does not freely absorb water and other solutions, but it has some power to absorb creams, oily and fatty substances, and heat. Such means as these are recommended to aid absorption:

1. To aid the absorption of fatty substances, such as oils, ointments and creams, use the red dermal light, infra-red lamp, or steam.

2. To aid the absorption of alcoholic solutions, such as most hair tonics, antiseptic or astringent face lotions, and bleaches, use steam. (Do not use a dry form of heat.)

Regulatory heat function of skin: By means of blood vessels and sweat glands, the skin **regulates the temperature of the body** to 98.6°F.

Excretory and secretory functions of skin:

1. The sweat glands in the skin excrete impurities.

2. The oil glands in the skin secrete oil (sebum).

Respiratory function of skin: A small amount of oxygen is taken in and a small amount of carbon dioxide is eliminated by means of the pores of the skin.

Source of skin nourishment: The contention that certain cosmetic preparations are food for the skin should be accepted with reservation. The main thing such preparations do is to soften and soothe the skin. The **true source of nourishment** for the skin is the blood stream.

Blood capacity of skin: The skin can contain from one-half to two-thirds of all the blood in the body at one time. This is significant in that blood is the true source of nourishment for the skin and in that the barber can stimulate circulation through scientific services.

Causes of wrinkles: Wrinkles are usually associated with senility, but they can develop pre-maturely. To reduce or help prevent wrinkles, the Rest Facial and such facial packs as Clay Pack and Egg and Honey are recommended. Contributing causes of wrinkles are:

1. Advancing age.
2. Worry.
3. Habitual squinting.
4. Retarded circulation.
5. Disease.
6. Poor metabolism.
7. Sluggish glandular activity.
8. Heredity.

PART II
Other Aspects of Skin

Histology: Histology is the study of the minute structure of tissues, such as the skin and hair.

Piliferous glands: These glands are better known as the "sebaceous" glands. They are located in the skin and most typically exist in relation to the hair follicles. These glands secrete a substance known as Cholesterol, which stimulates the growth of hair and provides lubrication for the skin. This fact should not be confusing when it is pointed out that sebum, a better known product of the sebaceous glands, contains cholesterol.

Perspiration: Perspiration is the product of the sweat glands. There are two kinds of perspiration.

1. Insensible perspiration is the kind one continually throws off and evaporates without one being aware of it.
2. Sensible perspiration is the type that appears on the skin in drops and is observable. This only happens when more perspiration appears on the skin than can be removed at once.
3. The amount of perspiration secreted during 24 hours varies according to one's size, his activity, his health, the amount of water he drinks, and the climate. The amount is estimated to average about 16 to 20 ounces.
4. Perspiration consists of 98% water and 2% organic substances.

Types of glands in body: There are two general types of glands in the body.
1. Duct glands.
   (1) These glands contain small tubes (ducts), through which their secretions are conveyed.
   (2) Examples of these glands are sebaceous, sudoriferous, and salivary glands.
2. Ductless glands. (Also called **endocrine** glands.)
   (1) These glands pass their secretions directly into the blood stream. They have no tubes or ducts.
   (2) Examples of these glands are the spleen, thymus, and thyroid glands.

Gland defined: A gland is an organ that secretes essential material to the system or excretes waste material. Examples: the sebaceous glands **secrete** an oily substance and the sudoriferous glands **excrete** sweat. These glands manufacture new substance from material extracted from the blood.

Finger nails: The finger nails are an appendage of the skin. They are composed of clear, horny cells of the epidermis, organized so as to form a solid structure. They grow by multiplication of the cells in the root.

The principal division of finger nails are:
1. Matrix—the bed of the nail. The cells of the nail originate in the matrix.
2. Lunula—the half-moon shaped marking at the base of the nail.
3. Cuticle—the overlapping part of the skin of the finger around the nail.
4. Nail body—the part of the nail between the Lunula and the free edge.
5. Free edge—the part that extends beyond the finger tip.

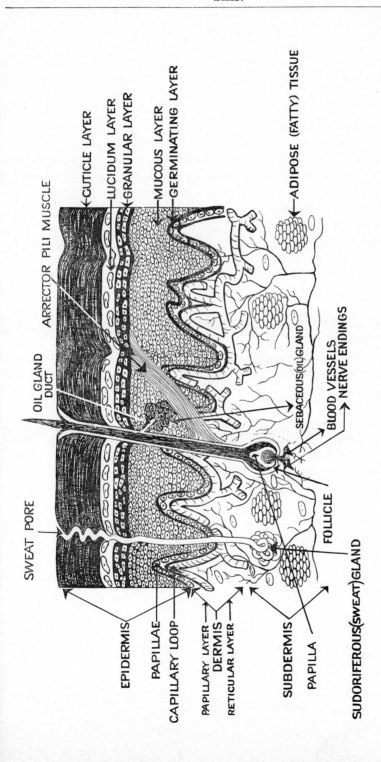

SWEAT PORE

CUTICLE LAYER
LUCIDUM LAYER
GRANULAR LAYER
MUCOUS LAYER
GERMINATING LAYER

ARRECTOR PILI MUSCLE

OIL GLAND DUCT

ADIPOSE (FATTY) TISSUE

SEBACEOUS (OIL) GLAND

BLOOD VESSELS
NERVE ENDINGS

EPIDERMIS

PAPILLAE

CAPILLARY LOOP

PAPILLARY LAYER
DERMIS
RETICULAR LAYER

SUBDERMIS

PAPILLA

FOLLICLE

SUDORIFEROUS (SWEAT) GLAND

Fig. 689
Anatomy of Skin
PART II

Diseases of the Skin and Hair

This study of the diseases of the skin and hair is limited to a brief discussion of the most common diseases of the skin of the neck, face, and scalp and of the hair. There are certain diseases of which the barber should have some knowledge. These are the diseases that he most frequently encounters in the practice of barbering. It is not properly within the scope of barbering to diagnose and treat all diseases—this belongs to the dermatologist or physician.

The most important thing for the barber to know about this subject is that he should not serve a customer who has a contagious skin disease. He thus safeguards his own health as well as that of his clientele. The barber may determine whether or not a condition is contagious either by recognition or by asking the customer. If neither he nor the customer knows, the customer should not be served until authorized by a physician, or until the condition disappears.

The barber should realize that the diagnosis and treatment of skin diseases are complicated and that even the best authorities are not always certain as to the immediate identity, cause, and proper treatments. Scarcely any of the diseases to be discussed in this chapter should be treated by the barber. He may treat some diseases in cooperation with and under the supervision of a physician. A prescription shampoo, ointment, or medicinal preparation for the scalp quite properly can be applied by a barber, with the permission of the physician. Then there are several skin conditions for which it is appropriate and desirable to give treatments. Such treatments are **soothing** and **alleviative**—these are for a tender, sensitive, slightly irritated skin, itchiness, dryness, oiliness, etc.

PART I
Aspects of Diseases of the Skin and Hair
Closely Related to Barbering

Barber's protection against disease: The barber may serve the public without fear of contracting diseases. The rigorous practice of sanitary measures supplemented with the help of nature makes the probability of contraction negligible:

1. The faithful practice of sanitation and sterilization in a shop is a good protection against diseases.

2. Nature has fortunately given the skin a natural protective agent and that is the cuticle layer of the epidermis. This horny layer of skin resists the invasion of disease germs. As long as the skin of the hands are unbroken and the cuticle is in good condition, one has a natural protection against germs. Many contagious diseases can be touched with the hands without fear of contagion. Should the barber have a break in the skin of his hands, he should cover it with "new-skin" or some other suitable protective.

Definition of disease: A disease is the opposite of health. (The term has been broken down to mean dis-ease (not at ease), but it has more serious connotation.) For practical purposes, in the present study "diseases," "ailments" and "disorders" will be used interchangeably to mean the same thing.

Barber shop treatments of skin and hair diseases classified:
1. Most of the treatments which the barber gives are known as **cosmetic.** They simply soothe, alleviate, and beautify. Such treatments may be given over some skin disorders such as those that are classified as non-contagious.
2. Some barber shop treatments are intended to **correct** or **help correct** certain disorders or undesirable conditions. Such treatments are **corrective** but are not to be construed as being therapeutic. Perhaps **alleviate** would be the preferable term for the barber to use.

Purposes of study:
1. To learn what to do and not to do with skin diseases.
2. To learn which skin diseases are or are not contageous.
3. To find out which skin disorders may be treated by the barber.

Some skin and hair disorders barber may treat:
1. Dandruff.
2. Itching scalp.
3. Excessive dryness.
4. Excessive oiliness.
5. Falling hair.
6. Simple pimples.
7. Blackheads.
8. Whiteheads.
9. Tender skin.
10. Sensitive skin.

An attempt will be made to familiarize the barber with the most common diseases with a minimum of technical terminology. Many of the technical terms will be studied later in the chapter. For the most part, the things about diseases that a barber should know are non-technical.

DANDRUFF

The most common abnormal condition that a barber encounters is dandruff. Dead cells are constantly being shed from the scalp, and this is normal as the study of cells reveals. When this shedding becomes excessive, the condition is known as dandruff. Dandruff is not restricted to the scalp, but when it is located there its technical name is **Pityriasis**. As such it is classified as a disorder which begins insidiously and without any symptoms. In only a few cases does the victim complain of slight itching. The initial signs are ill-defined patches of scaliness, but they enlarge and gradually cover the entire scaly except the extreme edges of the scalp. Scalp treatments, or shampoos and tonics may clear up the condition for a few days, and such treatments given twice a week may even keep it under reasonable control. "Dandruff removers" are popular on this basis. Dandruff—excessive scales—is easily removed from an otherwise normal scalp. Pityriasis may continue through the entire span of life. In many cases, however, in prolonged pityriasis, seborrhea develops and dandruff disappears. The simple type of dandruff is typically dry.

Definition of dandruff: Dandruff is dry or oily bran-like scales formed on an abnormal scalp. Soon these scales shed in the form of flakes.

Extent of dandruff: Practically the entire population is affected at one time or another with dandruff.

Course of dandruff: Dandruff is injurious only if it leads to some kind of dermititis or baldness. It has been charged with hastening baldness, but the fact is that countless people have dandruff all their lives and retain full heads of hair.

Types of Pityriasis: There are two general types of pityriasis, namely, **dry** and **oily**. The most widely used technical terms for these conditions are as follows:

1. **Pityriasis Capitis.** (Its alternate name is Pityriasis Simplex Capitis.) This is the **dry** type of dandruff.
2. **Pityriasis Steatoides.** This is the **oily** type of dandruff. In this type of dandruff the scales assume a sticky, oily character. The scalp is covered with a sticky mass of yellowish brown scales. The scales mat together and tend to clog the openings of the hair follicles and the pores of the skin. It is the more serious type of the two.

Dandruff characterized: Dandruff is characterized by powdery or flaky, grayish white dry scales, and sometimes itching. In prolonged cases, the hair becomes lusterless. Pityriasis is non-inflammatory and non-contagious. This is true partly because the scales result from a continual superficial exfoliation of the horny layer of the skin.

Causes of Pityriasis: Predisposing causes include family tendency and scalp neglect. It is the consensus that an indisputable cause has not been discovered, although the condition is associated with a disorder of the sebaceous glands. Even though it is a recurring condition, proper treatment will keep it under control. It should be borne in mind that dandruff has been with us even since the Pharaohs and still there is no sure cure, but rather control through treatment. Not even physicians can always be certain where normal shedding of dead cells ends and abnormal scaling begins. The line of demarcation is not always definite, since these small dry scales represent only a few of the millions of cells shed each day. Some contributing causes of dandrufl are:

1. Family trend.
2. Neglect of scalp and hair.
3. Disorder of oil glands.
4. Poor blood circulation.
5. Lack of thorough rinsing after shampoo.
6. Disease.
7. Systematic disturbances.
8. Improper cosmetics.
9. Strong irritating soaps.
10. Braiding of hair. The tight braiding of hair may cause too much tension on the roots of hair and cause the hair to fall out. If the hair dressing style is changed, the hair usually grows back.

Treatment of Pityriasis: There is no established cure for pityriasis. Some cases respond to treatment, although they may recur. Any skin disease of course can be cured if the causes are removed. Barber science treatments are worth while even if they only hold pityriasis under control or alleviate the condition. **Dandruff preparations often include** resorcin, sulphur, oil, alcohol, and salicylic acid. Oil shampoos and oil treatments, scalp ointment, and antiseptic scalp lotions and tonics are recommended.

FALLING HAIR

Falling hair or baldness is one of the principal concerns of the present study. **Efforts are directed mainly towards prevention,** since restoration borders on the impossible, at least at present. The **first indications** of baldness occur at the vertex or at both the vertex and the extreme frontal region. **Alopecia** is the technical name for baldness.

Definition of Alopecia:
1. Alopecia is the **abnormal loss of hair.**
2. Alopecia may be used to designate either a partial or generalized loss of hair regardless of the cause or on what part of the human body it occurs. In other words, irrespective of whether baldness is only a slight thinning out or a complete absence of hair, **whether it be temporary or permanent, whether it occurs on the scalp, on other places, or over the entire body, it is still alopecia.**

Causes of alopecia: Almost everything has been blamed for causing alopecia, including too frequent or too infrequent shampoos, wearing or not wearing hats, too much or too little exposure to the sun, etc.

How to regenerate hair has not definitely been discovered, although research reveals that the loss of hair is progressive on a man whose general health is good. Medical science has even included the injection of hormones, but this too is experimental. The following are some recognized causes:

1. Heredity. That is, baldness frequently runs in families. To explain heredity as a cause of baldness is a problem which has baffled authorities—they only know it happens.
2. Improper blood circulation. Unless the blood stream delivers food and oxygen to the papilla, the hair cannot live.
3. Improper diet. Diet must consist of the proper food elements, else the function of both blood circulation and the sebaceous glands are impaired and the hair will suffer accordingly.
4. Disorders of the sebaceous glands.
5. Diseases. (It is preferable to say "constitutional diseases.") Such diseases may bring bacteria to the follicles, toxins to the blood stream, and interfere with the functions of the various organs in the body. Some of these constitutional diseases are:
   (1) Pneumonia.   (4) Syphilis.
   (2) Typhoid fever.   (5) Influenza.
   (3) Diabetes.   (6) Nervous disorders.
6. Old age. The explanation of this cause centers around weakened regenerative powers, sagging tissues, and lack of vigorous physiological functions.
7. Lack of proper care of the hair. One primary factor is that the scalp and hair must be kept clean.

Treatments of Alopecia: The chief purpose of treatments is to remove the cause or causes. Treatments are worth while even if they merely slow down falling hair. (See chapter on Scalp Treatments.)

Major Types of Alopecia: There are FOUR major types of alopecia.

1. **Alopecia Adnata**—congenital baldness or baldness at birth. (Alternate name: Alopecia Congenital.)
2. **Alopecia Prematura**—baldness early in life or before the age of thirty-five.
3. **Alopecia Senilis**—baldness in old age. It is usually evident by the age of fifty.
4. **Alopecia Areata**—baldness in spots or patches.

Alopecia Adnata: Baldness at birth is treated only by a physician. This condition is usually temporary. Egg shampoo and Castile shampoo are often recommended. Adnata is due in part to an arrested development of hair follicles. It is **not** treated by the barber.

Alopecia Prematura: Nearly all scalp treatments designed for alopecia are for this particular condition. This type of baldness becomes evident around the age of 25 and is usually complete by the age of 35. In fact, it develops between the ages of 18 and 25. The frontal and vertex regions are affected. It is usually considered limited to males. There are two kinds of premature baldness:

1. **Alopecia symptomatica.** It occurs during acute or chronic illnesses such as severe anemia, influenza, scarlet fever, typhoid fever, pneumonia, and tuberculosis (Fig. 693). This kind of premature baldness might be called symptomatic baldness, meaning that it is caused by disease. It is usually temporary and responds to treatment very well. As soon as a person has recovered from the disease sufficient to attend a barber shop, recommend that he have several scientific scalp treatments. It would be ideal to contact the customer's physician and proceed under his instruction. Some cases of symptomatic baldness will clear up without treatments, but treatments will hasten recovery. Recommend general scalp treatment. (Refer to chapter on scalp treatments.) A physician should be consulted.

2. **Alopecia Idiopathic.** This is simply premature baldness. This kind of alopecia can be caused by neglect of the scalp, worry, poor blood circulation, heredity, etc. Its response to treatments is problematic. The barber can recommend treatments and suggest that a physician be consulted. (Refer to chapter on scalp treatments.)

Alopecia Prematura Idiopathic: This kind of premature baldness might be called regular premature baldness. Treatment consists of the following:
1. Correctly selected shampoo.
2. Scalp manipulation.
3. High frequency.
4. Scalp antiseptics.
5. Ointments.

Alopecia Areata (Fig. 690) :
1. This kind of alopecia means baldness in spots.
2. The bald areas are usually round or oval, and run from one to two inches in diameter.,
3. Areata may occur on either sex, both young and old.
4. Causes (no one cause for all cases) :
   (1) The exact causes for many cases have not been determined. It may result from systemic disorders or a disfunction of the papilla. It occasionally accompanies anemia.
   (2) It may develop from favus, fevers, erysipelas, or syphilis.
   (3) It may also be caused from **nerve injury or ringworms.**
5. **When caused by ringworm it is contagious** In such a case it is usually temporary. Refer all ringworm cases to a dermatologist.

6. Some cases of areata baldness are permanent and some temporary.

7. Some sources of alopecia areata are domestic animals—cats and dogs—contact with the disease, parasitic vegetable fungi, etc.

8. Treatments consist of egg shampoo, high frequency, sulphur ointment, oil of cade, and iodine.

9. The barber may treat alopecia areata due to ringworm only after the infection is checked by a dematologist. Treatments will hasten recovery and probably keep it from breaking out again.

0. The barber should treat alopecia areata only in cooperation with a dermatologist. Some cases clear up without any treatment whatsoever. (See chapter on Scalp Treatments.)

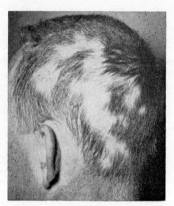

Fig. 690
Alopecia Areata

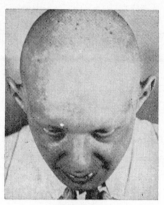

Fig. 691
Alopecia Totalis
(Courtesy Dr. Norman Tobias)

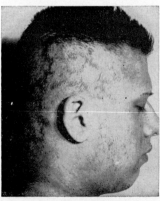

Fig. 692
Alopecia Syphilitica

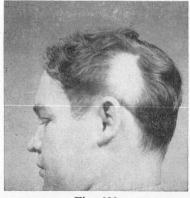

Fig. 693
Alopecia Symptomatica

Alopecia Adnata: This congenital type of baldness is very rare. It is traceable to a lack of development of the hair follicles, and is often accompanied with other development defects. The condition may be permanent. **Refer to a physician.** There is an **infantile** type of alopecia that is temporary. It occurs in many infants soon after birth. It affects the parietal and frontal areas. Shedding is gradual and, although a second crop is due normally about six months after birth, complete replacement may take as long as two years. Refer to a **physician.**

Alopecia Senilis: This is a diffuse type of baldness. It is associated with grayness and other indications of senility. It occurs around 50 years of age. Recommend a general scalp treatment. Treatments have been without avail.

Special forms of alopecia: These special forms of alopecia **should not be treated by the barber except** on recommendation of a physician. Even then, the barber will probably be restricted just to a shampoo. Each one of these is named after its cause.

1. **Alopecia Syphilitica.** This kind of baldness is due to syphilis. Syphilitic Alopecia usually affects the posterior part of the scalp. (The beard or eyebrows may also be involved.) The bald patches have a "moth-eaten" appearance but is noninflammatory. Regrowth can usually be assured. Refer to a physician. (Fig. 692).

2. **Alopecia Totalis.** This means complete baldness of the scalp (Fig. 691).

3. **Alopecia Universalis.** This is the disappearance of hair all over the body. It is usually hereditary.

4. **Alopecia Cachectic.** This kind of baldness is due to malnutrition. (Also known as Alopecia Cachecticorum.)

5. **Alopecia Neurotica.** This kind of baldness is due to disorder of the nerves. It may be caused by an injury to a nerve. It is also called **Alopecia Localis.**

What alopecia treatments may accomplish:

1. It is plausible that any form of alopecia can be corrected if the cause or causes are removed.

2. Both alopecia adnata and alopecia symptomatica are usually temporary and respond to treatment very well. When baldness at birth is accompanied by physical deformities, its correction is very slow if at all. By proper scalp treatments of symptomatic baldness, the barber may be reasonably sure of favorable results, but no miracle is possible. His treatments will be successful only by the assistance of nature which sponsors normal physiological functions. The chief merit of treatments is to assist nature; they simply hasten recovery.

3. Nothing much can be done as yet to correct alopecia senilis. The

frequent lack of normal physiological functions make its treatment an up-hill attempt.

4. Alopecia idiopathic affords the barber science barber his most attractive challenge. He can only apply the best barber science discoveries and hope for the best possible results. Three outcomes will characterize his attempts:

(1) In some cases, treatments will correct this type of baldness completely.

(2) In some cases, treatments will partially correct this kind of baldness.

(3) In some cases, treatments will have no noticeable results.

5. Never guarantee to cure any form of alopecia. Only recommend barber science treatments and assure him that scientific treatments embrace the only hope. (Associate with this point of view the following advice in "6".)

6. It is fitting and proper to suggest that the patron consult a dermatologist. Maximum results are possible only when the barber and dermatologist cooperate.

Two abnormalities of the hair:

1. **Trichoptilosis.** This is the technical term for split ends. Among the causes are excessive dryness, mechanical or chemical injury, overexposure to sun or wind, prolonged nervousness, use of excess alkaline cleansing agents, and disease. Recommend "terminal" cutting and oil treatments.

2. **Hypertrichosis.** This is the technical term for superfluous hair. This condition is regarded as hereditary.

Canities: This term means grayness or whiteness of hair. It is depigmentation of the hair. Why the hair loses its pigment and becomes gray or white is still not definitely known. In canities, hair never returns to its original color—there is no recovery. Premature canities is often observable in adolescence, and a "salt and pepper" effect may appear between the ages of 25 to 35. It is usually complete by 50. It is a benign condition.

1. Causes: The most widely accepted causes are (1) heredity and (2) senility. It often seems to be **accidental** when it follows nervous strain and prolonged illness or a terrific shock—this is only a presumption. Canities is still a mystery. It is certain, however, that the **immediate cause** is the **loss of natural pigment in the hair.**

2. Types of canities:

(1) Canities senilis—grayness from old age.

(2) Canities prematura—grayness before 35 years of age.

(3) Canities celeris—grayness from emotional disturbance (nerve disorders).

Matting of hair: The matting of hair is an abnormality, and a fertile place for disease. It is found mainly on long haired aged women who do not give their hair proper care. There is a so-called chignon fungus disease but it is rarely encountered today because of improved hygienic and sanitary conditions. Gross neglect of the hair becomes a breeding place for this fungus. Hair badly matted should be stripped with plain shears or thinned with thinning shears and reduced to a manageable length and shampooed. Spray oil on the hair before cutting or thinning.

Trichotillomania: This is the term for pulling out one's hair. This disorder is most common among pre-adolescents, but it has been noted at all ages, and both the sane and insane may have it. The causes of this inclination are not yet determined but it is associated with excessive excitement, prolonged mental strain, emotional upsets, intense itching, neurosis or just nervousness, pregnancy, idiosyncrasy, and disease. The duration of this disorder runs from several months to several years. Children frequently out-grow the tendency to pull out their hair. Ointments to relieve itching have been found helpful. In addition the hands can be attached to the sides while sleeping. Children thus affected should be kept occupied at hobbies and activities. An activity program removes the restlessness which is a major contributing factor. Painting the involved areas with collodion often causes the patient to refrain from pulling out hair in those particular areas. One practical remedy is to cut the hair very short. Have the hair cut weekly, and shampoo the head at least twice weekly. The epilation is usually confined to one portion of the scalp. Trichotillomania should be referred to a physician.

SOME NON-CONTAGIOUS SKIN DISEASES
FREQUENTLY ENCOUNTERED BY BARBER

Comedones: Comedones are blackheads. They are usually located on the forehead, sides of the nose, and cheeks. If they are allowed to remain,

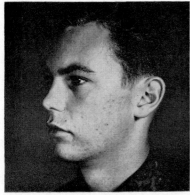

Fig. 694
Acne Vulgaris

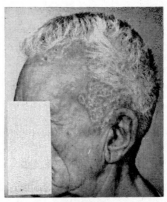

Fig. 695
Psoriasis

they may become pimples. **Blackheads are most common in teenagers.**
1. The alternate name for comedones is **Acne Comedo.**
2. Comedones are dark plugs of dried sebum lodged in the mouths of the ducts of the oil glands.
3. Principal causes:
   (1) Disorder of oil glands.
   (2) Digestive disturbance.
   (3) Excess of fatty substance in body.
   (4) Gross neglect of skin.
   (5) Systemic disturbances.
4. **Treatment.** Facials that include comedone extraction. If excessive, refer to a physician.

Milia: The alternate name is **Acne Albida.** It is non-contagious. Refer to a dermatologist, if excessive.
1. Milia or acne albida is the technical name for whiteheads.
2. Whiteheads are pearly knobs of hardened sebum. Their favorite site is around the eyes.
3. Whiteheads seldom recur.
4. Treatment: Any facial that includes extraction.

Acne Vulgaris: (Fig. 694). This is the technical term for common pimples. They occur mostly on teenagers. This condition is associated with an oily skin. It is **not contagious.** The alternate name is **Acne Simplex.** Contributory causes are:
1. Over-action of oil glands.
2. Systemic disturbances.
3. Fingering face.
4. Hygienic.

Shop treatment: Acne Facial. (Refer to dermatologist. Resulting pits can be reduced and sometimes removed by dermal or surgical planning.)

Psoriasis (Fig. 695):
1. This is a chronic **inflammatory** skin disease, characterized by dry, red round patches and silvery scales. It is **non-contagious.**
2. The barber should **not** treat Psoriasis. However, he may give soothing facials or shampoos over this condition.

Eczema:
1. Eczema is an **inflammatory** skin disease characterized by burning, redness, swelling, and sometimes itching.
2. It is the **most common skin disease.**
3. It is **not contagious.**
4. The barber may give a soothing facial or shampoo over this condition, but its actual treatment is administered by a dermatologist.

Seborrhea: Seborrhea is excessive secretion of sebum caused by an over-action of the oil glands.
1. Seborrhea exists in two forms:

(1) Seborrhea Oleosa. This form is excessive oiliness, especially about the forehead and nose.

(2) Seborrhea Sicca. This is dry seborrhea in the form of a coating of crusts and scales of sebum. (Some authorities use this term for **dandruff.**)

2. **Seborrhea Capitis** is seborrhea of the scalp.

3. **Seborrhea Faciei** is seborrhea of the face.

4. Treatment of Seborrhea Capitis: Tar shampoo, followed by menthol tonic or sulphur ointment.

Asteatosis: This is a deficiency of sebum, resulting in dry skin. Emollients soothe and relieve.

ACNES

Acne is an inflammatory skin disease of the sebaceous glands. In general is it characterized by pustules, papules and tubercles.

(1) A pustule is an inflamed pimple containing pus.

(2) A papule is a hard pimple containing no fluid.

(3) A tubercle is a hard pimple, but larger and more deep-seated than a papule.

There are more than fifty kinds of acne. They appear mostly on the face, back and chest. In many instances, as adolescence passes, acne vanishes.

Five acnes barber may treat: Treatments are qualified to mean soothing and alleviative facials.

1. **Acne Vulgaris.** Its alternate name is Acne Simplex. (Refer to Fig 694 and section on Acne Vulgaris.)

2. **Acne Rosacea.** (Refer to Section on Acne Rosacea.)

3. **Acne Comedo.** (Refer to section on Comedones.)

4. **Acne Albida**—whiteheads. (May be extracted.)

5. **Acne Artificialis**—reddish pimples caused by external irritants such as poor cosmetics. Recommend Acne facial.

Acne Rosacea: (Fig. 696). This is a complex type of acne marked by extreme redness or flushing of face, affecting chiefly the nose and cheeks. It is chronic, **non-contagious,** and inflammatory. There is usually no recovery. This disease is also known as "whisky nose" or "rum blossom." In its first stage, there is observable slight pinkness; in the second stage, the capillaries become noticeably dilated, and large oily pores and blackheads appear; and in the third stage, there is disfiguring. Contributory causes are:

1. Alcoholism.
2. Over-acidity.
3. Poor digestion.
4. Faulty elimination.
5. Faulty diet.
6. Disorder of oil glands.

Shop treatment: (Alleviative) **Acne Rosacea Facial.** (Refer to dermatologist.)

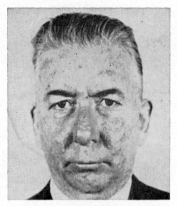

Fig. 696
Acne Rosacea
(Courtesy Dr. Norman Tobias)

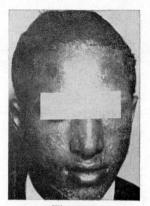

Fig. 697
Contact Dermatitis
From Hair Straightening
Preparation
(Courtesy Dr. Gerald A. Spencer)

Contact dermititis: Alternate name, **Dermititis Venenata.** This is an inflammation of the skin that can be caused by contact or application of certain substances, such as **some** medicated creams and shampoos, ointments, soaps, lotions, hair straightening agents and dyes to which a person has a skin **allergy.** Such dermatitis is more likely to occur on sore, irritated or erupted skin.

An inflamed eruption develops within 12 to 72 hours after contact. (Refer to a dermatologist.) (Fig. 697).

Dermititis: This is the name for inflammation of the skin.

Barber's Itch: (Fig. 698). This term is a misnomer, for there is no such disease. Unfortunately, there is a skin infection which was formerly known by this term because it was associated with shaving, but it may be contracted in barber or beauty shops or other public places, and also from animals. Scientific research reveals that such an infection is caused by the Staphylococcus Aurens which may gain entry in the follicles of the bearded region sensitized to this organism by openings in the skin and by low resistance. Too close shaving does weaken the power of the cuticle layer of the epidermis to resist pathogenic bacteria. This infection is a **ringworm condition,** characterized by inflammation, itching, and scaly patches. It is **contagious. Refer to a physician.** Many technical terms have been used for this condition. Here are a few:

1. **Tinea barbae.** This is perhaps the most widely accepted term for "barber's itch." (A ringworm condition).

2. Other acceptable terms for this condition are: (1) Tinea Sycosis and (2) **Sycosis Barbae.**

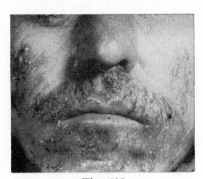

Fig. 698
Tinea Barbae

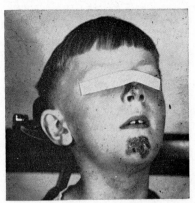

Fig. 699
Impetigo

Three diseases of beard:
1. Tinea Barbae (just explained, contagious).
2. Sycosis Barbae. (just explained, contagious.)
3. Eczema Barbae. (Eczema of beard, not contagious.)

Impetigo: It is an acute **contagious** skin disease that forms vesicles which rupture easily. It is commonest among children. It is easy to cure. The face is chiefly affected, but it may affect the nostrils, the chin, and the ears. It occurs mostly in summer months. Impetigo may be spread by touch and contaminated towels. Do not service a patron who has impetigo. Refer to a dermatologist. (Fig. 699).

Other Tinea diseases: Tinea means ringworm; it is contagious.
1. **Tinea Capitis** (also known as **Tinea Tonsurans).** This is ringworm of the scalp.
2. **Tinea Corporis.** This is ringworm of the body.
3. **Tinea Nodosa.** This is ringworm of the hair of the mustache.
4. **Tinea Barbae.** This is ringworm of the beard.

Eight non-contagious skin diseases:

1. Pityriasis.
2. Comedones.
3. Eczema.
4. Psoriasis.

5. Seborrhea Sicca.
6. Seborrhea Oleosa.
7. Acne Rosacea.
8. Acne Vulgaris.

Lentigo: This is the technical name for freckles.

1. Freckles are pigmented spots varying in color from yellowish to dark brown. They vary in size from that of a pea to a pinhead. They are **benign.**
2. Lentigo occurs chiefly on the face and back of the hands, but they may appear on any part of the body.
3. Lentigo is sometimes temporary. The dormant kind shows just for

a few days after exposure to the sun, especially on children and it may continue from early childhood through adolescence. The freckle age is from ten to twenty, although they may be permanent. They may appear on persons of advanced age as symptoms of senility.

4. Both sexes are equally subject to lentigo, but blondes and redheads are more subject.
5. Freckles crop out more in summer than in winter.
6. Lentigo is regarded as **hereditary.**
7. Clay Packs or Bleach Packs are recommended.

Albinism: This is the term for the absence of coloring matter in the skin and hair. In Latin it means "white." It is depigmentation—the absence of pigment grains.

1. Albinism is permanent and no treatment to restore melanin has been discovered.
2. The hair of an albino is either white or yellowish white. Such a person has a congenital deficiency of pigment in the hair, skin, and eyes.

Two disorders of sweat glands: For the following conditions, shampoos and facials bring only temporary relief. (Refer to a physician.)

1. Hyperidrosis—excessive sweating.
2. Anidrosis—insufficient sweating.

Urticaria: Its common name is "hives." This acute skin disorder is characterized by small reddish elevations that burn and itch. There is often generalized itching. It is caused by food allergies. Some get it from eating strawberries, fish, etc. Urticaria may last from 24 hours to 10 days. Its appearance or disappearance is sudden. Refer to a physician.

Labial Chancre: Chancre is the name of the sore-like sympton of syphilis. While it commonly appears on or about the genital organs, it may appear on other surfaces of the skin, especially on the lips where it is called labial chancre. This condition is contagious. The barber should not render a service over or near such a chancre. Refer to a physician.

PART II
Other Aspects of Diseases of Skin and Hair
Abnormalities of the hair:

1. **Pili Torti.** This is the technical name for twisted hair. It is a rare malformation of hairs.
2. **Trichonodosis.** This is the technical term for knotted hair. It is likely due to the inability of new hairs to grow normally from their follicles.
3. **Trichorrhexis Nodoso.** This is the technical term for brittleness of the hair and nodular swelling along the hair shaft. The hair shaft

has a tendency to fracture and split. (The alternate name is **Fragilitas Crinium.**)

4. **Monilethrix.** This is the technical term for beaded hair. It is an example of atrophy of the hair, resulting in alternate swellings of the shaft. This condition is characterized by excessive dryness and fragility.

5. **Trix annulata.** This is the technical term for ringed hair. The hair appears silvery gray in alternate dark and light bands.

Herpes Simplex: This is the technical name for "fever blisters" or "cold sores." It is an acute inflammation of the skin or mucous membrane characterized by a group of vesicles. Commonly recurrent. Due to a virus.

Herpes Facialis is the type of herpes simplex occurring on the face, usually about the lips. The condition usually persists from 6 to 10 days, during which antibodies develop. It is non-contagious. (Refer to a physician.)

Acnes barber should not treat: (These are non-contagious.)
1. **Acne Indurata.** Characterized by painful lesions chiefly on the back.
2. **Acne Decalvans.** Characterized by inflammation of hair follicle and sometimes the forerunner of baldness.
3. **Acne Hypertrophica.** Characterized by pits and scars.
4. **Acne Pustulosa.** Characterized by abcesses.
5. **Acne Medicamentosa.** Caused by excessive internal use of medications or drugs.

Steatoma. Alternate name: **Sebaceous Cyst or Wens.** It occurs usually on the scalp, the face, the lobe and posterior surface of the ear, and the back. As a rule it is a single lesion, round or oval in shape. Steatoma is painless. It's size ranges from that of a pea to an orange. It is caused by stoppage of the ducts of oil glands. (Refer to a dermatologist.)

Some disorders of sweat glands: (Refer to physician.)
1. Bromidrosis—foul smelling perspiration.
2. Uridrosis—perspiration with urine odor.
3. Hemidrosis—sweat containing blood.
4. Sudamen—sweat in small pearl-like vesicles.
5. Miliaria—prickly heat or heat rash.

Nevus: This is the name for a mole. Moles are benign growths. There are many kinds of nevi, and they vary in color and size. Nevus verricosus is a wart-like growth covered with hair. Nevus voscularis is the birthmark type.

Furuncle: This is the technical term for the common boil. It is an acute circumscribed inflammation in the sebaceous glands or hair follicle. A boil typically has pus which forms in a central mass or core. Boils are con-

tagious. Refer to a physician. Do not serve a patron who has an active boil on the scalp, face, or neck.

Carbuncle: A carbuncle is a widespread acute inflammation of the skin not circumscribed. Unlike the boil, it has many openings, and involves many hair follicles. Carbuncles are **contagious.** Refer to a physician. Do not serve a patron who has an active carbuncle on the scalp, face, or neck.

Verruca: Verruca is the technical name of a **wart.** It is a growth from the papillary layer of the skin. There are several varieties of warts. The common wart is called **Verruca Vulgaris.** It is usually grayish in color, pinhead to pea in size, and has a warty surface. This variety of warts occurs chiefly on the hands and fingers but occasionally on the face and scalp. Refer to a dermatologist.

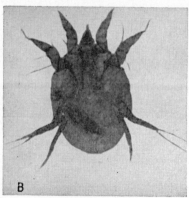 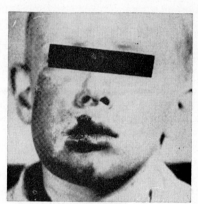

Fig. 700   Fig. 701
Itch Mite (Causes Scabies)   Erysipelas on Rige Side of Face
(Courtesy Dr. Norman Tobias, "Essentials of Dermatology."
J. P. Lippincott Co., Pub.).

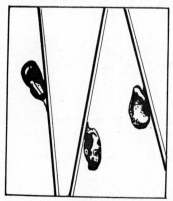 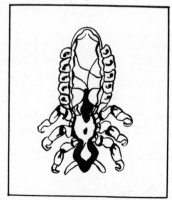

Fig. 702   Fig. 703
Nits   Pediculosis Capitis

Favus: Its common name is "honeycomb ringworm" (Tinea Favosa). It is a chronic **parasitic** skin disease characterized by diffuse scaly areas, round or oval elevated yellow pustular patches. They are covered with thick concrete-like crusts. Favus may persist for twenty or more years. It is extremely rare in the U.S., except on immigrants from Europe. In Favus pustules are found around hair follicles. It may lead to permanent but not complete baldness. Refer to a dermatologist.

Scabies: Its common name is the "seven year itch." It is a **contagious** disease caused by the itch mite. It is characterized by night itching, red papules, and scratching. (Refer to a dermatologist.) (Fig. 700).

Erysipelas: It is commonly known as "St. Anthony's Fire." It is an acute infectious skin disease, characterized by burning, **redness,** swelling, and sometimes vesicular lesions. It is localized to a given area. It is associated with fever, chills, and nausea. Recovery is possible within 10 days. It is **contagious.** (Refer to a dermatologist.) (Fig. 701).

Pediculosis: This is a skin disease due to the infestation of lice. Head lice are known as **pediculosis capitis. Nits** on the hair shaft are simply oval-shaped eggs laid by lice. These eggs are cemented very firmly to the hair shafts by a chitinous secretion. A head louse never invades other regions of the body since it has neither mandible nor mouth and it never bites. These parasites invade first the occipital region and then move on to the parietal regions. The chief symptom is intolerable itching caused by the sucking of the parasites. A person who complains of excessive itching of the scalp in the occipital and retro-auricular regions may have Pediculosis Capitis. Once this condition is discovered by the barber, he should refer the patron to a physician. A crusting and oozing, itchy scalp may have lice. A head louse is about 2mm. long, with a gray slender shape marked with black spots on the border of its stomach. Neglect can lead to folliculitis and abscesses of the scalp. Do not serve a person with head lice. (Refer to a physician.) (Figs. 702-703).

Vitiligo: This is a skin disease characterized by the **absence of pigment.** The affected areas are depigmented. It begins as white spots around the mouth, nostrils, eyes, and ears, and may extend to other parts of the body. It is **non-contagious.** It is believed to be hereditary. It can be permanent, but it has been known to disappear spontaneously. The barber should not treat this condition. (Fig. 704) .

Leucoderma: Leucoderma is the name of acquired white spots or blotches. It may follow a disease such as ringworm or injury such as burns and cuts. It is **non-contagious.** It is usually not permanent. The barber should not treat this condition. (Fig. 705).

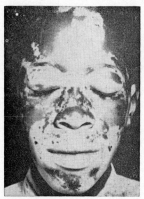

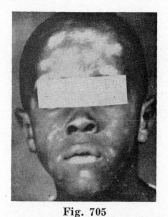

Fig. 704
Vitiligo
(Absence of Pigment)

Fig. 705
Leucoderma
(Causes by Ringworm)

(Courtesy Dr. Gerald A. Spencer, "Cosmotology in the Negro."
Arlain Printing Co., N. Y. C.).

Some terms used in the study of diseases: An attempt has been made to select the most used terms.

1. **Acute** means more or less violent, but temporary—brief but severe.
2. **Chronic** means of long duration—mild but recurring.
3. **Congenital** means present at birth.
4. **Parasitic** means caused by vegetable or animal parasites. They are responsible for lice, scabies, and ringworm. Parasites live off living
5. **Systemic** means to arise from functional disturbance of internal glands.
6. **Allergy** means sensitivity to normally harmless substances.
   (1) Some causes of skin allergy are certain cosmetics, plants, dyes, medicines, and certain foods.
   (2) Some symptoms of a skin allergy are itching, redness, swelling, blisters, scaling, and eruptions.
7. **Symptoms** are manifestations, such as abnormal appearances or sensations. There are two kinds of symptoms:
   (1) **Objective** symptoms. These are easily observable, such as redness, swelling, pimples, etc.
   (2) **Subjective** symptoms. These are known and felt only by the person affected and include burning, itching, and pain.
8. **Etiology** is the study of the causes of diseases.
9. **Inflammation** is characterized by redness, swelling, pain and heat.
10. **Diagnosis:** This means recognizing a disease from symptoms.
11. **Prognosis:** This means the prediction of the duration or termination of a disease—the course of the disease—**probable outcome.**
12. **Dermatitis** is any inflammatory condition of the skin. (**Derm** refers to the skin and **itis** denotes inflammation.)

13. **Dermatosis** is the general term of any disease of the skin.
14. **Benign** means not malignant—not endangering to health or life— not harmful.
15. A **pathogenic disease** is one caused by pathogenic bacteria such as staphylococci and streptococci.
16. A **systemic disease** is one due to the disturbance of internal glands.
17. A **congenital disease** is one that is present at birth.
18. **Fungus:** A fungus is a vegetable parasite. In Latin, it means "mushroom". It is a spongy growth of diseased tissue on the body. For example, ringworm is a fungus infection.

Lesions: A lesion is a structural tissue change usually from injury or disease. The skin takes on abnormal appearance. (Allergies and functional disturbances may cause lesions.) Skin diseases are characterized by lesions. Sores and pimples are lesions. There are **three** general types of lesions; teritary, which are found in cancer, will not be discussed, and the other two are:
1. Primary lesions. (These are due to manifestations of the disease itself.)
2. Secondary lesions. (These are due to another infection, to scratching, or to the irritation of a primary lesion.)

Primary lesions:
1. Pustule: An elevation of the skin containing pus. It is usually yellow or greenish in color.
2. Papule. A small solid elevation of the skin without fluid. In color it may be pink, red, yellow, brown, or black.
3. Tubercle: (Pimple) A solid elevation, similar to a papule, only larger and deep-seated.
4. Nodule: A large tubercle, but more deep-seated.
5. Vesicle: (Blister) A pea-sized elevation, blister or cyst, containing watery fluid.
6. Macule: (Spot) A small non-elevated spot such as occurs from freckles and vitiligo.
7. Tumor: A large elevation—abnormal swelling of the skin, varying in size, shape, and color.
8. Bulla: (Bleb or blister) An elevation containing watery fluid, similar but larger than a vesicle.
9. Wheal: A temporary elevation or ridge such as occurs from hives, an insect bite, or from the blow of a whip. (Alternate name: Pomphus.)
10. Comedone: A blackhead.

Secondary lesions:
1. Scales: (Squamae) Dry or greasy exfoliations of the skin. Scales may be branny or shiny, white or yellow, or gray, thin or thick,

and occur in small surfaces or large sheets.

2. Crust: (Scab) A hard mass composed of dried secretions, such as blood, pus, or serum.

3. Ulcer: An open lesion with pus.

4. Fissure: A crack in the skin, penetrating into the dermis, as observed in chapped hands or lips. A fissure may be caused by diseases or injury.

5. Scar: The tissue formed after the healing of a wound.

6. Excoriation: (Abrasions) A raw surface due to scratching or excessive friction. It may result from injury.

7. Pigmentation: A discoloration of the skin, such as may remain after the disappearance of moles, freckles, or certain diseases. It is due to a deposit of melanin.

Hair

Hair is the chief subject with which the barber is concerned. He should have a great deal of knowledge of the hair in order that he may serve the public well and take advantage of his opportunity to establish a source of income from hair treatments. The public has become hair-conscious; consequently, the modern barber must know something more than how to trim and shape hair; he should also know its proper care and treatment. The barber who has knowledge of the structure, functions, and characteristics of hair, and understands its growth and regrowth, has the foundation for the care and treatment of hair.

Unlike the other chapters on theory, **this chapter is not in two parts,** because all the phases of the subject presented here are **closely related to barbering.**

Purposes of this study:
1. To determine the fundamental requirements of hair.
2. To determine what the barber can do to help nature supply these fundamental requirements.
3. To determine the characteristics of healthy hair.
4. To determine the characteristics of unhealthy hair.
5. To determine the causes of unhealthy hair.
6. To learn the structure of hair.
7. To learn the functions of hair.
8. To study the growth and regrowth of hair.

Fundamental requirements of hair:
1. **Nourishment.** The hair must have adequate nourishment. This primary need can be met by the proper function of the circulatory system.
2. **Lubrication.** The primary lubricant for the hair can be provided by the proper function of the sebaceous glands. This vital need, however, can be met by lubricating agents, such as hair oils and hair creams.
3. **Cleanliness.** The hair must be kept clean. This can be accomplished by combing, brushing, and shampooing.

Aids to fundamental requirements of hair:
1. Shampooing.
2. Massaging.
3. Antiseptics.
4. Ointments.
5. Scalp treatments.
6. Advice on care of hair.

General basis for healthy hair: Although the hair has its fundamental needs which can be met by nature and scientific barber services. Nevertheless, the hair depends in general on two factors. These factors are:

1. The health of the body.
2. The health of the scalp. (Here lies the field in which the barber has duties and opportunities.)

Characteristics of healthy hair:

1. Glossiness.
2. Elasticity.
3. Normal quantity.
4. Free from trichoptilosis.
5. Normal growth.
6. Proper color.

Characteristics of unhealthy hair: Unhealthy hair lacks all the characteristics of healthy hair.

1. Lack of sheen.
2. Brittleness.
3. Excessive oiliness.
4. Excessive dryness.
5. Excessive split ends.
6. Abnormal shedding.
7. Dullness of color.
8. Excessive thinness.

Some causes of unhealthy hair:

1. Neglect.
2. Insufficient circulation.
3. Disorder of oil glands
4. Diseases.
5. Mechanical or chemical irritation.

Locations of hair growth:

Hair grows on the entire surface of the body except on the palms of the hands and the soles of the feet. (This is a generally accepted statement because it is substantially true. It is to be noted, however, that no hair grows on the eyelids, on the dorsal surfaces of the terminal phalanges of the fingers and toes, nor on the lips.)

Definition of hair: Hair is a thread-like appendage of the skin tapered to a fine point at the free end.

Trichology: This is the technical term for the study of hair. (**Trich** refers to hair, and **ology** refers to study or science.)

Purposes of hair: Hair has three recognized uses or purposes.

1. Protective agency.
2. Promoter of adornment. (It enhances appearance.)
3. Preservative of heat. (It helps keep body at normal temperature.)

How hair is protective agency:

1. Scalp hair protects the scalp against falls or blows and excesses of heat and cold
2. Hair of the nostrils serve as filters against foreign particles.
3. Ear-hairs check the entrance of foreign bodies.
4. Eyelashes help protect the eyes from light glare and flying particles.

Varieties of hair: There are three varieties of hair.
1. **Long hair** of the scalp and face.
2. **Short hair** of the eyebrows and eyelashes.
3. **Lanugo.** This is the fine, soft, downy hair of the forehead and cheeks. It also is found on certain areas of the body.

Hair of eyebrows and eyelashes: These hairs are of the short bristly type. The average life span of these hairs is from four to five months.

Layers or cross-sections of hair: The hair has three layers, except the medulla layer is usually absent in Lanugo. The **cortex layer is the bulk and chief part of the hair shaft,** consisting of about 75% of it.
1. Cuticle Layer. This is the **outermost** layer of the hair.
2. Cortex Layer. This is **between** the cuticle and medulla.
3. Medulla Layer. This is the **inmost** layer of the hair.

Noteworthy points on layers of hair: The Cuticle is referred to as the **outer flat covering** of the hair—it contains scales; the Cortex as the **Body** or **pigment layer;** and the Medulla as the **central pith** layer. The Medulla has **air spaces** between its cells, and it is thought that such spaces affect the **color** of hair.

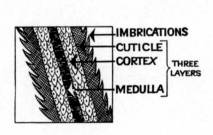

Fig. 706
Layers of Hair and Imbrications

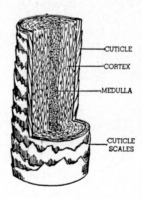

Fig. 707
Cuticle Scales and Layers of Hair

Shapes of hair cells: The cells in the **cuticle** layer are **flat;** in the **cortex, long, spindle** shaped; and in the **medulla** layer, **round, coin shaped.**

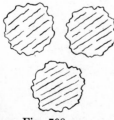

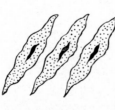

Fig. 708
Cells of Cuticle

Fig. 709
Cells of Cortex

Fig. 710
Cells of Medulla

Hair cells: From the cells that grow **on** the papilla the bulb of the hair is formed. Hair grows from the multiplication of cells **in the bulb.** They multiply by mitosis (indirect cell division). The cells just above the papilla of course are the **youngest** and the cells at the point of the hair shaft are the **oldest.** The origination of hair cells has been pin pointed with respect to the various layers of the hair. It is held that the cells of the medulla grow from the top of the papilla; those of the cortex originate from the sloping sides of the papilla; and the cuticle cells originate where the outer rim of the bulb lies along the base of the papilla. In short, hair cells originate in the portion of the bulb that fits over the top and sides of the papilla.

Imbrications: The cells in the cuticle layer of the epidermis overlap like shingles on a roof. These formations are called **imbrications.** Five cells, with the free ends, overlap one another in the length of one. These overlapping scales (cells) of the cuticle layer are needle point projections. Heat as well as peroxide, cause these imbrications to loosen up and permit absorption.

Shapes of individual hairs. Hairs have three general shapes (Fig. 711).
1. **Round.** This shape of hair is straight.
2. **Oval.** This shape of hair is wavy.
3. **Flat.** This shape of hair is curly and kinky.

CUTICLE CORTEX MEDULLA

KINKY HAIR   STRAIGHT HAIR   WAVY HAIR

Fig. 711
Different Shapes of Hair

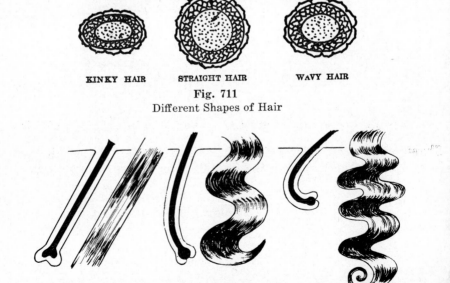

Fig. 712
Influence of Follicles on Shapes of Hairs

Shapes of individual hairs determined by follicles: (See discussion of follicle.) The pouch-like tube in which the hair grows is called the follicle. Whether a hair is round, oval, or flat, is determined by the follicle. The shape of the follicle is set by **heredity.**

Directions and angles of follicles: (Fig. 712).
1. The direction of the follicle immediately above the papilla is the point where the tendency to straightness or curliness is imparted. Hair in the straight follicles is inclined to be straight; hair in slightly curved follicles is inclined to be wavy; and hair in decidedly curved follicles is inclined to be curly or kinky. If hair emerges from the skin at right angles, the follicles are at right angles to the skin.
2. The angles of follicles to the skin of the face and scalp set the "grain" of the beard and the hair streams of the scalp. Such angles run according to areas set by nature, and this is why hair emerges from the skin slanting in a given direction.

Kinds of hair in different races:
1. **Straight, coarse, dark** hair is most common with Indians and the Yellow race.
2. **Wavy, soft, light** hair is most common with Caucasians.
3. **Curly, kinky** hair is most common with Negroes.

Lengthwise divisions of the hair: Broadly, the lengthwise divisions are the Shaft and Root. But for the sake of accurate reference the hair has been divided into four divisions. (Fig. 713).
1. **Bulb.** This is the lower end of the hair that fits over the papilla. It is **club-shaped.**
2. **Root.** This is the portion of the hair enclosed within the follicle.
3. **Shaft.** This is the portion of the hair that extends above the surface.
4. **Point.** This is the tapered end of the upper end of the shaft.

Follicle—noteworthy points:
1. The follicle is the funnel-shaped depression in the skin containing the root of the hair.
2. The **size, shape, and direction of hair are determined by the follicle.**
3. Hair follicles vary in length from 1/12 to 1/4 of an inch.
4. From one to six oil glands are attached to each hair follicle.
5. The funnel-shaped mouths of hair follicles are favorite lodging places for dirt and germs. Hence, the importance of cleanliness.
6. Attached to almost every hair follicle is an arrector pili muscle. This muscle is located on the side toward which the follicle slopes. The action of this muscle encourages the flow of blood by making a suction effect.

Papilla: The papilla is the **cone-shaped elevation at the bottom of the hair follicle.** (It is not an actual part of the hair.) It is through the papilla

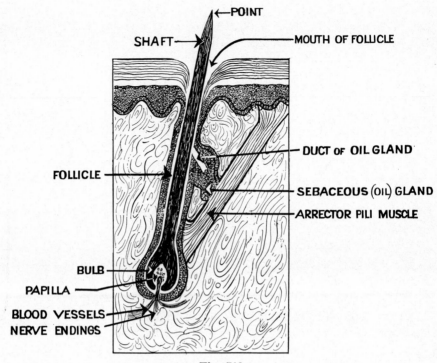

Fig. 713
Follicle and Closely Related Structures to Hair

that nourishment reaches the hair bulb. (There are no blood vessels in the hair.) The papilla is really the **productive organ** of the hair, since it has the ability to produce hair cells. As long as the papilla functions, the hair will grow. Hair cannot grow and neither can new hair cells be formed without the papilla. (Fig. 713).

Number of hairs on head:
1. The average number of hairs on the head is 120,000.
2. The average number of hairs per square inch on the head is 1000.
3. The number of hairs on the head varies according to color and texture: Red hair is estimated at 90,000; blond hair at 140,000; brown and black at about half way between these numbers.
4. In diameter, blond hair is the **smallest** (1/1500 to 1/500 of an inch), and black hair is the **largest** (1/450 to 1/140 of an inch).
5. Hairs are more numerous or thickest at the crown.

Pigment of Hair: Pigment means coloring matter.
1. The tiny pigment grains in the cells of the cortex layer comprise the coloring matter of hair. These cells originate in the bulb.
2. The color of hair depends on the color and amount of **pigment grains.**

3. The source of pigment has not been determined, but it is largely racial and hereditary.
4. The coloring matter of hair is called **melanin,** and the more melanin the darker the hair.

Chemical composition of hair:
1. Hair consists of Carbon, Oxygen, Hydrogen, Nitrogen and Sulphur.
2. Each of these elements is known by its first letter. The keyword is the name COHNS. (C. O. H. N. S.)
3. The largest per cent is Carbon and the smallest Sulphur.
4. Per cent of Chemical Elements in hair:
   (1) Carbon (50%).   (3) Hydrogen (6%).
   (2) Oxygen (21%).   (4) Nitrogen (18%).
                        (5) Sulphur (5%).

Keratin in hair: The chief ingredient of hair is keratin. It is a protein that contains Carbon, Oxygen, Hydrogen, Nitrogen and Sulphur. (It is the principal constituent of the cuicle layer of the epidermis.) While keratin is readily dissolved by alkalies, it will withstand pepsin and hydrochloric acid.

Average maximum length of head hair: The maximum length of hair varies according to race and sex. On the white race, the average length will be given according to consensus:
1. On women: From 18 to 24 inches.
2. On men: From 12 to 16 inches.

Texture of hair: Texture means the degree of fineness. coarseness, **or** softness of individual hairs. The texture varies according to races.
1. On the white race, hair is typically fine to medium in texture.
2. On the yellow race, hair is typically coarse in texture.
3. On the black race, hair is typically fine in texture. However, hair on Negresses is often medium to coarse and wiry.

Hair stream: A hair stream means that all hair within the same area slopes in the same direction.

Part natural: A natural part is where two hair streams extend in opposite directions from a common line.

Crown: The crown is where hair slopes in all directions from a definite point.

Whorl: A whorl is formed at the crown where the natural part ends; and at the forehead where the part ends at the hairline a "cowlick" is formed. A "whorl" is a coiled effect, and a "cowlick" is a tuft of hair turned upward as if licked by a cow.

Scalp hair from birth to puberty: The scalp is the first region of the body to have hair. At birth a few lanugo hairs are present, but these are replaced in from two to six months with a second generation of fine silky hair which is pigmented. Hair becomes coarser and more pigmented during childhood. It is not until puberty that hair is medullated, fully pigmented, and grown to its full size and length. Only about 85 per cent of the scalp hair ever becomes full fledged hair with all three layers; the remaining 15 per cent, even in old age, remains downy hairs.

Elasticity of hair: This means a rubber-like ability of the hair to stretch and return to its original position without breaking. A healthy hair can be stretched from 1/8 to 1/5 of its length. The cuticle layer gives hair its elasticity.

Effect of climate on hair:
1. Heat causes hair to expand and absorb moisture.
2. Cold causes hair to contract and become dry.
3. Slight dampness activates hair to be wavy or curly.

Life span of hair: Authorities have not yet agreed upon the exact life span of hair. Some determining factors have been discovered, such as age, sex, type of hair, and individual peculiarities. It is reasonably close to set the average life span of hair at **four years,** recognizing the probability that some hairs live only two years while others live six years.

Nostril Hair: The unsightly long hairs protruding from the nostrils should be CUT on the OUTSIDE of the nostrils with clean shears. A special shear is made for this purpose; it has blunt points. Never attempt to snip them inside the nose; and never pull them out. Hair-in-the-nose cutting can be fatal. If the delicate mucous membrane inside the nose is snipped, "facial erysipelas" and even "cavernous sinus thrombosis" might result. The pernicious habit of pulling hairs from the nostrils by the fingers or tweezers is likewise risky. Nostril hairs are filters that protect the nostrils from the invasion of bacteria.

Ingrown Hair: An ingrown hair is a recurved hair that grows underneath the skin or reenters the skin and causes a papule (a solid-like pimple). The papule is a lump or bulge of the skin in which the deranged hair is visible. If such a papule is grossly inflamed, the patron should be referred to a dermatologist; otherwise, the barber may extract the ingrown hair with a sterilized tweezer. To avoid breaking the hair, pull it upward in line with its uncurved portion. Be sure to saturate the point of extraction with peroxide or some oher aniseptic.

Singeing of hair: Singeing is a process of burning the ends of hair with a singeing taper. It was formerly contended that singeing closes the ends of freshly cut hair and thus stops the escape of sebum and in this way prevents split ends. But the hair is not hollow. It consists of a solid mass of cells and has no tube or duct. **Singeing has been discontinued on scientific grounds.**

How hair grows:

1. Hair grows as a result of the multiplication of the soft cells on the papilla. From these cells the bulb of the hair is formed. These "hair cells" actually give birth to the hair. THE PAPILLA IS REALLY THE PRODUCTIVE ORGAN OF THE HAIR. The forming of hair cells, their multiplication and growth depend upon proper nourishment and oxygen which only the blood stream can supply. The function of blood therefore is indispensable to the life and health of hair. It is noteworthy that the cells born on the papilla become elongated and finally flattened as they form the cuticle layer of the hair. (The **bulb,** which fits over the papilla, **is composed of soft growing cells.**)

2. Normally, cast-off hairs are replaced by new ones. When a hair completes its life span it releases itself from the papilla and moves to the middle region of the follicle and remains there until it is pushed out by new hair formed below. As new hair grows and moves upward from the papilla it literally pushes out the old hair. Some old hair thus suspended in the follicles may fall out from combing or brushing. The new hair, normally, lives its predestined life and then follows the same routine as its predecessor.

3. It takes from 41 to 72 days for new hair to grow from the papilla to the surface of the scalp.

Rate of growth: The rate of growth has been reasonably well established. The rate varies somewhat according to sex, race, variety of hair, and general body health. The length of rest periods of growth has not been definitely determined. It is even contended that hair growth on the scalp of men and women is practically continuous. **From ⅜ to ¾ of an inch a month** has been advanced as the **rate of growth.**

Rest periods of growth. The length of rest periods of growth is still not definitely established. Some authorities regard as negligible the whole theory of rest periods, but all agree that after the bulb detaches itself from the papilla, the papilla takes a rest period before becoming active again. **After shedding, a new hair begins to form within 21 to 42 days.** Since different hairs, even in the same area, have different life cycles, as well as different starting and ending cycle dates, constantly some hairs are being shed, some new hairs are being formed, and some hairs are growing. While there is no consensus of the duration of rest periods, there is consensus that **hair does have alternate periods of growth and rest.** Rest periods in the scalp are regarded as shorter.

Normal shedding: Hairs shed daily. They make way for new hair, produced at the bottom of the follicle on the papilla. Authorities differ on the average number of hairs shed normally each day. An attempt has been made to arrive at a figure which represents their varying deductions, and so the average daily shedding is estimated at 50 to 80 hairs. All the **hair of the head with which a child is born falls out** almost entirely in from **two to six months after birth** and it is replaced by new hair. The shedding or falling out of hair gives no sense of feeling or pain, and this is why baldness creeps upon a person almost unawares.

Porosity of hair: Porosity means that hair has pores or spaces through which it can absorb moisture or liquid preparations. The pores or overlapping spaces of the cuticle layer allows such absorption. Bleached, tinted or damaged hair is most porous and most readily absorbs moisture or chemicals. If hair wets readily, feels extremely soft, cuts very easily when dry, or feels rough to the finger tips, it is very porous. If hair feels smooth and hard and springs back into place upon release from fingers, or has natural luster, it is not especially porous.

Hygroscopic ability of hair: The ability of hair to absorb moisture makes it hygroscopic. It is made more readily hygroscopic by such agents as steam and chemicals. In hair coloring, the hair is made more absorbent degree. It is water proof in almost the same way as wood, the wood used by peroxide. Hair does not normally absorb water beyond a negligible to make boats.

Answers to eight often asked questions about hair:

1. Does hair grow after death? No. The shrinking of tissues causes the hair to project above the skin, giving the illusion of growth.

2. Is it harmful to shampoo the hair every day? Not necessarily, but use a soothing shampoo.

3. Will a hair tonic cure dandruff? No. But a tonic helps to control and alleviate dandruff.

4. Can hair bleed? No. It contains no blood vessels.

5. Is salt water injurious to hair. No. Salt water contains no injurious ingredients.

6. Can hair receive food by external means? No. The hair receives food only from the blood.

7. Will the extraction of one hair be replaced by two or more hairs? No. Only one hair grows in a follicle.

8. Does shaving the scalp make hair grow? No. If it did, the problem of baldness would be solved.

STUDENT PROJECT
PART I
To Be Answered in Writing Before Completing 200 Hours

1. Define sanitation.
2. Why is it important for the barber to practice sanitation?
3. Itemize ten points in the practice of shop sanitation.
4. What is an antiseptic?
5. Name two disinfectants and explain how to mix them.
6. What is the best time to disinfect implements?
7. How are the implements of barbering classified?
8. List five structural parts of shears.
9. What are the two types of shear grinds?
10. What are two types of plain shears?
11. How are the sizes of shears indicated?
12. Most combs are made from what material?
13. What are the two types of electric clippers?
14. Name five structural parts of hand clippers.
15. What are the two general grinds of razors?
16. Name five structural parts of a razor.
17. How are the sizes of razors indicated?
18. What is meant by the **finish** of a razor?
19. How are hones classified?
20. From what animals are strops made?
21. Shell strops come mainly from which animals?
22. How are the sizes of lather brushes indicated?
23. What are the two types of electric vibrators?
24. Name the six standard kinds of hair cuts.
25. Define feathering.
26. List five shapes of heads.
27. Explain a natural part.
28. At what angle or angles to the scalp should hair be cut?
29. Where should the neck edge be on a very long neck?
30. How is a normal neck-line indicated?
31. Name two methods of topping a head of hair.
32. What is another name for Medium Brush Cut?
33. Is it ever correct to cut the top hair first?
34. Describe a good taper on a Long Hair Cut.
35. Define slithering.
36. Name two types of women's neck-edges.
37. Name five types of beards.
38. What constitutes a shaving stroke?
39. What are the four shaving strokes?
40. Sketch the fourteen sections of the face.
41. What are two purposes of lathering for a shave?

42. What are two purposes of steaming face for a shave?
43. Name three types of shampoos.
44. Name three types of shampoo movements.
45. Outline the standard procedure of a liquid soap shampoo.
46. What are the two methods of shampooing?
47. Give the name, purpose, and procedure of three shampoos.
48. How are tonics classified?
49. Name five brands of tonics.
50. What are five scalp conditions which the barber may treat?
51. Outline a scalp treatment for dry dandruff.
52. Outline a scalp treatment for falling hair.
53. What are some ingredients which an ointment for an oily scalp should contain?
54. Give the name, purpose and procedure of five facials.
55. Name five types of massage movements and manipulations.
56. Make ten statements about salesmanship.
57. What are ten ways of building up business?
58. What would you do as first aid for the patron who faints?
59. What are the dangers of expressing yourself freely on all subjects before customers?
60. Make five statements on ethics in barbering.

PART II

To Be Answered in Writing 30 Days Prior to Graduation

1. On the history of barbering, state five important dates and explain what happened on each one.
2. Define metabolism.
3. Why are pathogenic bacteria undersirable?
4. In what ways may bacteria enter the body?
5. What are three kinds of hygiene?
6. Define protoplasm.
7. How can metabolism be activated?
8. What are two functions of the blood?
9. What is composition of blood?
10. How can the barber increase circulation in the scalp?
11. Name four arteries of the scalp.
12. Name purposes of the high frequency.
13. What are two uses of the red dermal light?
14. List five muscles of the face.
15. What is the history of massaging muscles?
16. What is the insertion of a muscle?
17. Name ten substances studied in cosmetic chemistry and state the effects of each on the skin or hair.
18. Name the principal nerve points of the face?
19. What are three symptoms of prolonged nervous tension?

20. What are four characteristics of healthy skin?
21. Name the three layers of the skin.
22. Make ten statements on the structure and function of skin.
23. Define dandruff.
24. List five contagious skin diseases.
25. Name five acnes.
26. What are comedones?
27. What are three layers of hair?
28. What are two characteristics of healthy hair?
29. What are three varieties of hair?
30. What is the hair follicle?
31. What are the major types of alopecia?
32. Name the five chemicals hair contains.
33. How are hair dyes classified?
34. List ten points in the barber law of your state.
35. Outline the Acne Facial.
36. What are two functions of the cells?
37. How do cells multiply?
38. Name the three blood vessels.
39. What are the functions of the blood?
40. How does blood become purified?
41. What percent of the body's weight is blood?
42. What are five sensations nerves convey?
43. What are two barber shop services that relax nerves?
44. What is meant by the term "dermatologist"?
45. Describe the sebaceous glands.
46. What are three causes of wrinkles?
47. Describe the cuticle layer of the epidermis.
48. Where does hair get nourishment?
49. What are two causes of greyness?
50. What is the essence of Hippocrates' theory of massaging?

Pronunciation Of Selected Words and Terms

Key to the Symbols of Pronunciation

ā as in āte   â as in câre   ī as in īce   ô as in lôrd
ă as in ădd   ē as in ēve   ĭ as in ĭll   ū as in cūbe
à as in America   ĕ as in mĕt   ō as in ōld   ŭ as in ŭp
ä as in ärm   ẽ as in makẽr   ŏ as in ŏdd   û as in ûnite
å as in våcation ê as in êvent   ô as in ôbey   û as in ûrn

The symbol ′ marks accent

abducens (ăb dū′ sĕnz)
abrasion (ăb rā′ zhŭn)
acne (ăk′ nĕ)
acne albida (ăl bĭ′ då)
acne artificialis (är tĭ fĭsh′ ĭ ăl ĭs)
acne cacheticorum
        (kå kĕk′ tĭ cō rŭm)
acne hypertrophica
        (hī pẽr trŏf′ ĭ kå)
acne indurata (ĭn dū råt′ å)
acne rosacea (rŏ zā′ shĕ å)
acne vulgaris (vŭl gā′ rĭs)
adnata, alopecia (ăd nåt′ å)
afferent (ăf′ ẽr ĕnt)
ala (ā′ lå)
albinism (ăl′ bĭ nĭz′m)
albino (ăl bĭ′ nō)
alopecia (ăl′ ô pē′ shĭ å)
alopecia adnata (ăd nåt′ å)
alopecia areata (ā rĕ å′ tå)
alopecia prematura (prē mă tū′ ră)
alopecia senilis (sĕ nĭl′ ĭs)
alveola (ăl vē′ ô lå)
anabolism (à năb′ ô lĭz′m)
anatomy (à năt′ ô mĭ)
anidrosis (ăn′ ĭ drō′ sĭs)
aniline (ăn′ ĭ lĭn)
anthrax (ăn′ thrăks)
antiseptic (ăn′ tĭ sĕp′ tĭk)
aorta (å ôr′ tå)
aponeurosis (ăp′ ô nŭ rō′ sĭs)

arrector pili (ă rĕk′ tŏr pī lĭ)
arrectores pilorum
        (ăr′ ĕk tō′ rēz pī lō′ rŭm)
arterial (är tēr′ ĭ ăl)
artery (är′ tẽr ĭ)
asteatosis (à stē′ à tō′ sĭs)
astringent (ăs trĭn′ jĕnt)
atrium (ā′ trĭ ŭm)
auditory (ô′ dĭ tō′ rĭ)
auricle (ô′ rĭ k′l)
auricular (ô rĭk′ û lẽr)
bacillus (bà sĭl′ ŭs)
bacteria (băk tēr′ ĭ å)
bactericide (băk tēr′ ĭ sīd)
bacteriology (băk tēr′ ĭ ŏl′ ô jĭ)
bacterium (băk tēr′ ĭ ŭm)
beriberi (bĕr′ ĭ bĕr′ĭ)
blood vascular system
        (blŭd′ văs′ kû lẽr sĭs′ tĕm)
bromidrosis (brŏ′ mĭ drŏ′ sĭs)
buccinator (bŭk′ sĭ nā tẽr)
canities (kà nĭsh′ ĭ ēz)
capillary (kăp′ ĭ lẽr′ ĭ)
carotid (kà rŏt′ ĭd)
catabolism (kà tăb′ ô lĭz′m)
cataphoresis (kăt′ à fŏ rē′ sĭs)
cerebellum (sĕr′ ĕ bĕl′ ŭm)
cerebrospinal system
        (sĕr′ ĕ brŏ′ spī′ năl)
cerebrum (sĕr′ ĕ brŭm)
cervical (sûr′ vĭ kăl)

chlorine (klō′ rēn)

cholesterin; cholesterol
(kô lĕs′ tēr ĭn) (kô lĕs′ tēr ōl)

citric acid (sĭt′ rĭk ăs′ ĭd)

clavicle (klăv′ ĭ k′l)

coagulate (kô ăg′ ủ lāt)

coiffure (kwä fūr′)

comedo (kŏm′ ē dō)

comedone (kŏm′ ē dōn′)

congenital (kŏn jĕn′ ĭ tăl)

contagious (kŏn tā′ jŭs)

contractible (kŏn trăk′ tĭ b′l)

contractile (kŏn trăk′ tĭl)

corneum (kŏr′ nĕ ŭm)

coronoid (kŏr′ ô noid)

corpuscle (kôr′ pŭs′l)

corrosive (kô rō′ sĭv)

corrugator (kŏr ủ gā′ tēr)

cortex (kôr′ tĕks)

cranial (krā′ nĭ ăl)

cranium (krā′ nĭ ŭm)

cuticle (kū′ tĭ k′l)

cytoplasm (sī tô plăz′m)

deodorant (dē ō′ dēr ănt)

depressor alae nasi
(dĕ prĕs′ ôr ā lē nā′ sī)

depressor anguli oris
(ăng′ gủ lī ō rĭs)

depressor labii inferioris
(lā′ bĭ ĭ ĭn fē′ rĭ ŏr ĭs)

dermis (dûr′ mĭs)

dermatitis (dûr′ mả tī′ tĭs)

dermatologist (dûr′ mả tŏl′ ô jĭst)

dermatology (dûr′ mả tŏl′ ô jĭ)

dermatosis (dûr′ mả tō′ sĭs)

dermis (dûr′ mĭs)

desquamation (dĕs′ kwả mā′ shŭn)

diagnosis (dī′ ăg nō′ sĭs)

digestion (dĭ jĕs′ chŭn)

disinfectant (dĭs′ ĭn fĕk′ tănt)

eczema (ĕk′ zĕ mả)

efferent (ĕf′ ēr ĕnt)

electrode (ê lĕk′ trōd)

emollient (ê mŏl′ ĭ ĕnt)

endocrine (ĕn′ dô krīn)

enzyme (ĕn′ zīm)

epicranius (ĕp′ ĭ krā′ nĭ ŭs)

epidermis (ĕp′ ĭ dûr′ mĭs)

erythema (ĕr′ ĭ thē′ mả)

ethmoid (ĕth′ moid)

etiology (ē′ tĭ ŏl′ ô jĭ)

exfoliation (ĕks fō′ lĭ ā′ shŭn)

faradic current
(fă răd′ ĭk kŭr′ ĕnt)

faradism (făr′ ả dĭz′m)

follicle (fŏl′ ĭ k′l)

folliculitis (fô lĭk′ ủ lī′ tĭs)

foramen (fô rā′ mĕn)

formaldehyde (fôr măl′ dê hīd)

frontal (frŭn′ tăl)

frontalis (frŏn tā′ lĭs)

fulguration (fŭl′ gủ rā′ shŭn)

galvanic current
(găl văn′ ĭk kŭr′ ĕnt)

galvanism (găl′ vả nĭs′m)

ganglion (găng′ glĭ ŭn)

gastric (găs′ trĭk)

germicide (jûr′ mĭ sīd)

germinative layer
(jûr′ mĭ nā′ tĭv lā ẽr)

glandular (glăn′ dủ lẽr)

glossopharyngeal
(glŏs′ ô fả rĭn′ jê ăl)

glycerine (glĭs ẽr ĭn)

hair (hâr)

halitosis (hăl′ ĭ tō′ sĭs)

hamamelis (hăm′ ả mê′ lĭs)

hemoglobin (hē′ mô glō′ bĭn)

histology (hĭs tŏl′ ô jĭ)

hydrogen (hī′ drô jĕn)

hygiene (hī′ jēn)

hyperemia (hī′ pẽr ē′ mĭ ả)

hyperidrosis (hī pẽr ĭd rō′ sĭs)

hypertrichosis (hī′ pẽr trĭ kō′ sĭs)

hypoglossal (hī′ pô glŏs′ ăl)

imbrication (ĭm′ brĭ kā′ shŭn)

immerse (ĭ mûrs′)

impetigo (ĭm′ pê tī′ gō)

implement (ĭm′ plê mĕnt)

inflammation (ĭn′ flă mā′ shŭn)

infra-orbital (ĭn′ frả ôr′ bĭ tăl)

infra-red (ĭn′ frả rĕd′)

ingredient (ĭn grē′ dĭ ĕnt)

insertion (ĭn sûr′ shŭn)

intestinal (ĭn tĕs′ tĭ năl)

involuntary muscle
(ĭn vŏl′ ŭn tẽr′ ĭ mŭs′l)

iodine (ī' ŏ dēn)
irritant (ĭr' ĭ tănt)
keratin (kĕr' a tĭn)
kneading (nēd' ĭng)

labial (lā' bĭ ăl)
labii (lā' bĭ ī)
lachrymal (lăk' rĭ măl)
lanolin (lăn' ŏ lĭn)
lanugo (la nū' gō)
lentigo (lĕn tī' gō)
leucocyte (lū' kŏ sīt)

levator anguli oris
     (lĕ vā' tēr ăng' gŭ lī ō' rĭs)
levator labii superioris
     (lĕ vā' tēr lā' bĭ ī
      sŭ pē' rĭ ō' rĭs)
levator palpebrae (păl' pĕ brē)
ligament (lĭg' a mĕnt)
light therapy (līt thĕr' a pĭ)
linear (lĭn' ĕ ēr)
litmus (lĭt' mŭs)
lubricant (lū' brĭ kănt)
lucidum (lū' sĭ dŭm)
lustreless (lŭs' tēr lĕs)
lymph (lĭmf)
lymphatic (lĭm făt' ĭk)

malar (mā' lēr)
malpighian (măl pĭg' ĭ ăn)
mandible (măn' dĭ b'l)
mandibular (măn dĭb' ŭ lēr)
manipulation (ma nĭp ŭ lā' shŭn)
massage (ma säzh')
masseter (mă sē' tēr)
mastication (măs' tĭ kā' shŭn)
matrix (mā' trĭks)
maxilla (măk sĭl' a)
maxillary (măk' sĭ lĕr' ĭ)
medulla (mĕ dŭl' a)
melanin (mĕl' a nĭn)
mentalis (mĕn tā' lĭs)
menthol (mĕn' thōl)
metabolism (mĕ tăb' ŏ lĭz'm)
miliaria (mĭl' ĭ ā' rĭ a)
mitosis (mĭ tō' sĭs)
motor oculi (mō' tēr ŏk' ŭ lī)
mucous (mū' kŭs)
muscular (mŭs' kŭ lēr)

naris (nā' rĭs)
nasalis (nă sā' lĭs)
neuritis (nŭ rī' tĭs)
neutralize (nū' trăl īz)
nitrogen (nī' trŏ jĕn)
non-pathogenic (nŏn păth' ŏ jĕn' ĭk)
non-striated (nŏn strī' āt ĕd)
nucleus (nū' klĕ ŭs)
nutriment (nū' trĭ mĕnt)
nutritive (nū' trĭ tĭv)
occipital (ŏk sĭp' ĭ tăl)
occipitalis (ŏk sĭp' ĭ tā' lĭs)
occipito frontalis
     (ŏk sĭp' ĭ tŏ frŏn tā' lĭs)
oculomotor (ŏk' ŭ lŏ mō' tĕ)
oleosa (ō lē ō' sá)
olfactory (ŏl făk' tŏ rĭ)
omohyoid (ō' mŏ hī' oid)
ophthalmic (ŏf thăl' mĭk)
optic (ŏp' tĭk)
oris (ôr' ĭs)
osmosis (ŏs mō' sĭs)
oxygen (ŏk' sĭ jĕn)
palate (păl' ĕt)
palatine (păl' a tīn)
palpebra (păl' pĕ brá)
palpebrarum (păl pē brā' rŭm)
papilla (pá pĭl' a)
papillae (pá pĭl' ē)
papillary (păp' ĭ lĕr' ĭ)
papule (păp' ūl)
parotid (pá rŏt' ĭd)
pathogenic (păth' ŏ jĕn' ĭk)
pediculosis (pĕ dĭk' ŭ lō sĭs)
percussion (pĕr kŭsh' en)
pericardium (pĕr' ĭ kär' dĭ ŭm)
periosteum (pĕr' ĭ ŏs' tĕ ŭm)
petrissage (pā' trĕ säzh')
phagocyte (făg' ŏ sīt)
pharmacology (fär' má kŏl ŏ jĭ)
phenol (fē' nōl)
physiological (fĭz' ĭ ō lŏj' ĭ kăl)
pilocarpine (pī' lŏ kär' pēn)
pityriasis (pĭt' ĭ rī' a sĭs)
pityriasis capitis (kăp' ĭ tĭs)
pityriasis steatoides (stē ă toy' dēz)
plasma (plăz' má)
platysma (plá tĭz' má)

posterior (pŏs tēr' ĭ ēr)
posterior auricular (ô rĭk' û lēr)
procerus (prô sē' rŭs)
prognosis (prŏg nō' sĭs)
protoplasm (prō' tô plăz'm)
psoriasis (sȯ rī' à sĭs)
pterygoid (tĕr' ĭ goid)
pulmonary (pŭl' mō nĕr ĭ)
pustular (pŭs' tû lēr)
pustule (pŭs' tūl)
pyramidal (pĭ răm' ĭ dăl)
quadratus labii superioris
    (kwŏd rā' tŭs lā' bĭ ī
    sū pē rĭ ôr' ĭs)
quinine (kwī' nīn)
reproductive (rē' prô dŭk' tĭv)
respiratory (rê spīr' à tō' rĭ)
resorcin (rĕz ôr' sīn)
reticular (rê tĭk' û lēr)
rheostat (rē' ô stăt)
risorius (rĭ sō' rĭ ŭs)
salicylic acid (săl ĭ sĭl' ĭk ăs' ĭd)
salivary gland (săl' ĭ vĕr' ĭ glănd)
sanitation (săn' ĭ tā' shŭn)
scabies (skā' bĭ êz)
sebaceous (sê bā' shŭs)
seborrhea (sĕb' ŏ rē' à)
seborrhea oleosa (ō lē ō' sà)
seborrhea sicca (sĭk' à)
seborrheic (sĕb' ŏ rē' ĭk)
sebum (sē' bŭm)
senile (sē' nīl)
senility (sē' nĭl' ĭ tĭ)
sheath (shēth)
spatula (spăt' û là)
sphenoid (sfê' noid)
sphincter (sfĭngk' tēr)
spirillum (spī rĭl' ŭm)
staphylococcus (stăf' ĭ lô kŏk' ŭs)
steatoma (stē' à tō' mà)
steatosis (stē' à tō' sĭs)
sterile (stĕr' ĭl)
sterilization (stĕr' ĭ lĭ zā' shŭn)
sterilize (stĕr' ĭ līz)
sternocleidomastoideus
    (stûr' nô klī' dô măs' toid ê ŭs)
stimulate (stĭm' û lāt)
streptococcus (strĕp' tô kŏk' ŭs)

styptic (stĭp' tĭk)
subcutaneous (sŭb' kû tā' nê ŭs)
subdermis (sŭb dûr' mĭs)
sublingual (sŭ lĭng' gwăl)
sudamen (sŭ dā' mĕn)
sudoriferous (sū' dēr ĭf' ēr ŭs)
supraorbital (sū' prà ôr' bĭ tăl)
suture (sū' tûr)
sycosis (sī kō' sĭs)
sycosis barbae (bär' bē)
sympathetic (sĭm' pà thĕt' ĭk)
symptomatica alopecia
    (sĭmp tŭm ăt' ĭ kā
    ăl' ŏ pē' shĭ à)
systemic (sĭs tĕm' ĭk)
tapotement (tà' pôt män')
technical (tĕk' nĭ kăl)
temporal (tĕm' pô răl)
temporalis (tĕm' pô rā' lĭs)
tendon (tĕn' dŭn)
theory (thē' ô rĭ)
therapeutic (thĕr' à pū' tĭk)
tinea (tĭn' ê à)
tinea barbae (tĭn' ê à bär' bē)
tinea tonsurans (tŏn sū' rănz)
trapezius (trà pê' zĭ ŭs)
triangularis (trī ăng' gû lā' rĭs)
trichology (trĭ kŏl' ô jĭ)
trichophytosis (trĭ kŏf' ĭ tō' sĭs)
trichoptilosis (trĭ kŏp tĭ lō' sĭs)
trichotillomania (trĭk ô tĭl ô mā' nĭà)
tricuspid (trī kŭs'pĭd)
trifacial (trī fā' shăl)
trigeminal (trī jĕm' ĭ năl)
urticaria (ûr' tĭ kā' rĭ à)
vascular (văs' kû lēr)
vaso-constrictor
    (văs' ô kŏn strĭk' tēr)
vaso-dilator (văs' ô dī lā' tēr)
vena cava (vē' nà kā' và)
ventricle (vĕn' trĭ k'l)
vertebra (vûr' tê brà)
vertex (vûr' tĕks)
vomer (vō' mēr)
vulgaris (vŭl gā' rĭs)
zinc sulphate (zĭngk sŭl' făt)
zygomatic (zī' gô măt' ĭk)
zygomaticus (zī' gô măt' ĭ kŭs)

Bibliography

Behrman, Howard T., The Scalp in Health and Disease. C. V. Mosby Co., 1952.

Behrman and Levin, Your Skin and Its Care. New York: Emerson Books, Inc.

Blakiston's, New Gould Medical Dictionary, 1949.

Blumbarten, Aaron Sawvel, Textbook of Materia Medica and Therapeutics. New York: The MacMillan Co., 1935.

De Zemler, Charles, Once Over Lightly, New York, 1939.

Gray, Goss, Gray's Anatomy, Philadelphia: Lea & Feiberg, 1959.

Greisheimer, Esther M., Physiology and Anatomy. Philadelphia: Lippincott Co., 1950.

Journeyman Barbers' Textbook of Practical and Scientific Barbering, J.B.H.C.P.I.U.A., Indianapolis.

Kibbee, Constance V., Standard Textbook of Cosmetology. New York: Milady Publishing Corp., 1959.

Kimber, Gray, Leavell and Stackpole, Textbook of Anatomy and Physiology, New York: The MacMillan Co., 1961.

Kozlay, Hazel L., Beauty Shop Compendium. Chicago: American Hairdresser.

Le Clair, MMe. Le Clair on Beauty Culture, Milwaukee, 1935.

Levin, Oscar L., Save Your Hair, New York: Greenberg Publishers, 1926.

McCarthy, Lee, Diseases of the Hair. St. Louis: C. V. Mosby Co., 1940.

Master Barbers' Textbook, Standardized Textbook of Barbering. Chicago: A.M.B.B.A., 1961.

Meyer, William, Cosmetiste. Chicago: The William Meyer Co., 1930.

Moler, A. B., The Barber's Manual. 1962.

Murray, Anne, Theory of Cosmetology. Hollywood: Anne Murray Publishing Co., 1942.

Pillsbury, Shelly, Kligman, Dermatology, W. B. Sauunders Co., Philadelphia, London, 1947.

Pusey, William Allen, The Care of the Skin and Hair. New York: Appleton-Century Co., 1934.

Reno's Scientific Method of Blue Print Curly Cutting, 1960.

Savill, Agnes, The Hair and Scalp. London: Edward Arnold (Publishers Ltd.) 1952.

Spencer, Gerald A., Cosmetology in the Negro. New York: Milady Publishing Co., 1944.

Stingley, Glendora, Progressive Manual on Cosmetology, Box 146, Maywood, Calif., 1960.

Sullivan, Ethel M., Sullivan Beauty Manual, Los Angeles, 1963.

Thorpe, S. C., Practice and Science of Standard Barbering, New York: Milady Publishing Corp., 1955.

Tobias, Norman, M.D., Essentials of Dermatology. J. B. Lippincott Company, 1956.

Trusty, L. Sherman, Questions and Answers on Barbering, 1963.

Trusty, L. Sherman, Workbook on Barbering and Related Sciences, 1964.

Van Dean Manual, Professional Training for Beauticians. New York: Milady Publishing Corp., 1960.

Wilkinson, Clark, Green, McLaughlin, Modern Cosmeticology, Chemical Publishing Co., Inc., New York, N. Y., 1962.

Index

SANITAS